MANAGEMENT
AND LEADERSHIP
for Nurse Administrators

SEVENTH EDITION

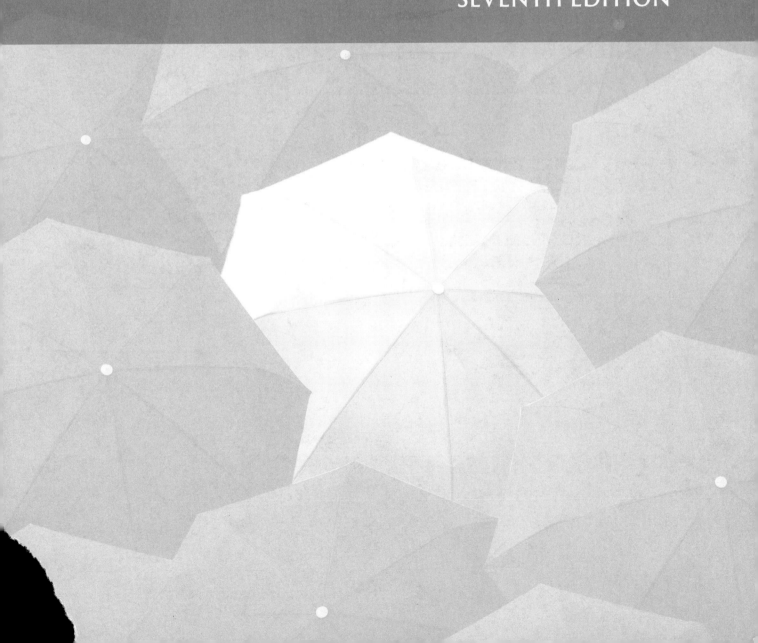

The Pedagogy

Management and Leadership for Nurse Administrators, Seventh Edition drives comprehension through various strategies that meet the learning needs of students, while also generating enthusiasm about the topic. This interactive approach addresses different learning styles, making this the ideal text to ensure mastery of key concepts. The pedagogical aids that appear in most chapters include the following:

CHAPTER 5

Transformational Leadership in an Era of Healthcare Reform

Lisa Mestas, Rita Stockman, Patricia Thomas, and Linda Roussel

LEARNING OBJECTIVES

1. Describe attributes of transformational leadership that promote contemporary care models.
2. Envision how nurse leaders position the discipline for success.
3. Acknowledge contributions of all team members in achieving organizational imperatives.

AONE KEY COMPETENCIES

I. Communication and relationship building
II. Knowledge of the healthcare environment
III. Leadership
IV. Professionalism
V. Business skills

AONE KEY COMPETENCIES DISCUSSED IN THIS CHAPTER

I. Communication and relationship building
II. Knowledge of the healthcare environment
III. Leadership
IV. Professionalism

I. **Communication and relationship building**
   - Effective communication
   - Relationship management
   - Influence of behaviors
   - Ability to work with diversity
   - Shared decision making
   - Community involvement
   - Medical staff relationships
   - Academic relationships

Learning Objectives Each chapter includes learning objectives that help you to identify and discuss important concepts from the text.

AONE Key Competencies AONE Key Competencies are outlined at the start of each chapter, focusing student attention and providing a framework for nurse leaders.

II. Knowledge of the healthcare environment
- Clinical practice knowledge
- Patient care delivery models and work design knowledge
- Healthcare economics knowledge
- Healthcare policy knowledge
- Understanding of governance
- Understanding of evidence-based practice
- Outcomes measurement
- Knowledge of, and dedication to, patient safety
- Understanding of utilization and case management
- Knowledge of quality improvement and metrics
- Knowledge of risk management

III. Leadership
- Foundational thinking skills
- Personal journey disciplines
- Ability to use systems thinking
- Succession planning
- Change management

IV. Professionalism
- Personal and professional accountability
- Career planning
- Ethics
- Evidence-based clinical and management practices
- Advocacy for the clinical enterprise and for nursing practice
- Active membership in professional organizations

FUTURE OF NURSING: FOUR KEY MESSAGES

1. Nurses should practice to the full extent of their education and training.
2. Nurses should achieve higher levels of education and training through an improved education system that promotes seamless academic progression.
3. Nurses should be full partners with physicians and other health professionals in redesigning health care in the United States.
4. Effective workforce planning and policy making require better data collection and information infrastructure.

Introduction

Nurse administrators utilize many leadership styles, such as situational, motivational, transformational, and servant leadership, to drive change and sustain success. Today's healthcare environment requires transformational leaders to inspire necessary culture shifts within healthcare systems as they move forward. In 2010, the Affordable Care Act (ACA) was passed by Congress with the intent of creating a more affordable, accessible healthcare system while improving

---

Future of Nursing: Four Key Messages Four key messages focused on the nurse's role and practices appear at the beginning of each chapter to help guide the student as they read.

Introductions Important concepts and topics covered in each chapter are highlighted at the beginning of the chapter to help focus students' attention on the essential material.

Reflective Questions Reflective questions appear at the end of each chapter to engage the reader by asking them to apply the principles they have just learned.

---

t Messaging

- carry cell phones and have them turned on.
- Ubiquity: Most people have a mobile device with text capability.
- Immediacy: Recipients are likely to read a text message as soon as they receive it.
- Communication: Two-way communication capability provides opportunities for direct engagement.
- Monitoring: Text messaging can be used to monitor or report symptoms.
- Measurability: Results can be tabulated and measured.
- Dissemination: Text messages can be used for emergency alerts and announcements.
- Multimedia: Texts can include links to audio, video, or websites.

Source: Adapted from Terry, 2008.

SUMMARY

In the rapidly evolving technological and complex healthcare system, nurse leaders need to be proactive and armed with skills that will allow forward thinking. Processes to enhance nursing tasks and the overall functions of the healthcare system are essential. Nurse leaders will need to have the ability to manage highly skilled nurses as technology continues to advance. Knowing how to prepare themselves and those they manage is imperative and can be demanding if they lack a new way of thinking. The four basic skills of leadership, professionalism, business, and communication have evolved to a new level, and organizations need to focus on developing employees that can meet and manage the goals of the strategic plan. Nurse leaders have a critical role in the adoption of technology by being change agents and empowering their staff to be partners through a shared governance structure. Nurses use technology more than any other discipline, and their knowledge, experience, and input can and should be considered when making IT-related decisions. For IT adoption to occur and have the intended positive consequence, nurse leaders must hold nurses accountable for using technology correctly.

REFLECTIVE QUESTIONS

1. Consider ways a nurse leader can promote education in this advancing technological healthcare environment that are not already in place. What do you see for the future?
2. What evidence do we have of the effectiveness of e-communication for health?
3. To what extent will nurses play a role in deciding which technologies will be used? Do you think nurses and nurse leaders have a significant say in how technologies are used? Why or why not?

Case Studies Case Studies provide real-life scenarios for the student to consider the nurse's role in the future of nursing.

CASE STUDY 11-1   Using Information Technology to Improve Work Flow (Continued)

3. Create a diagram that represents the new work flow for nursing staff since the test version of the preoperative nursing documentation flow sheet went live. Create a clear and logical process that the board members will be able to follow.
4. Create a chart using a word processing program, such as Microsoft Word, to demonstrate both positive and negative views of how nurses are responding to the new work flow process on the unit. An example is as follows:

	Positive Nursing Views	Negative Nursing Views
1. Go Live Training and Education		
2. Transition and Support		
3. Nursing Views and Opinions		
4. Compliance with New Process		

Wade Forehand

Sam is a nurse manager on a busy neurosurgical intensive care unit (NICU). Sam is logged in to one of the computer workstations in the hallway of the unit and is working on weekly audits. He soon notices that a commotion is occurring at the end of the hallway. The patient in this room is decompensating and is about to go into cardiac arrest. Sam rushes to the room to assist his staff with the critical patient. Because he is in a hurry, Sam forgets to exit the computer workstation and leaves the documentation system open. Sally, a volunteer in the hospital, is walking by the computer station and realizes that the system has not been shut down. She approaches the workstation to close it. Upon reaching the computer, she notices that the screen is displaying the name of her friend within her senior community center. Before she closes the computer, Sally hovers over the patient's name to discover why he is in the hospital. After reading the information, Sally closes the computer and returns to her volunteer post. Later that evening, Sally called her friends from the senior center to talk about the information she learned.

Several days after the information was shared, the hospitalized patient discovers that Sally was involved. He decided to report this incident to hospital administrators. An investigation by the HIPAA compliance officer is initiated.

Case Study Questions

1. Begin by exploring what ethical principles have been compromised by both Sam and Sally.
2. What role, if any, did technology play in this situation?
3. From the perspective of a nursing leader, how should this investigation be handled?
4. Should disciplinary action be pursued for either Sam or Sally? Explain your answer for both individuals.

CASE STUDY 6-3   Culture of Safety

- Rapid cycle improvement collaborative
- Crucial conversations training
- Safety coach training

How did the nurse leader put it all together? 1900 for about 5 minutes that includes reviewing data, current status (census, watchers, staffing, regulatory visitors), a look back (any concerns fr

Another example is standardization of the s checking the patient's ID bracelet, review of fl and edit of the patient plan of care.

Another component of the safety culture is information obtained from nurses by the charge nurse, including RN concerns, family concerns, and unclear orders. In addition, the resident meets with family members or assesses patients as needed. The patient and family remain at the center of all decision making, leading to better patient outcomes.

Case Study Questions

1. How would knowledge of marketing influence the creation of this safety culture?
2. What additional outcome measures could the point-of-care nurse leader use to ensure sustainability of the culture?
3. How does the nurse leader know when evidence updates need to be incorporated into the next change?

References This section outlines additional material that is referenced throughout the text.

REFERENCES

Allen, S. R. (2013). *An ethnonursing study of the cultural meanings and practices of clinical nurse council leaders in shared governance* (Unpublished dissertation). University of Cincinnati, Ohio.

American Association of Critical-Care Nurses. (2015). *AACN Healthy Work Environment Initiative*. Retrieved from http://www.aacn.org/wd/hwe/content/hwehome.pcms?menu=hwe

American Nurses Association. (2009). *Nursing administration: Scope and standards of practice*. Silver Spring, MD: Author.

American Nurses Association. (2012). *Nurse's essential role in care coordination*. Silver Spring, MD: Author.

Aricca, D., Van Citters, B. K., Larson, K. L., Carluzzo, J. N., Gbemudu, S. A., Kreindler, F. M., … Fisher, E. S. (2012). *Four health care organizations' efforts to improve patient care and reduce costs*. Retrieved from http://www.commonwealthfund.org/publications/case-studies/2012/jan/four-health-care-organizations

Betbeze, P. (2014, May 13). Presidents, CEOs, and the new leadership model. Retrieved from http://www.healthleadersmedia.com/content/MAG-304260/Presidents-CEOs-and-the-New-Leadership-Model

Drucker, Peter F. (1999). *Management challenges for the 21st century*. New York, NY: HarperBusiness.

Porter, M. E., & Teisberg, E. O. (2006). *Redefi competition on results*. Cambridge, MA

Porter, M. E., & Teisberg, E. O. (2007). H health care. *Journal of the American Medica*

Porter-O'Grady, T., & Malloch, K. (2015 *healthcare innovation* (4th ed.). Burling

Rittenhouse, D. R., & Shortell, S. M. (20 Will it stand the test of health reform? *Jour tion, 301*(19), 2038–2040. doi:10.1001/j

Rock Island County. (n.d.). Health Departi Health LINK. Retrieved from http:/. /SchoolHealthLINK.aspx

Schoen, C., How, I. W., Weinbaum, I., Cr views on shaping the future of the U.S. health system. Retrieved from http://hagel.senate.gov/index.cfm?FuseAction=News.HealthCareCommission

Stacey, R. (2010). *Complexity and organizational reality: Uncertainty and the need to rethink management after the collapse of investment capitalism* (2nd ed.). New York, NY: Routledge.

Stiefel, M., & Nolan, K. (2012). *A guide to measuring the triple aim: Population health, experience of care, and per capita cost* (IHI Innovation Series white paper). Cambridge, MA: Institute for Healthcare Improvement.

The Joint Commission. (2008). National patient safety goals. Retrieved from http://www.jointcommission.org/PatientSafety/NationalPatientSafetyGoals

TIGER Initiative. (2007). TIGER summary report. Retrieved from http://www.thetigerinitiative.org/

Vlasses, F. R., & Smeltzer, C. H. (2007). Toward a new future for healthcare and nursing practice. *Journal of Nursing Administration, 37*(9), 375–380.

Selected Websites Refer to online resources for timely information relevant to content in the text.

SELECTED WEBSITES

Agency for Healthcare Research and Quality

www.ahrq.gov

The Agency for Healthcare Research and Quality funds, conducts, and disseminates research to improve the quality, safety, efficiency, and effectiveness of health care. The information gathered from this work and made available on the website assists all key stakeholders—patients, families, clinicians, leaders, purchasers, and policy makers—to make informed decisions about health care.

American Association of Critical-Care Nurses

www.aacn.org

The American Association of Critical-Care Nurses provides leadership and resources to their members to improve health care for critically ill patients and their families. The core concepts of patient- and family-centered health care are integrated throughout their practice guidelines.

MANAGEMENT AND LEADERSHIP
for Nurse Administrators

SEVENTH EDITION

EDITED BY

LINDA ROUSSEL, PhD, RN, NEA-BC, CNL
Professor
University of Alabama, Birmingham
Birmingham, Alabama

PATRICIA L. THOMAS, PhD, RN, NEA-BC, ACNS-BC, CNL, FACHE
Vice President of Clinical Quality & Transformation, Chief Nursing Officer
Trinity Home Health Services
Livonia, Michigan

JAMES L. HARRIS, PhD, APRN-BC, MBA, CNL, FAAN
Professor
University of South Alabama
Mobile, Alabama

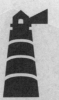

JONES & BARTLETT
LEARNING

World Headquarters
Jones & Bartlett Learning
5 Wall Street
Burlington, MA 01803
978-443-5000
info@jblearning.com
www.jblearning.com

Jones & Bartlett Learning books and products are available through most bookstores and online booksellers. To contact Jones & Bartlett Learning directly, call 800-832-0034, fax 978-443-8000, or visit our website, www.jblearning.com.

Substantial discounts on bulk quantities of Jones & Bartlett Learning publications are available to corporations, professional associations, and other qualified organizations. For details and specific discount information, contact the special sales department at Jones & Bartlett Learning via the above contact information or send an email to specialsales@jblearning.com.

07840-4

Production Credits

VP, Executive Publisher: David D. Cella	VP, Manufacturing and Inventory Control: Therese Connell
Executive Editor: Amanda Martin	Composition: Cenveo® Publisher Services
Associate Acquisitions Editor: Rebecca Myrick	Cover Design: Kristin E. Parker
Editorial Assistant: Lauren Vaughn	Rights & Media Research Assistant: Wes DeShano
Senior Production Editor: Nancy Hitchcock	Cover Image: © blackdovfx/iStock/Thinkstock
Senior Marketing Manager: Jennifer Scherzay	Printing and Binding: Edwards Brothers Malloy
Media Development Assistant: Shannon Sheehan	Cover Printing: Edwards Brothers Malloy

Library of Congress Cataloging-in-Publication Data
Management and leadership for nurse administrators / [edited by] Linda Roussel, James L. Harris, and Tricia Thomas. -- 7.
    p. ; cm.
Includes bibliographical references and index.
ISBN 978-1-284-06762-0
I. Roussel, Linda, editor. II. Harris, James L. (James Leonard), 1956- , editor. III. Thomas, Patricia L., 1961- , editor.
[DNLM: 1. Nursing, Supervisory. 2. Nurse Administrators. WY 105]
RT89
362.17'3068--dc23
                                                       2015009930

6048

Printed in the United States of America
20 19 18 17   10 9 8 7 6 5 4

Dedication

We are most appreciative to our contributors and their staff, patients, families, and students: Thank you for your commitment, tireless work, and passion for safe, quality healthcare environments for our consumers and for those entrusted to our care. What we hope for all nurse leaders, irrespective of setting, is that you will find yourself and engage in the sense-making in the challenges we face in health care.

Contents

CHAPTER 3   Professional Practice: A Prototype Linking Nursing in Interprofessional Teams   **49**

Gay Landstrom and Donald D. Bignotti

CHAPTER 4   Professional Development: An Imperative for Leadership in Nursing and Healthcare Organizations   **65**

Patricia L. Thomas, Micki McMillan, Patricia A. Barlow, and Lesa Becker

PART II   Leading the Business of Health Care: Processes and Principles

CHAPTER 7   Strategic Planning and Change Leadership: Foundations for Organizational Effectiveness

Patricia L. Thomas and Roland Loup

CHAPTER 10   Managing Performance   251

Kathryn M. Ward-Presson

CHAPTER 11   Information Management and Knowledge
Development as Actions for Leaders   283
Donna Faye McHaney and Miriam Halimi

PART III   Leading to Improve the Future Quality and Safety of Healthcare Delivery

CHAPTER 12   Laws, Regulations, and Healthcare Policy Shaping Administrative Practice   325
Carolyn Dolan and James L. Harris

CHAPTER 13   Anticipating and Managing Risk in a Culture of Quality, Safety, and Value   361
Shea Polancich and Marylane Wade Koch

Foreword

Although management and leadership concepts cross all sectors of the economy, the reality is that, by its very nature, health care in the United States is complex. The skills and knowledge that are needed to manage and lead healthcare providers and the services they deliver are constantly evolving. In its seventh edition, *Management and Leadership for Nurse Administrators* provides a comprehensive picture of the areas of knowledge that are foundational for nurse executives. In addition, the text provides helpful strategies for developing one's skills as an effective leader. For example, chapter 4 focuses on professional development, which is an ongoing process for all leaders, irrespective of whether one is a novice or an experienced leader.

A number of drivers will impact health care in the immediate future and for years to come. Grounded in an era of healthcare reform, nurse executives must be agile and proficient while also being politically savvy, resourceful, and responsive to stakeholders. Chapter 5 showcases how changes to organizational structures and systems require that transformational leaders understand and use tools such as action research, variation, and getting outside the C-suite mentality to successfully navigate in uncertain environments.

The healthcare industry will continue to be highly regulated and have a strong emphasis on policy development. Chapter 8 addresses nurse executives' roles in this area and includes concepts such as value-based purchasing, brokering healthcare services, and accountable care organizations. Having a baseline understanding of these concepts is critical for working effectively with other healthcare executives to shape how health care is delivered.

Nurse executives must also be able to manage human capital, including fostering healthy work environments (chapter 9) and enhancing the performance of others, while providing opportunities for professional growth and building loyalty to the employer (chapter 10). Risk management is another growing area of importance for organizational leaders. Chapter 12 discusses legal perspectives that will assist managers to identify potential strategies and initiate actions that reduce litigation.

Nurse executives practice across a continuum of healthcare settings and bring a voice to the work of nursing, whether as a single discipline or, increasingly, within the concept of team-based care. The final chapter illustrates the multiple stakeholders that rely on nurse executives to champion the profession and the practice in the public domain.

To each of you who are expanding your knowledge and skills to be more effective nurse leaders, thank you for your unwavering commitment to lifelong learning. To the editors, congratulations on providing a comprehensive picture of the critical work of nurse executives. *Management and Leadership for Nurse Administrators* has been, and will continue to be, a rich resource within nursing education and for nurse executives who are shaping not only their practice, but also the professional growth of other nurses who are on the leadership journey.

Jane Marie Kirschling, PhD, RN, FAAN
Dean and Professor, University of Maryland School of Nursing
University Director, Interpersonal Education
Past President, American Association of Colleges of Nursing (2012–2014)

Preface

This new edition is framed around the American Organization of Nurse Executives (AONE) competencies, the American Nurses Association's (ANA) *Scope and Standards for Nurse Administrators*, the Institute of Medicine's (IOM) *Future of Nursing* report, and current trends in healthcare management and leadership. The American Nurses Credentialing Center's (ANCC) focus on magnetism is also integrated, specifically, the components of transformation leadership, structural empowerment, exemplary professional practice, new knowledge, innovation, improvement, and quality. Quality, safety, evidence-based practice, and improvement science are threaded throughout this new edition. *Management and Leadership for Nurse Administrators, Seventh Edition* is suitable as an introductory course in nursing administration graduate programs. This text can be used in upper-level baccalaureate programs in which traditional and accelerated students and registered nurses may obtain a bachelor's or graduate degree. Due to the integrative perspective of this text, doctor of nursing practice programs may also find this text useful in their organizational, leadership, and systems core courses that provide essential content in culture, improvement science, and change theory. Faculty and students will find this text to be an essential resource in basic courses pertaining to management and leadership. Staff development nurse managers in service settings can access this reference when mentoring and developing staff, specifically from a quality improvement and evidence-based practice perspective. This reference can also serve as an important resource to the advanced generalist role of clinical nurse leaders, who consider change, microsystems, complexity, systems thinking, collaboration, and leadership as core work in their programs of study. Doctor of nursing practice faculty and students will find this resource important to their understanding of organizational and systems leadership to improve patient and healthcare outcomes. Doctoral-level knowledge and skills in these areas can be reinforced as students review content relative to organizational, political, cultural, and economic perspectives. The theory and principles of *Management and Leadership for Nurse Administrators, Seventh Edition* apply to the entire spectrum of healthcare institutions and settings.

Management and Leadership for Nurse Administrators, Seventh Edition provides theoretical and practical knowledge that will aid professional nurses in meeting the demands of continually changing patient care services managed within complex adaptive systems. Because the demand for nurses in some specialties and geographical areas exceeds supply, it is essential that management processes create a culture of innovation, creativity, improvement, productivity, and greatness. Financial considerations and technology have increasingly dominated the healthcare industry, making the job of managing costly human and material resources urgent. Resource management that considers human, financial, physical, emotional, and social capital are strongly emphasized and woven throughout this new edition. Time is of the essence in application and translation of best practices in leadership and management science.

Healthcare institutions have been restructured, demassed, and decentralized along with other business and industrial institutions. This text has been revised to provide the best management and leadership concepts and theories of business that are available from the fields of generic management and nursing management sources. Application and translation underpin all chapters through the use of reflective questions and dynamic case studies.

Chapters have been updated, streamlined, and synthesized to reflect high-level evidence and best practices in leadership and administration. New chapters reflect changing markets and trends and address the critical need to collaborate, innovate, translate science, and work with clinical and academic partners. Chapters discussing topics of trends, executive summary and portfolio development, risk management, and a culture of magnetism have been revised or added to this new edition.

Contributors

Elizabeth Anderson, MSN, RN

Chief Executive Officer
University of South Alabama Medical Center
Mobile, Alabama

Patricia A. Barlow, BA, MCC

President and Founding Partner, Blue
Mesa Group
Fort Collins, Colorado

Lesa Becker, PhD, RN, PCC

Leadership Coach and Consultant, Blue
Mesa Group
Graduate Adjunct Faculty, Boise State
University
Cascade, Idaho

Donald D. Bignotti, MD

Senior Vice President, Chief Medical Officer
Trinity Health
Livonia, Michigan

Denise Danna, DNS, RN, NEA-BC, FACHE

Louisiana State University Health Sciences
Center
School of Nursing
New Orleans, Louisiana

Carolyn Dolan, RN, JD, MSN, FNP-BC, PNP-BC

Professor of Nursing
University of South Alabama
Mobile, Alabama

Val Gokenbach, DM, RN, MBA, NEC-A, RWJF

Dr. Val Leading Leaders, Leadership
Consultant, Executive Coach, Professional
Speaker
Grosse Pointe, Michigan

Miriam Halimi, DNP, MBA, RN-BC

Vice President, Chief Nursing Informatics
Officer
Trinity Health
Livonia, Michigan

James L. Harris, PhD, APRN-BC, MBA, CNL, FAAN

Professor of Nursing
University of South Alabama
Mobile, Alabama

Cynthia King, PhD, NP, CNL, FAAN

Professor and Nurse Scientist
Queens University
Charlotte, North Carolina

Gay Landstrom, PhD, RN, NEA-BC

Chief Nursing Officer
Dartmouth-Hitchcock Health
Lebanon, New Hampshire

Anne Longo, PhD, MBA, RN-BC

Sr. Director, Center for Professional
Excellence/Education
Cincinnati Children's Hospital Medical Center
Cincinnati, Ohio

Roland Loup, PhD

Principal and Owner, Roland J. Loup
Organization Consultant
Ann Arbor, Michigan

Donna Faye McHaney, DNP, BSCS, ARNP, RN, NP-C

National Consultant, Clinical Affairs
ITT Technical Institute
Henderson, Nevada

Micki McMillan, MEd, MCC

CEO and Founding Partner, Blue Mesa Group
Fort Collins, Colorado

Lisa Mestas, MSN, RN

Chief Nursing Officer
University of South Alabama Medical Center
Mobile, Alabama

Shea Polancich, PhD, RN

Assistant Professor
University of Alabama at Birmingham
School of Nursing
Birmingham, Alabama

Carol Ratcliffe, DNP, RN, NEA-BC

Associate Professor
Samford University
Birmingham, Alabama

Linda Roussel, PhD, RN, NEA-BC

Professor
University of Alabama Birmingham
School of Nursing
Birmingham, Alabama

Rita Stockman, MSA, BSN, RN

System Director, Accreditation & Regulatory
Services
Trinity Health
Livonia, Michigan

*Patricia L. Thomas, PhD, RN, NEA-BC, ACNS-BC,
CNL, FACHE*

Vice President Clinical Quality &
Transformation, Chief Nursing Officer
Trinity Home Health Services
Livonia, Michigan

Marylane Wade Koch, MSN, RN, CNA

Instructor
Loewenberg School of Nursing
University of Memphis
Memphis, Tennessee

Kathryn M. Ward-Presson, DNP, RN, NEA-BC

Healthcare and Leadership Consultant
Ward Consulting Partners, LLC
Jonas Scholar in Veterans Healthcare Alumni
Raleigh, North Carolina

CASE STUDY CONTRIBUTORS

Susan Allen, PhD, RN-BC

Assistant Vice President, Center for
Professional Excellence/Education
Cincinnati Children's Hospital
Cincinnati, Ohio

Darla Banks, MS, RN, CCRN, CNL

Director of Clinical Nurse Leader Program
Texas Health Resources
Fort Worth, Texas

Patricia A. Barlow, BA, MCC

President and Founding Partner, Blue
Mesa Group
Fort Collins, Colorado

Lesa Becker, PhD, RN, PCC

Leadership Coach and Consultant
Blue Mesa Group Graduate Adjunct Faculty
Boise State University
Cascade, Idaho

Stephanie Burnett, DNP, RN, CRRN

University of Alabama Medical Center
Birmingham, Alabama

Sheree C. Carter, PhD, RN

University of Alabama in Huntsville
Huntsville, Alabama

Sergül Duygulu, PhD, RN

Associate Professor
Hacettepe Üniversitesi Hemşirelik Fakültesi
Hacettepe University Faculty of Nursing
Samanpazari, Ankara, Turkey

Kathleen E. Ebert, MS, RN NEA-BC

Nursing Excellence and Quality Outcomes
NEA-BC
Ohio Health
Columbus, Ohio

Jennifer L. Embree, DNP, RN, NE-BC, CCNS

Clinical Assistant Professor
Indiana University School of Nursing-IUPUI
Indianapolis, Indiana

Debbie R. Faulk, PhD, RN, CNE

Professor of Nursing
Auburn University Montgomery
Montgomery, Alabama

Wade Forehand, DNP, RN-BC

Troy University, School of Nursing
Troy, Alabama

James L. Harris, PhD, APRN-BC, MBA, CNL, FAAN

Professor of Nursing
University of South Alabama
Mobile, Alabama

Kristen Herrin, DNP, RN

University of Alabama Huntsville
Huntsville, Alabama

Lisa Keegan, EJD, MSM, MED, BSN, NE-BC

Chief Nurse Medical Care
Veterans Administration Hospital
Cincinnati, Ohio

Cynthia R. King, PhD, NP, MSN, RN, CNL, FAAN

Principal & Consultant
Special Care Consultants
New Hartford, New York

Gay Landstrom, PhD, RN, NEA-BC

Chief Nursing Officer
Dartmouth-Hitchcock Health
Lebanon, New Hampshire

Lori Lioce, DNP, FNP-BC, CHSE, FAANP

University of Alabama Huntsville
Huntsville, Alabama

Anne Longo, PhD, MBA, RN-BC, NEA-BC

Maineville, Ohio

Micki McMillan, MEd, MCC

CEO and Founding Partner, Blue Mesa Group
Fort Collins, Colorado

Jennifer Melvin Pifer, DNP, MBA, RN, CNOR, CM

Associate Chief Nursing Service
Department of Veterans Affairs
Durham, North Carolina

Arlene H. Morris, EdD, RN, CNE

Professor of Nursing
Auburn University Montgomery
Montgomery, Alabama

Kristen Noles, MSN, RN, CNL

University of Alabama Medical Center
Birmingham, Alabama

Terri Poe, DNP, RN, NE-BC

Chief Nursing Officer
University of Alabama Medical Center
Birmingham, Alabama

Shea Polancich, PhD, RN

Assistant Professor
University of Alabama at Birmingham
School of Nursing
Birmingham, Alabama

Kathryn G. Sapnas, PhD, RN-BC, CNOR

Director of Clinical Strategic Planning and
Measurement
Department of Veterans Affairs
Washington, District of Columbia

Patricia L. Thomas, PhD, RN, NEA-BC, ACNS-BC, CNL, FACHE

Vice President Clinical Quality & Transformation, Chief Nursing Officer
Trinity Home Health Services
Livonia, Michigan

Abigail Veliquette, PhD

Special Assistant Professor and Leadership Coach
Colorado State University
Fort Collins, Colorado

Joseph White, DNP, RN

University of Alabama Medical Center
Birmingham, Alabama

Kerri Wilhoite, DNP, RN, NEA-BC

Associate Director of Patient Care Services/Nurse Executive
Northern Arizona Veterans Healthcare System
Prescott, Arizona

Lonnie K. Williams, MSN, RN

Educational Consultant
Washington, District of Columbia

Joyce Young, PhD, MS, RN, CENP

Vice President Patient Care Services/CNO
St. Joseph Mercy Ann Arbor and Livingston
Ypsilanti, Michigan

INTERVIEW CONTRIBUTORS

Velinda J. Block, DNP, RN, NEA-BC

SVP, System Chief Nursing Officer
KentuckyOne Health
Louisville, Kentucky

Anne Marie Dooley, DNP, MBA/HCM, BN, RN

Director, Medicine, Neurosciences Nursing
King Fahad Specialist Hospital—Dammam
Kingdom of Saudi Arabia

Nancye R. Feistritzer, DNP, RN

Vice President Patient Care Services
Chief Nursing Officer
Emory University Hospital
Atlanta, Georgia

Jessica Hardy, DNP, RN

Executive Director
Alabama Department of Public Health
Office of Women's Health Director
Montgomery, Alabama

Pam Jones, DNP, RN, NEA-BC

Associate Professor
Senior Associate Dean
Clinical and Community Partnerships
Nashville, Tennessee

Gay Landstrom, PhD, RN, NEA-BC

Chief Nursing Officer
Dartmouth-Hitchcock Health
Lebanon, New Hampshire

Lisa Mattox, MSN, RN

Nurse Manager
University of Alabama Medical Center
Birmingham, Alabama

Lisa Mestas, MSN, RN

Chief Nursing Officer
University of South Alabama Medical Center
Mobile, Alabama

Elizabeth Murphy, BSN, MSBA, RN, NEA-BC, FACHE

VP Patient Care Services/CNO
Mercy Health Saint Mary's
Grand Rapids, Michigan

Margaret Nadler Moore, DNP, RN

Manager of Student-Run Clinic
University of South Alabama
Mobile, Alabama

Kristen Noles, MSN, RN, CNL

Nurse Manager
University of Alabama Medical Center
Birmingham, Alabama

Terri Poe, DNP, RN, NE-BC

Chief Nurse Executive
University of Alabama Medical Center
Birmingham, Alabama

Soha Sahwan, MSN, RN

Nurse Manager
HHC/Apheresis/Family Medicine/Rehab/
 Stoma & Wound Service
King Fahad Specialist Hospital—Dammam
Kingdom of Saudi Arabia

Barbara Samson, MS, MBA, RN, CHC, CRRN

Director of Clinical Services
Trinity Home Health Services
Livonia, Michigan

Joseph White, DNP, RN

Nurse Manager
University of Alabama Medical Center
Birmingham, Alabama

Lori Wightman, DNP, RN, NEA-BC

VP Patient Care Services/CNO
Saint Agnes Medical Center
Fresno, California

Joyce Young, PhD, MS, RN, CENP

Vice President Patient Care Services/CNO
St. Joseph Mercy Ann Arbor and Livingston
Ypsilanti, Michigan

Nursing Leadership Matters: Managing in the New Age of Health Care

Linda Roussel, Patricia L. Thomas, and James L. Harris

CONCEPTS

The concepts included in this text are as follows: controlling, evaluating, measuring, standards, transformation, information age, quantum leadership, microsystems, failure mode effect analysis, root cause analysis, Gantt chart, performance evaluation and review technique, benchmarking, evidence-based management, and quality awards.

The past decade in the U.S. healthcare system saw unprecedented challenges and opportunities for improvement and innovation. Current healthcare delivery evolved from the industrial age of the late 18th and early 19th centuries, when separate and distinct departments were formed with defined roles and tasks. The command and control style of management and leading aligned with this mechanistic approach to organizational work. Departments and services were typically arranged in silo structures that increased barriers to interprofessional collaboration, and inefficiencies were commonplace, leading to prolonged hospital stays, medical specialization, and inflated cost for care (Wiggins, 2008). From the 1990s to today, caregivers and managers are challenged to consider multiple strategies to manage complex situations due to biomedical and information technology advances, increases in patient morbidity and mortality, shorter hospital stays, escalating costs, and demands for quality and access (Aiken, Clark, Slone, Sochalski, & Silber, 2002; Long, 2004). Of notable interest are historical markers that continue to impact the healthcare industry, including hospital ratings on technology and safety; the introduction of 10 starter set core measures by The Joint Commission; the Malcolm Baldrige National Quality Award first awarded to a hospital; the Centers for Medicare and Medicaid Services launch of hospital comparisons; the introduction of transforming care at the bedside; the passage of healthcare reform legislation; and the release of the *Future of Nursing* report by the IOM.

Four generations that have different approaches and work-related behaviors are operating in tandem within healthcare organizations:

1. Veterans (1922–1943): This generation defines the workplace based on military or church hierarchy and respect for authority with clear privileges given to each level in the organization. They expect and deliver no-nonsense performance.

2. Baby boomers (1943–1960): Self-esteem and happiness are driving forces for this group, driven by passion and the need to make a difference. They desire social or team environments with personal recognition for their hard work. If they believe in the vision of an organization, they will give 110% of themselves in hours and commitment; this generation invented the 60-hour work week.

3. Generation X (1960–1980): This generation desires independence and hands-off management. They demand a balance between their personal lives and careers. Individuals see themselves as equal players to *all* ages and want to be evaluated based on merit, not seniority. Respect comes from competency, not hierarchy.

4. Nexters (1980–current): Nexters expect economic prosperity and recognize that they are in high demand because there are not enough of them. They are used to a global world and are technologically very savvy with their ability to quickly access and use information and knowledge. This group values new knowledge and fast-paced environments (Leitschuh, 2011).

Coupled with potential conflicts and differences that may arise in today's workforce from generational differences, work behaviors, and challenges that are inherent in reforming health care, nurse managers must use a variety of approaches. Managers must be armed with skill sets that are different from those of past decades. Logic, predictability, cause and effect, and linear reasoning are no longer enough. A new way of approaching work is required for success and survival in a chaotic, changing, and evolving healthcare environment.

ORGANIZATIONAL SYSTEM: CONTEXT FOR CHANGE

Today's nurse managers must position themselves to manage in chaotic and staccato-paced environments. The forces and pressures that require change as an imperative, not an option, coupled with a quest for quality, safety, efficiency, and customer satisfaction require managers to consider alternatives to past practices and techniques. Talents such as critical thinking, insight, problem solving, and sharp analytic and imagination skills are in great demand. They require organizational climates and cultures to create space so these talents can come together and emerge with innovative solutions. The pursuit of quality, safety, and efficiency consumes enormous amounts of time and requires different ways of thinking about work. Likewise, developing and adopting new care delivery models is necessary to address financial constraints and is an instrument for change (Morjikian, Kimball, & Joynt, 2007). The multiplicity and complexity of increasing demands that are being placed on nurse managers can result in leadership blind spots, where the manager is not able to serve the patient population or be the best steward of the organization. Robinson-Walker (2008) asserts that leadership blind spots are significant aspects of institutional life, whereby individuals fail to exercise their best judgment and discrimination. Often nurse managers find themselves in new leadership roles without adequate formal education and support, contributing to a lack of awareness of leadership blind spots. It is imperative that nurse managers possess exceptional organizational agility to know and understand how organizations work, how to get things done, the reasoning behind policy and practice, the value of evidence to guide best practice, and an organization's culture (Lombardo & Eichinger, 2004). Thus, leadership blind spots can be minimized.

Management in times of chaos and proposed healthcare reform requires a new way of thinking and responding to mandates. Managing in light of intense demands for greater quality, improvement, efficiency, and effectiveness of patient care necessitates consideration of alternatives to usual business practices. The unusual becomes the usual; the ordinary becomes the extraordinary. Both have a place in managing and leading organizations and deserve to be considered. Nurse leaders need to be armed with new skills sets to move teams toward increased accountability and transparency. Creating a just culture requires the best thinking available.

Stacey (1996) distinguished ordinary from extraordinary management. Ordinary management considers a logical analytic process to daily operations using data analysis, goal setting, weighing available options against goals, rationality, implementation, and evaluation, which are generally accomplished through hierarchical monitoring. Control is at the center of ordinary management. Cost-effective performance is the measure by which effective and efficient systems are valued and judged.

According to Stacey (1996), extraordinary management is also essential if the organization is to transform itself in situations of open-ended change. Stacey posits that extraordinary management supports the integration of teams from diverse units within a system, encouraging engagement of creative problem solving and decision making from inside and outside the organization. Establishing a culture of openness allows for an exchange of information and social capital through informal structures that develop as needed. The informal structures become the infrastructure in which issues and problems can be readily addressed.

Innovative strategies that are grounded in structure, process, and outcome measures are needed in today's environment. In the old model, organizations dominated by overly rationalist thinking machines are driven by predictability, but complexity and chaos theorists posit that the natural world does not operate this way. Stacey purports that the creative disorder in the universe needs to be an integral part of nurse managers' activities. The consequences of creative disorder turn management practices upside down. Considering complexity theory and organizations as complex adaptive systems, Stacey (1992) postulates the following points:

- Analysis loses its primacy.
- Contingency (cause and effect) loses its meaning.
- Long-term planning becomes impossible.
- Visions become illusions.
- Consensus and strong cultures become dangerous.
- Statistical relationships become dubious.

The list could be endless. Any organization attempting to achieve stable relationships within an unpredictable environment is a recipe for catastrophe. Organizations seeking and expecting linear and predictable outcomes may lag behind others as they continuously engage in work processes that had previously worked. Successful organizations emerge from complex and continuing interactions among people. According to Stacey (1993), the dominant 1980s approach to strategy, which distanced itself from the strategic planning paradigm of preceding decades, still managed to maintain the aim of strategic management as its intent. Theorists of complexity management underscore process flow; instead, they embrace openness to what may happen, serendipity, and synchronicity.

Innovation and creative approaches in nursing management are required more today than in the past. Thinking differently will require individuals to try new ideas, learn from failures, and embrace a willingness to function in an often ambiguous and uncertain environment. This is an essential skill set for nurse managers.

COMPLEX SYSTEMS: REVISITING MENTAL MODELS TO EFFECT CHANGE

Healthcare environments challenge the most skilled managers and often lead them to question their ability and approach to effect change at the micro, intermediate, or macro level. Change resides at the heart of leadership. Appreciative inquiry enhances a system's capacity to apprehend, anticipate, and heighten positive potential (Cooperrider & Whitney, 2011).

The emergence of complexity science offers alternative leadership and management strategies for the chaotic and complex healthcare environment. Survey data reveal that healthcare leaders intuitively support principles of complexity science. Leadership that uses complexity principles offers opportunities in the chaotic healthcare environment to focus less on prediction and control and to focus more on fostering relationships and creating conditions in which complex adaptive systems can evolve to produce creative outcomes (Stacey, 1996).

Zimmerman, Lindberg, and Plsek (1998), in their work with complex adaptive systems, note that this theory has much in common with general systems thinking, the learning organization, quality, empowerment, gestalt theory, organizational development, and various other approaches. Conceptualizing complex adaptive systems asserts an understanding of how things work in the real world. The authors provide a number of principles in their work with complex adaptive systems that include working with paradox and tension; being cooperative and competitive in tandem; using chunking to make sense of large projects and information; and being good enough in order to take action.

Plsek (2001) stresses that mental models often are so ingrained in one's thinking that it is difficult (without reflection and examination) to embrace other perspectives and viewpoints. Without this much-needed work, it is likely that fads and gimmicks will be espoused without real change; thus, new ways of doing business are not likely to last, add value, and spread throughout an organization. Nurse managers have a moral obligation to embrace divergent thinking, stay informed of impending legislation, and lead the dialogue of reform beyond fads and gimmicks that are here today and gone tomorrow.

Change is inevitable in health care. Arming oneself with knowledge and engaging others in meaningful activities will result in prolonged and sustainable change. Being open to new venues and embracing differing perspectives drive success and engender collaboration among all healthcare team members.

CREATING INNOVATIVE ENVIRONMENTS TO SUSTAIN CHANGE AND ADD VALUE

In an era of healthcare reform and the quest for quality, safe, and efficient care, creating and sustaining innovative environments where staff function at their highest potential and add value to an organization is pivotal to ongoing success. The two sides of reform span coverage expansion proposals and payment reform proposals. For example, coverage expansion includes an individual mandate for coverage and no preexisting condition exclusions, to name two. Payment reform proposals include, but are not limited to, no pay for never events, pay for performance, readmission penalties, and bundled payments.

With the advent of the IOM *Future of Nursing* report, a blueprint was created that positions nursing to lead and effect change, partner with others in redesigning health care in the United States, be transformative, and create environments for lifelong learning while adding value within organizations and communities of interest. The four key messages included in the IOM report include the following:

1. Nurses should practice to the full extent of their education and training.
2. Nurses should achieve higher levels of education and training through an improved education system that promotes seamless academic progression.
3. Nurses should be full partners, with physicians and other health care professionals, in redesigning health care in the United States.
4. Effective workforce planning and policy making require better data collection and an improved information infrastructure (Institute of Medicine [IOM], 2011, p. 14).

Eight recommendations were also outlined in the report:

1. Remove scope-of-practice barriers. Advanced practice registered nurses should be able to practice to the full extent of their education and training.
2. Expand opportunities for nurses to lead and diffuse collaborative improvement efforts. Private and public funders, health care organizations, nursing education programs, and nursing associations should expand opportunities for nurses to lead and manage collaborative efforts with physicians and other members the health care team to conduct research and to redesign and improve practice environments and health systems. These entities should also provide opportunities for nurses to diffuse successful practices.
3. Implement nurse residency programs. State boards of nursing, accrediting bodies, the federal government, and healthcare organizations should take actions to support nurses' completion of a transition-to-practice program (nurse residency) after they have completed a prelicensure or advanced practice degree program or when they are transitioning into new clinical practice areas.
4. Increase the proportion of nurses with baccalaureate degrees to 80 percent by 2020. Academic nurse leaders across all schools of nursing should work together to increase the proportion of nurses with a baccalaureate degree [from] 50 to 80 percent by 2020. These leaders should partner with education accrediting bodies, private and public funders, and employers to ensure funding, monitor progress, and increase the diversity of students to create a workforce prepared to meet the demands of diverse populations across the lifespan.
5. Double the number of nurses with a doctorate by 2020. Schools of nursing, with support from private and public funders, academic administrators and university trustees, and accrediting bodies, should double the number of nurses with a doctorate by 2020 to add to the cadre of nurse faculty and researchers, with attention to increasing diversity.
6. Ensure that nurses engage in lifelong learning. Accrediting bodies, schools of nursing, healthcare organizations, and continuing competency educators from multiple health [professions] should collaborate to ensure that nurses and nursing students and faculty continue their education and engage in lifelong learning to gain the competencies needed to provide care for diverse populations across the lifespan.
7. Prepare and enable nurses to lead change to advance health. Nurses, nursing education programs, and nursing associations should prepare the nursing workforce to assume leadership positions across all levels, while public, private, and governmental health care decision[s] should ensure that leadership positions are available and filled by nurses.

8. Build an infrastructure for the collection and analysis of inter-professional healthcare workforce data. The National Health Care Workforce Commission, with oversight from the Government Accountability Office and the Health Resources and Services Administration, should lead a collaborative effort to improve research and the collection and analysis of health data on healthcare workforce requirements. The Workforce Commission and [Health] Resources and Services Administration should collaborate with state licensing boards, state nursing workforce centers, and the Department of Labor in this effort to ensure that the data are timely and publicly accessible (IOM, 2011, p. 32).

Meeting the recommendations in the IOM report will require actions and engagement by Congress, state legislators, the Centers for Medicare and Medicaid Services, the Office of Personnel Management, the Federal Trade Commission and the Antitrust Division of the Department of Justice, governmental agencies, professional organizations, communities, accrediting bodies, organizations that are supportive, all stakeholders, nursing programs, and the nursing profession.

In an envisioned future in which healthcare environments continuously adapt to change and reform and are responsive to individuals' desires and needs through patient-centered care, innovation will become the hallmark of sustainment and value. Primary care and prevention, interprofessional collaboration, healthy work environments, and affordable, quality care for all will be the norm, not the exception. To ensure the vision is realized, several drivers are framing meaningful strategies and are the linchpins for success. The drivers are timely and central to the efforts required by all nursing leaders, administrators, and stakeholders. The following text identifies and overviews each of the drivers.

There are a number of industries that are error prone, where the slightest mistake can be catastrophic. Health care is not exempt. Although multiple efforts have focused on quality improvement, high-reliability organizations is the next step. A high-reliability organization demonstrates performance at high levels of safety over time (Chassin & Loeb, 2011).

Although the introduction of Medicare improved the access to care, the quality of care was not directly improved. What followed were utilization review committees, experimental medical care review organizations, professional standards review organizations, peer review organizations, and multiple improvement activities. Practice guidelines were later developed and adopted in an effort to prompt providers to rely on scientific evidence in providing care. However, Balas and Boren (2000) found that it takes an average of 17 years for research to reach practice.

During the 1990s, a shift from practice guidelines to standardized quality measures and public reporting of the resulting data emerged (Kizer, 2001). Now more than ever there is a requirement for improvements in quality and safety, and nurse managers play a role in this effort. Frankel, Leonard, and Denham (2006) identify three requirements for achieving high reliability: leadership, a culture of safety, and robust process improvement. Each requirement will guide actions by all members of the healthcare team and offer opportunities for nurses to guide processes and evaluate outcomes. This is supported by evidence-based practice, where nurses are positioned to influence and shape care decisions and improve the delivery of quality care. Newhouse, Dearholt, Poe, Pugh, and White (2007) define evidence-based practice as "a problem-solving approach to clinical decision making within a healthcare organization that integrates the best available scientific evidence with the best available experiential (patient and practitioner) evidence" (p. 27). Nurse managers can coach staff to use the best available evidence to guide practice. This supports the notion that nursing is a science and an applied discipline. Accountability continues to be the vanguard leading to high quality, safe, and efficient care, and it can be achieved through translating evidence into practice.

Building on initiatives that Medicare implemented in prior years, accountable care organizations are another model set forth to address the inadequacy of the U.S. healthcare system. An accountable care organization is characterized by provider groups that are willing to take responsibility for improving the overall health status, efficiency, and healthcare experience for a defined population (DeVore & Champion, 2011). The success of accountable care organizations will be supported by collective efforts with other healthcare reforms that include support for primary care, comprehensive performance measurement, and interfacing with other payment reforms (McClellan, McKethan, Lewis, Roski, & Fisher, 2010). Additionally, other activities that will support and advance accountable care organizations include the following:

- Executive sponsors and participation
- Payer partners
- Data transparency
- Aligned physician networks
- Savvy contracting
- Adequate population base
- Acceptance of common cost and quality metrics
- Data infrastructure
- People-centered foundation
- Leadership
- Population health data management

In 2011, the U.S. Department of Health and Human Services launched an incentive, the Hospital Value-Based Purchasing program, to adjust Medicare reimbursement based on how well hospitals were performing on 12 clinical process measures and 9 patient experience measures relative to a baseline performance period. Hospitals are scored for each measure between an achievement threshold and a benchmark. The achievement threshold is the minimum performance level, and the benchmark is based on the highest level of performance among hospitals during the baseline period. The financial incentives of the Value-Based Purchasing program are not the most significant characteristic; the most important feature is the measurement tools it provides. Many hospitals are concerned about meeting and maintaining performance measures, thus increasing the likelihood of reduced operating revenue (Shoemaker, 2011). However, gains in value that are secondary to the program can be realized from prevention, early intervention, and ambulatory management of patients versus emergency department visits and hospital admissions and readmissions (Tompkins, Higgins, & Ritter, 2009). Such gains are supported by nursing activities through patient management and inclusiveness of patients in all care decisions.

The evolving Patient Centered Medical Home model of care is another innovative driver to effect change and add value (Clancy, 2011). The model has two primary goals: to treat patients in the lowest-cost setting and proactively manage the treatment of patients to prevent acute care episodes. The Patient Centered Medical Home model is an interdisciplinary team approach whereby staff members work to the full scope of their practice and expertise, focus care on holistic health, and enhance access to enable more frequent communication between patients and team members. Patient Centered Medical Homes maximize the capabilities of existing staff to support the care model. This is another avenue where nurse managers can have a significant impact on enhancing care delivery and placing the patient at the center of care and decision making.

Last, nurses have an opportunity in the creation of a standardized, scientifically reliable method to document, measure, and disseminate nursing contributions to safe and efficient patient outcomes in support of healthcare information technology. During the upcoming years, the U.S. government will be developing standards for a national electronic medical record. Meaningful use will guide the process, criteria, and terms to direct the collection, recording, and reporting of clinical data in the electronic medical record. Criteria defining meaningful use will roll out in three stages through 2015; mechanisms will be framed to allow the exchange of key information among the healthcare team, as well as elements related to privacy and security (Bolla, 2011; Halamka, 2009).

Meaningful use and information are the cornerstone of problem solving and making good decisions. Asking better questions leads to better decisions. Diversity and conflict can be used in creating strategic alliances. Heffernan (2015) proffers that rich debate and argument are essential activities; if well done, they generate ideas and surface any fears and doubts. Heffernan (2015) provides a list of questions that serve to facilitate lively debate and discussion:

- Who needs to benefit from our decisions? How?
- What else would we need to know to be more confident of this decision?
- Who are the people affected by this decision? Who has the least power to influence it?
- How much of this decision must we make today?
- Why is this important? And what's important about *that*?
- If we had infinite resources—time, money, people—what would we do? What would we do if we had no resources?
- What are all the reasons this is the right decision? What are all the reasons it is the wrong decision?

SUMMARY

Change in health care is inevitable, and the various forces affecting care delivery require innovative approaches. Understanding and responding to organizational dynamics and mandates necessitate that nurse managers approach business from different perspectives and engage others to arrive at decisions. Using evidence to guide actions will accentuate success and result in sustained change that is valued by organizations, employees, and stakeholders. The health and welfare of Americans are entrusted to all managers and providers. True healthcare reform will be accomplished through knowledge attainment and engagement in activities that promote learning environments.

REFERENCES

Aiken, L. H., Clark, S. P., Slone, D. M., Sochalski, J., & Silber, J. H. (2002). Hospital nurse staffing and patient mortality, nurse burnout, and job satisfaction. *Journal of the American Medical Association, 288*, 1987–1993.

Balas, E. A., & Boren, S. A. (2000). Managing clinical knowledge for health care improvement. In J. Bemmel & A. McGray (Eds.), *Yearbook of medical informatics: Patient centered systems* (pp. 65–70). Stuttgart, Germany: Schattauer.

Bolla, Y. (2011). Meaningful use 101. *Nursing Management, 42*(8), 18–22.

Chassin, M. R., & Loeb, J. M. (2011). The ongoing quality improvement journey: Next stop, high reliability. *Health Affairs, 30*(4), 559–568.

Clancy, T. R. (2011). Improving processes through evolutionary optimization. *The Journal of Nursing Administration, 41*(9), 340–342.

Cooperrider, D. L., & Whitney, D. (2011). *A positive revolution in change: Appreciative inquiry.* Retrieved from http://appreciativeinquiry.case.edu/intro/whatisai.cfm

DeVore, S., & Champion, R. W. (2011). Driving population health through accountable care organizations. *Health Affairs, 30*(1), 41–50.

Frankel, A. S., Leonard, M. W., & Denham, C. R. (2006). Fair and just culture, team behavior, and leadership engagement: The tools to achieve high reliability. *Health Services Research, 41*(4 part 2), 1690–1709.

Halamka, J. (2009). Making smart investments in health information technology: Core principles. *Health Affairs—Web Exclusive, 28*(2), w385–w389.

Heffernan, M. (2015). *Beyond measure: The big impact of small changes.* New York, NY: Simon and Schuster.

Institute of Medicine (IOM). (2011). *The future of nursing: Leading change, advancing health.* Washington, DC: National Academies Press.

Kizer, K. W. (2001). Establishing health care performance standards in an era of consumerism. *Journal of the American Medical Association, 286,* 1213–1217.

Leitschuh, C. (2011). *Understanding generational differences.* Retrieved from http://ezinearticles.com/?Understanding-Generational-Differences&id=503459

Lombardo, M., & Eichinger, R. (2004). *For your improvement (FYI): A guide for development and coaching.* Minneapolis, MN: Lominger International.

Long, K. A. (2004). Preparing nurses for the 21st century: Reenvisioning nursing education and practice. *Journal of Professional Nursing, 20*(2), 82–88.

McClellan, M., McKethan, A. N., Lewis, J. L., Roski, J., & Fisher, E. S. (2010). A national strategy to put accountable care into practice. *Health Affairs, 29*(5), 982–990.

Morjikian, R. L., Kimball, B., & Joynt, J. (2007). Leading change. The nurse executive's role in implementing new care delivery models. *The Journal of Nursing Administration, 37*(9), 399–404.

Newhouse, R. P., Dearholt, S. L., Poe, S. S., Pugh, L. C., & White, K. M. (2007). *Johns Hopkins nursing: Evidence-based practice model and guidelines.* Indianapolis, IN: Sigma Theta Tau.

Plsek, P. E. (2001). Appendix B: Redesigning health care with insights from the science of complex adaptive systems. In IOM Committee on Quality of Health Care in America (Ed.), *Crossing the quality chasm: A new health system for the 21st century* (pp. 309–322). Washington, DC: National Academies Press.

Robinson-Walker, C. (2008). Leadership blind spots. *Nurse Leader, 6*(4), 10–11.

Shoemaker, P. (2011). What value-based purchasing means to your hospital. *Healthcare Financial Management Association,* August: 61–68.

Stacey, R. D. (1992). *Managing the unknowable: Strategic boundaries between order and chaos in organizations.* San Francisco, CA: Jossey-Bass.

Stacey, R. D. (1993). *Strategic management and organizational dynamics.* London, England: Pitman.

Stacey, R. D. (1996). *Complexity and creativity in organizations.* San Francisco, CA: Berrett-Koehler.

Tompkins, C. P., Higgins, A. R., Ritter, G. A. (2009). Measuring outcomes and efficiency in Medicare value-based purchasing. *Health Affairs, 28*(2), w251–w261.

Wiggins, M. S. (2008). The challenge of change. In C. Lindberg & S. Nash (Eds.), *On the edge: Nursing in the age of complexity* (pp. 149–190). Bordentown, NJ: Plexus.

Zimmerman, B., Linderberg, C., & Plsek, P. (1998). Nine emerging and connected organizational leadership principles. In B. Zimmerman & C. Linderberg (Eds.), *Edgeware: Lessons for complexity science for health care leaders* (pp. 292–305). Dallas, TX: VHA.

Leading in Times of Complexity and Rapid Cycle Change

CHAPTER 1

Forces Influencing Nursing Leadership

Linda Roussel

LEARNING OBJECTIVES

1. Discuss current trends in healthcare management and their impact on quality, safety, and value-added care (care delivery).
2. Envision care delivery systems for the future.
3. Discuss major influences—specifically, Institute of Medicine (IOM), Agency for Healthcare Research and Quality (AHRQ), Institute for Healthcare Improvement (IHI), Magnet, Baldrige, and other major stakeholders—in healthcare systems.
4. Identify how ethics relates to managing healthcare services.

AONE KEY COMPETENCIES

I. Communication and relationship building
II. Knowledge of the healthcare environment
III. Leadership
IV. Professionalism
V. Business skills

AONE KEY COMPETENCIES DISCUSSED IN THIS CHAPTER

II. Knowledge of the healthcare environment
III. Leadership
IV. Professionalism

II. Knowledge of the healthcare environment
- Clinical practice knowledge
- Patient care delivery models and work design knowledge
- Healthcare economics knowledge
- Healthcare policy knowledge
- Understanding of governance
- Understanding of evidence-based practice
- Outcomes measurement
- Knowledge of, and dedication to, patient safety

- Understanding of utilization and case management
- Knowledge of quality improvement and metrics
- Knowledge of risk management

III. Leadership

- Foundational thinking skills
- Personal journey disciplines
- Ability to use systems thinking
- Succession planning
- Change management

IV. Professionalism

- Personal and professional accountability
- Career planning
- Ethics
- Evidence-based clinical and management practices
- Advocacy for the clinical enterprise and for nursing practice
- Active membership in professional organizations

FUTURE OF NURSING: FOUR KEY MESSAGES

1. Nurses should practice to the full extent of their education and training.
2. Nurses should achieve higher levels of education and training through an improved education system that promotes seamless academic progression.
3. Nurses should be full partners with physicians and other health professionals in redesigning health care in the United States.
4. Effective workforce planning and policy making require better data collection and information infrastructure.

Introduction

Health care is a moving target with forces for change impacting outcomes for quality, safety, and value-added care. These forces include shifting population demographics, finance reform, consumerism, and personalized medicine. Quality, safety, and translational science are at the heart of future trends, focusing on interprofessional teams and patient-centered care. Based on the evidence, health-care systems have made limited progress in improving the patient experience and meeting the IHI triple aims (Stiefel & Nolan, 2012).

In the past decade, health care has experienced dramatic swings, including a change in social demographics, advancements in medical technologies, heightened consumer awareness, and greater demand for high-quality, efficient, and cost-effective care. This consumer-driven, competitive environment proclaims a transformation that all healthcare organizations must embrace to succeed and be sustainable. Quality improvement, evidence-based practice, translational science, the patients' experience, and systems thinking are essential to sustaining a competitive edge. The traditional hierarchical, bureaucratic, and insulated organizational models no longer make sense in this new business of health care. An evolving model needs to be flat, innovative, nimble, just in time, and responsive to change. If a healthcare organization is to survive at today's frenetic pace, greater flexibility and the ability to deal with ambiguity are essential (Porter-O'Grady & Malloch, 2015).

Being great, or going from good to great, takes the courage of one's convictions, vision, and energy, according to *Good to Great: Why Some Companies Make the Leap…and Others Don't*, a management book by James C. Collins. We are charged with keeping up with trends that affect short- and long-term planning. Collins (2001) contends that visionary companies have better management development and succession planning than comparable companies, thereby ensuring greater continuity in leadership talent grown from within. Collins's research contends that Level 5 leadership does matter.

According to Collins (2001), a Level 5 leader is a person who harmonizes extreme personal humility with intense resolve. In his 5-year research study, Collins discovered that Level 5 leaders combined traits that served as catalysts for transforming a good company into a great one. Using Level 5 as the highest level in a hierarchy of executive capabilities, Levels 4, 3, 2, and 1 follow in this leveling process. Leaders in the four other levels can have some measure of success, however, not enough to move from mediocrity to sustained greatness. Collins contends that a company cannot go from good to great without Level 5 leadership (*Executive*) at the helm. To better understand Level 5 leaders (builds greatness), it is useful to understand Levels 1 through 4.

Level 4 is described as an *effective leader* who is able to stimulate teams to high-performance standards by demonstrating commitment to aggressive pursuit of a compelling vision. Level 3 has been identified as a *competent manager* able to effectively and efficiently organize people and material resources using stable objectives, often predetermined by executive leaders. Level 2 illustrates a *contributing team member* able to add to the achievement of team objectives and to demonstrate effective group work in a variety of cultures and settings. Level 1 leaders are identified as *highly capable individuals* who demonstrate the productive activity through talent, knowledge, skills, and good work habits. Collins (2015) contends that individuals do not proceed sequentially through each level of the hierarchy to reach the top; however, fully evolved Level 5 leadership does require the capabilities of Levels 1 through 4, along with special characteristics of Level 5 (humility, resolve).

Visioning and futuristic thinking embrace an openness to change. In the 21st-century workplace that is driven by innovation and technological transformation, new knowledge, skills, and abilities are demanded from everyone. New roles to address the demands are critical. A high level of trust, encouraging the heart, authentic leadership, and relationship-based care are important in balancing safe and quality health care, efficiency, and costs.

According to Kouzes and Posner (2003), encouraging the heart is about keeping hope alive by setting high standards and by demonstrating authentic interest and optimism about the employee's capacity to achieve meaningful goals. High-performing managers are approachable and embrace diversity through timely feedback and by sharing their thoughts, feelings, and perceptions. Kouzes and Posner go on to describe seven essentials to encouraging the heart and include setting clear standards, expecting the best, paying attention, personalizing recognition, telling the story, celebrating together, and setting positive examples. Telling the story can serve to clarify standards and gives examples of best practices. "Stories are essential means of conveying that we are making progress.... Stories put a human face on success" (p. 105).

There is a different emphasis and skill set for nurse administrators today than those that dominated the past century. Logic, predictability, and linear reasoning were the order of the day and gave some measure of success in a stable environment. These skills alone are not enough and no longer serve us well in our complex, complicated systems (Porter-O'Grady & Malloch, 2015).

ORGANIZATIONAL SYSTEM: CONTEXT FOR TRENDS AND CHANGE

Considering trends in light of organizations and systems propels the nurse administrator to consider different, innovative ways to structure and redesign processes and outcomes that are necessary to transform care delivery. Organizations must move away from domination by an overly rational thinking machine that is focused on predictability; theorists of complexity and chaos show us that the natural world does not operate this way. Stacey (2010) purports that this revelation of the role of creative disorder in the universe needs to be taken to heart by managers. The consequences, as Stacey summarizes, turn management practices upside down. Considering complexity theory and organizations as complex adaptive systems (CAS), Stacey postulates the following points (2010):

- Analysis loses its primacy.
- Contingency (cause and effect) loses its meaning.
- Long-term planning becomes impossible.
- Visions become illusions.
- Consensus and strong cultures become dangerous.
- Statistical relationships become dubious.

The list continues to change. An organization seeking stable relationships within an unpredictable environment is a recipe for failure. An organization expecting predictable outcomes by focusing on its strengths, continuing what it does best, and making limited adjustments will likely be left in the dust by its innovative rivals. Successful strategies, in the long run, do not come by fixing organizational intention and circling around it; they emerge from complex and continuing interactions among people. According to Stacey (2010), the dominant 1980s approach to strategy, which distanced itself from the strategic planning paradigm of preceding decades, still managed to maintain the aim of strategic management as its intent. Theorists of complexity science emphasize the essential nature of openness to accident, coincidence, and serendipity. The emerging resultant is strategy.

Management in times of chaos requires a new way of thinking and being in the world. Managing in light of intense demands for greater quality, safety, efficiency, and effectiveness of patient care necessitates consideration of alternatives to business as usual. The unusual becomes the usual; the ordinary becomes the extraordinary. Both have a place in managing and leading organizations. Safety has become first and foremost at the center of healthcare delivery.

Results measurement emphasizes analyzing outcomes to evaluate the value of care. In this model, competition is value based and therefore focused on outcomes. As a result, process measures and evaluations of specific procedures and episodes of care are not useful unless they provide knowledge to improve outcomes. Value can be determined only if outcomes are measured across the care cycle based on healthcare systems and medical conditions. The principles of value, results measurement, system restructuring, and value-based competition provide a promising framework for transforming health care. Value, rather than procedures, becomes the basis for reimbursement, which eliminates unhealthy competition and cost shifting. Effective outcomes are determined based on the care cycle rather than the episode.

PRINCIPLES TO CREATE FUTURE CARE MODELS

Value-Based Competition

To develop future healthcare models, value-based competition is one of the first principles that needs to be addressed. The concept of value-based competition was introduced by Porter and Teisberg (2006) as an alternative to what they describe as failed incremental changes in both the healthcare system and financing structure. They contend that competition has promoted progress in other industries, but not in health care. Health care has fallen victim to zero-based competition, which is defined as winning at the expense of another, and operating in a system where cost shifting has benefited neither providers nor patients. Vlasses and Smeltzer (2007) set forth three interrelated principles to drive healthcare transformation:

- Positive-sum competitors
- System restructuring
- Rewards management

A transition to positive-sum competition in health care is based on value or health outcomes per dollar spent. Positive-sum competition incentivizes improved results based on clinical outcomes, as opposed to volume or length of stay. To restructure the healthcare system, Porter and Teisberg (2007) proposed a system organized around medical conditions and care cycles rather than provider specialties such as cardiology or endocrinology. Medical conditions reflect the set of sequelae commonly seen with a particular diagnosis that is addressed in an integrated way. An integrated care unit is then equipped to deliver care along the continuum based on the patient's experience of the disease.

Safety: Where Are We Now?

Safety and quality go hand in hand, with greater incentives to reduce adverse events and improve the patients' experiences. A study in the *New England Journal of Medicine* reported data from North Carolina hospitals that showed there had been minimal progress in reducing harm from unsafe medical care between 2002 and 2007 (Landrigan et al., 2010). In another study, James (2013) found that between 200,000 and 400,000 Americans die each year from unsafe medical care, making it the third leading cause of death in the United States behind heart disease and cancer. Additional evidence was noted in an eye-opening November 2011 report on adverse events in hospitals. The Office of Inspector General (OIG) in the U.S. Department of Health and Human Services found that 5% of Medicare patients suffered an injury in a hospital that prolonged their stay or caused permanent harm or death. Another 13.5% of Medicare patients suffered temporary harm, such as an allergic reaction or hypoglycemia. Taken together, the evidence purports that more than one in four hospitalized Medicare beneficiaries suffer some type of injury during their inpatient stay, much higher than previous rates. The OIG report also noted that unsafe care contributes to 180,000 deaths of Medicare beneficiaries each year, and that Medicare pays at least $4.4 billion to treat these injuries. Despite all the focus on patient safety, it seems we have not made much progress at all (Committee on Health, Education, Labor, and Pensions, 2014).

Although this is not good news, there are areas in which we have made notable gains, most notably with healthcare-associated infections. These gains have been attributed to the work of Dr. Peter Pronovost, of Johns Hopkins University, and the Centers for Disease Control and Prevention (CDC). Pronovost created a simple five-item checklist that was tested in more than 100 intensive care units in Michigan to reduce rates of central line infections. Pronovost found that each of these infections can incur up to $50,000 in treatment costs, necessitating an average of 7 additional days in the hospital. While central line infection is complex and expensive, Pronovost's checklist intervention is simple by comparison. Using the checklist, the hospitals involved in the project reduced their central line infection rates to essentially zero in 3 months. Individual providers were not the focus; rather, the system was the primary focus for improvement. The checklist improved the care delivery system by notably reducing the number of infections. The checklist program was disseminated to more than 1,100 intensive care units across the country and is saving lives and resources daily (Brody, 2008).

The CDC is the other major player in the improvement effort. It established the National Healthcare Safety Network (NHSN), which is a voluntary online system that tracks healthcare-associated infections nationwide. Through the NHSN, the CDC established standard metrics for assessing and reporting healthcare-associated infections (HAIs), affording providers the opportunity to track their own data and report it anonymously and directly to the CDC. These efforts have been instrumental in helping providers, healthcare executives, and policy makers keep up with infection rates and ensure that requisite preventive procedures are carried out. The NHSN allows hospital leaders to benchmark their facilities against others to determine where improvement is critical to better outcomes. The NHSN purports that good metrics, offered in a timely way, make a significant contribution to provider performance. Rates of central line infections from 2008 to 2012 decreased by 44%. Specifically, rates of infection in the 10 most common surgical procedures fell by 20%. All told, there has been progress in reducing infection rates caused by the healthcare system. In a number of ways, the problems described here do not tell the story of medical errors. Although much attention has focused on acute hospitals, there has been relatively limited attention paid to discharged patients and care transition. In another report, the OIG found that 22% of Medicare beneficiaries in skilled nursing facilities (SNFs) experienced a medical injury that increased their length of stay or caused death or permanent harm. The same report found that an additional 11% suffered a temporary medical injury. The OIG estimates that adverse events cost Medicare roughly $2.8 billion per year, and about half these events are preventable. The OIG report is concerning given that about 20% of hospitalized Medicare patients go to an SNF after discharge. There is a clarion call to improve patient safety as a national priority (Conway, 2013).

With safety front and center, what additional forces and trends can we anticipate as we navigate the future of health care? Forces to consider include technology, healthcare finance, personalized medicine, population, social networking, and consumerism.

Technology

Technology has far-reaching implications for reform because it affects both processes of care and the way organizations work. Technology also empowers consumers. Although some new technology may increase the cost of care up front, it has the potential to improve health and eventually decrease healthcare costs.

Among the broad-based effects of technology are the development of health information systems and the genomics that are contributing to biotechnical advances in care. Health information systems are increasingly being used to decrease healthcare costs by standardizing and improving data capture to support both billing practices and care decisions. Information systems can potentially reduce the rate of increase in healthcare costs, which were predicted to reach 19% of the gross national product by 2014. Information systems enable leaders to more effectively capture cost and quality indicators that are used to improve practice and reward performance, thereby improving the efficiency and efficacy of health care. Users of healthcare services and the technology of health care will progressively interface. Connections between providers and patients will have more virtual and seamless interactions, with supporting technology enabling the provision of clinical services to patients remotely (Porter-O'Grady & Malloch, 2015). Just as technology is increasingly assisting caregivers with diagnosis and treatment, it also enables patients to assume more ownership of their health. Personalized medicine, which will become personalized health care over time, is one of the most exciting aspects of future health care. The continued development of personalized medicine will require not only a time commitment from nurse executives and their colleagues but also a paradigm shift from consumer as patient to consumer as partner.

Automation

Administrators and physician owners who are focused on preparing for the future do not dwell on today's healthcare problems. Although they still see reimbursement cuts and increased administrative tasks, they do not allow these issues to consume their work. Technology can provide greater efficiency. For example, a provider must consider the time it takes to standardize a process and then find the technology to automate the task.

Imaging Technology

New devices make imaging more portable and accessible to patients. For example, the Vscan from GE Healthcare can allow patients to take an ultrasound image of their heartbeat from home and send the visuals to their physician for review. Or a surgeon in a surgery center can use an ultrasound device over a patient's heart and will be able to determine abnormal rhythms or other anomalies in real time. This changes the meaning of a visit. Additionally, surgery centers can regularly monitor a patient's condition remotely and provide timely alarms that could reduce risks and improve quality of life. In the same vein, data about a patient's weight or physical activity could be assessed through a device, such as an Internet-enabled scale or pedometer, and sent directly to the patient's records. Scans and radiological images could also be tracked and stored in the patient's health record.

Electronic Health Records

Electronic health records (EHRs) are mainly used as digital storage systems for patient records. Currently, EHRs do not have strong analytical capabilities, but in the future they could assist healthcare providers by analyzing patient data and assisting in the process of care. The big data movement is upon us and will provide greater continuity of care and a smoother transition of care delivery. The use of big data sets could potentially connect the dots between patients and conditions and provide new insight to clarify the healthcare picture.

EHR implementation is a huge expense and takes time and energy for staff members to fully integrate the system into the healthcare center. However, the technology makes it easier to report quality data and serves as the basis for evolving toward the level of care coordination that is necessary to treat patients. As the learning curve decreases, healthcare providers will be able to engage with their patients and health records at the same time by capturing videos and pictures for future review.

Robotic Technology

The precision that can be achieved with robotic technology allows physicians to transition more complex surgeries into outpatient procedures. The da Vinci Surgical System, which is used for several types of general and urological surgery procedures, has made a big impact on the field. Robotic technology requires a large capital investment, and a significant number of surgery centers have not taken the leap, especially since the robot does not bring higher reimbursement from insurance companies. Surgery centers that have invested in robotic technology have business models that attract high-acuity cases to their centers so they can maintain profitability and provide quality care.

Healthcare Finance

Considering the preferred future in health care, financial reform must be part of the conversation. Healthcare costs continue to rise, and cost shifting is occurring among employers, healthcare providers, workers, and insurers. The number of uninsured persons in the United States is reaching the nation's capacity to provide care. Cost, access, and quality will continue to be the triple charge that guides healthcare system redesign. Preventing medical errors and positioning higher safety standards also impact financial commitments and cost constraints. The rapid pace of healthcare changes will affect how work is done. Community and outpatient care will dominate the healthcare market, with services moving out of the hospital at greater rates. Hospitals will no longer be the main point of care as services continue to be decentralized (Porter-O'Grady & Malloch, 2015).

Personalized Medicine

Personalized medicine is the development and treatment of disease, and disease propensity, with interventions based solely on a person's genetic profile. Making personalized medicine a reality will improve patient outcomes and necessitate changes in health care given the advances in genomic, pharmacokinetic, and computer technology. Personalized medicine underscores a growing consumer expectation that health care in general should be tailored and custom fitted to the individual. Consumers are demanding individualized services.

According to the report *The New Science of Personalized Medicine: Translating the Promise into Practice* (2015), the market for personalized medicine in the United States is already $232 billion and projected to grow 11% annually. Targeting individualized treatment and care based on personal and genetic variations is the focus of personalized medicine. This is disruptive innovation, and it is also creating a booming market with opportunities and challenges for traditional and emerging market participants. PricewaterhouseCoopers forecasts that a more personalized approach to health and wellness will expand to as much as $452 billion by 2015. This estimate goes beyond pharmacological innovation and devices, along with low-tech products and services. These changes are focused on consumers' greater awareness of health promotion and greater recognition of an individual's own health risks (PricewaterhouseCoopers Scientific Advancement, 2015).

With personalized health care, consumers take a more active role in their care. The Internet has had a significant impact on the trend toward self-help, with the growth of home diagnostics, advances in monitoring, and easy access to health information (Harvard-Partners Center for Genetics and Genomics, 2007).

Personalized medicine also implies that treatment will be customized, a trend that is already under way. Patients are expected to participate in the planning process for their health and share a plan of action for their own health care. Ideally, patients receive and evaluate information about their care before office visits. In a study of 12,878 participants, it was found that uninsured individuals with chronic disease were more likely than those who were privately insured to use the Internet for information (Vlasses & Smeltzer, 2007).

Population-Based Health Care

Population-based health care has always been important, and now more than ever, with social determinants of care, it has a greater impact. We know that factoring in social determinants makes care coordination more comprehensive and sustainable. An aging and increasingly diverse population is one major factor with immediate consequences for health care because it increases the demand for care and taxes the diminished workforce. The aging population requires chronic disease management, which incurs added costs for managing multiple disease processes and care transitions. With limited numbers of nurses, physicians, and other allied health professionals, healthcare leaders are charged with redesigning both systems and roles (Vlasses & Smeltzer, 2007).

Social Networking

Social networking techniques are most commonly associated with sites such as Facebook and MySpace, but social networking can have applications within health care. Health-related social networking, such as DailyStrength (http://www.daily strength.org/), PatientsLikeMe (http://www.patientslikeme.com/), and Flu Wiki (http://flu.wikia.com/wiki/Flu_Wiki), led the CDC and the American Cancer

Society, among other healthcare institutions, to use Second Life (http://www .secondlife.com), a popular virtual world site. Their presence on Second Life promoted awareness of disaster planning, good nutrition, cancer prevention, and other healthy behaviors. Social networking technologies can help providers as well as patients. An example of how social networking can be effective includes the LINK, which is a comprehensive school-linked health clinic with the capacity to provide preventive medical care, acute medical care, referrals, and health education in the schools as needed. Healthcare services through the LINK impact children's and adolescents' health (http://www.rockislandcounty.org/HealthDept /SchoolHealthLINK.aspx).

The Nursing and Midwifery Electronic Community of Practice (E-CoP), also known as the Global Alliance for Nursing and Midwifery (GANM), provides an example of community ownership and interactivity within the nursing social networking space. The E-CoP has more than 1,800 members in 132 countries, and its site contains a robust knowledge base of culturally sensitive and specific tools that members contributed. The site also includes open-source literature, a platform where members can interact to reduce isolation, and mechanisms to enhance access to online education.

Consumerism

Consumerism can be described in a variety of ways. It is at first a way of organizing means of individuals, groups, and governmental agencies to protect consumers from activities, policies, and practices that may violate their rights to fair trade and business practices. It has also been described as the ongoing and increasing consumption of goods and services which forms the basis of a sound economy. It can also be described by the continuation of acquiring goods and services and the wants and needs that drive this desire (Business Dictionary, 2015).

The future trend of consumerism in health care is about protection of consumers rights as well as the understanding of how accelerating innovation to adapt to increasing consumption impacts individual deals, societal demands, and quality, safety, and financial viability of meeting healthcare needs. Partnerships, collaboration, and cooperation enhance and promote consumerism and advance evidence-based processes and outcomes. An example of accelerating innovation can be found in the Forum on Health Care Innovation. The Forum on Health Care Innovation is a collaboration between Harvard Business School (HBS) and Harvard Medical School (HMS). The purpose of the Forum is to bring together leading executives, academics, and policy makers in a cross-disciplinary inquiry of innovative actions serving to improve quality, reduce costs, and most importantly increase value in the healthcare industry. Proceedings from the first conference in 2014 identified five imperatives for addressing healthcare innovation challenges: making value the central objective; promoting novel approaches to process improvement; making *consumerism* really work; decentralizing approaches to problem solving; and integrating new approaches into established organizations (Chin, Hamermesh, Hickman, McNeil, & Newhouse, 2014). For example, making value the central objective focuses on collaborative efforts of stakeholders. A value proposition must be made for care coordination and shared information strategies to reduce costs and improve patient and systems outcomes. Promoting novel approaches to process improvement encourages problem solving that considers the environment and culture in which the work (care delivery) is happening and invites failure as part of the process. Consumer incentives to encourage healthy behavior ranked last among 11 possible innovations in terms of their ability to increase value, with 44.6% of respondents indicating that it would have only a minimal or slight impact on improving quality and 43.9% noting its minimal or slight potential for controlling cost (Chin, Hamermesh, Hickman, McNeil, & Newhouse, 2015). Key insights identified as part of the consumerism as an imperative include sharing responsibility for a complex problem (healthcare delivery system) and putting patients first. In putting patients first care processes and structures are centered around patient, family, and community needs, and not the providers or caregivers.

Making consumerism really work also requires attention to strategies that enhance patient engagement and self-care management. Providers and caregivers become facilitators and coaches. Porter-O'Grady and Malloch (2015) describe responsibility and accountability, a shift from 20th-century to 21st-century thinking, with accountability of consumers and providers being focused on results, outcomes, accomplishment, fit, and sustainability and being internally generated. Decentralizing approaches to problem solving involve facilitating the movement of care delivery and healthcare innovation from centralized centers of expertise out to the microsystem engaging a greater number of providers, innovators, and patients in a collaborative effort to improve outcomes. Integrating new approaches to established healthcare systems involves understanding our history, building on successes, and embedding evidence-based strategies into relevant and value-added work.

Nursing takes great pride in being the 24-hour patient advocate at all points in the healthcare continuum. Nursing's social contract is centered on a patient–family relationship of providing holistic care throughout the care continuum. In our current environment, technology, communication, and consumer knowledge will continue to raise consumer expectations and underscore nursing's capability to fulfill the social contract. With consumerism comes the mandate to envision creative options to traditional care delivery. Core practices of all the professions have been significantly altered. Consumers are choosing high-intensity interventions in primary care settings instead of hospitalization. They are also becoming more engaged in their own health. This shift will change how healthcare professionals provide health care. They will have the essential work of helping to transfer the locus of control for medical decision making and life management to patients, who have never had this responsibility and are sometimes at a loss to know what to do for their own care (Porter-O'Grady & Malloch, 2015). Patients have voiced their negative experiences about receiving timely care, the cost of care, and paperwork related to care and billing practices. They conveyed their problems and challenges in navigating the healthcare system.

As patients become more knowledgeable about their health care, the time pressure on providers can be expected to increase. In 2004, the reported median time physicians spent with patients during an office visit was 14.7 minutes. The challenge for providers is to apply their expertise in collaborations with consumers so they can evaluate Internet information and up-to-date scientific evidence. Berry and Edgman-Levitan (2012) noted that the Picker Institute carried out a multiyear research project that identified eight characteristics of care as the most important indicators of quality and safety. This work was done in partnership with patients and families. From the perspective of patients, the following characteristics were identified: respect for the patient's values, preferences, and expressed needs; coordinated and integrated care; clear, high-quality information and education for the patient and family; physical comfort, including pain management; emotional support and alleviation of fear and anxiety; involvement of family members and friends, as appropriate; continuity, including through care-site transitions; and access to care. These eight characteristics will not be successfully carried out unless patients and families are involved in designing, implementing, and evaluating care delivery systems.

NURSING-SENSITIVE INDICATORS, SAFETY STANDARDS, AND QUALITY INDICATORS

Maas, Johnson, and Morehead (1996) used the phrase nursing-sensitive indicators to reflect patient outcomes influenced by nursing practice. Needleman and colleagues noted that nursing-sensitive indicators may be a more comprehensive term focusing on the relationship of nursing with negative or adverse patient outcomes, such as medication errors, patient falls, and nosocomial infections (Needleman, Buerhaus, & Mattke, 2001). These authors note that there is less evidence examining the relationship of nursing and positive patient outcomes. They attribute the use of negative outcomes to the fact that adverse patient outcomes are more readily available in medical records and administrative data sets.

Needleman and colleagues refer to outcomes that are potentially sensitive to nursing (2001) recognizing nursing contributions in the clinical care delivery process; their reluctance points to the struggle in determining attribution when care delivery processes are interwoven. The reporting of nursing-sensitive information to the Centers for Medicare and Medicaid Services (CMS) is forthcoming. Starting in October 2010, hospitals were required to inform CMS of their plans to report nursing measures electronically.

The National Database of Nursing Quality Indicators (NDNQI) serves as a repository for translating data to aid the delivery of high-quality care. The American Nurses Association (ANA) pushed through efforts to collect and evaluate nursing-sensitive indicators in the early 1990s, providing ongoing support for database development activities through the National Center for Nursing Quality. The University of Kansas School of Nursing, which ranks among the top nursing schools in the nation for nursing research funded by the National Institutes of Health, continues to provide ongoing nursing-sensitive indicator consultation and research-based expertise to the NDNQI, which was recently sold to Press Ganey. The school conducts research primarily on clinical and health policy topics in two areas: healthcare effectiveness and health behavior. The NDNQI continues to grow and is a powerful tool for nurse executives. This national database program has two primary goals (American Nurses Association [ANA], 2004):

- Provide comparative information to healthcare facilities for use in quality improvement activities
- Develop national data on the relationship between nurse staffing and patient outcomes

According to the ANA, the database is growing and contains hundreds of participating healthcare facilities and various kinds of data. For example, patient outcome and nurse staffing data are being collected on critical care, step-down, medical, surgical, medical–surgical, pediatric, psychiatric, and rehabilitation units. Nurse satisfaction data are being collected from a wide variety of nursing units and across the organization. The data are collected according to strict standards; collaboration has been a key component in the growth of the NDNQI. Participants can be part of the development process if they so choose.

The NDNQI provides the capacity to trend data by providing participants with quarter-by-quarter and unit-by-unit comparisons of nursing care, thus eliminating isolated and perhaps misleading snapshots of performance. The NDNQI data allow nurse executives to mark progress, understand and improve patient care and nursing work environments, avoid costly complications, and assist in marketing the quality of nursing leadership's efforts. The NDNQI can also serve as a valuable tool for nursing staff retention and recruitment of potential employees (ANA, 2004).

In a similar vein, reports from the IOM's quality initiative brought public attention to the urgent need for understanding, measuring, improving, and ensuring the quality of health care in the United States. These quality initiatives, which are focused on important aspects of healthcare quality, such as revealing serious healthcare systems errors and patient safety concerns, recommended a taxonomy of quality attributes for the healthcare system. Recommendations were further proposed to enhance quality initiatives by coordinating quality-related efforts in six government programs. They offered strategies for interdisciplinary education in the health professions and identified needed changes in the nursing work environment to improve patient safety. These major initiative reports represent a systematic effort to focus on quality and patient safety concerns in health care and to advance critical healthcare quality efforts in the United States.

In addition, macro-level quality initiatives in the public and private sectors are ongoing. For example, within the federal government the Quality Interagency Coordination Task Force was formed, bringing together independent initiatives within various governmental agencies that relate to or affect healthcare quality. Another example is the National Healthcare Quality Report, developed by the AHRQ, which presented data on the quality of services for seven clinical conditions and included a set of performance measures that serve as a baseline for the quality of health care.

Private groups, such as the Leapfrog Group, the National Quality Forum, The Joint Commission, and the IHI, are also proposing efforts and recommendations for improving and ensuring high-quality health care (Institute for Healthcare Improvement, 2008; Leapfrog Group, 2008; National Quality Forum, 2008; The Joint Commission, 2008). Many of these initiatives attempt to move closer to the point of care delivery. As reported, professional organizations and provider groups, such as the ANA, the American Medical Association, and the Veterans Health Administration, also proposed quality surveillance activities aimed at identifying and capturing provider- and profession-specific clinical quality indicators. Public reporting of healthcare quality data can drive quality improvement and expand the potential value of quality indicators.

Another example comes from the AHRQ, which identifies quality indicators to measure healthcare quality by using available hospital inpatient administrative data. Patient safety indicators are tools to help health system leaders identify potential adverse events occurring during hospitalization (Hussey, Mattke, Morse,

& Ridgely, 2006). The AHRQ quality indicators expanded the original Healthcare Cost and Utilization Project quality indicators. The first set of AHRQ quality indicators (the prevention quality indicators) was released in November 2001. The second set (the inpatient quality indicators) was released in May 2002 and in March 2003. In February 2006 the fourth quality indicator module (the pediatric quality indicators) was added as the pediatric population was removed from the other modules (Agency for Healthcare Research and Quality, 2002).

Innovative Care Delivery Models

Most innovations in health care involve only specific aspects of care or system processes and are not based on our current model of aligning financial incentives. Consider that the implementation of electronic health records often does not result in a beneficial transformation if the records simply reflect the current state of care delivery. These types of changes alone do not respond to patient-centered care. As noted by futurists, the U.S. healthcare system needs either dramatic, transformational change or complete re-visioning.

New models and principles for care delivery are surfacing. They are focusing the point of care on the primary care environment and redefining the timing of interventions based on genetic makeup. The hospital is no longer the center of the healthcare universe.

Healthcare consumers are seeking continuity of care, with attention paid to interprofessional collaboration and smooth handoffs in transitions of care. Evidence-based transitional care models are gaining traction and engage patients and their support systems in all aspects of their health (Coleman, Parry, Chalmers, & Min, 2006; Naylor et al., 2004). Care coordination must be a standard that becomes second nature to all passages in the healthcare delivery system. Examples of models that address care coordination—the medical home and the ambulatory intensive care unit—are described in the following sections. As a result of their study of more than 1,000 randomly selected U.S. citizens, Schoen and colleagues offered clear direction for the future based on evidence from their current healthcare system experience (Schoen, How, Weinbaum, Craig, & Davis, 2006). These researchers found that customers want value. They want well-coordinated care that is provided through one source, with access to both their medical record and information regarding quality and cost. Yet studies indicate that patients are more likely to have short-term relationships with physicians and minimal, if any, access to their medical record. The gap between what customers want and reality is considerable. In Schoen and colleagues' study, 42% of the participants reported that they experienced inefficiencies in care, poor coordination of care, or unsafe care in the previous 2 years.

Medical Home

The patient-centered medical home model is an evidence-based framework for integrated health care (Rittenhouse & Shortell, 2009). The idea of the medical home, sometimes referred to as an advanced medical home concept, was developed by the American Academy of Pediatrics as a model for the care of children with chronic illnesses. The American Academy of Family Physicians, the American Academy of Pediatrics, the American College of Physicians, and the American Osteopathic Association (2007) recently published a joint article with their consensus definition of a medical home. A medical home is patient-centered care focused on prevention, health promotion, and coordinated care across the life span. This model incorporates all aspects of the care continuum and focuses on care coordination and active disease management (Rittenhouse & Shortell, 2009). Essential components of the medical home integrate expectations from both consumers and healthcare professionals. Although variations can be found in the literature, the patient-centered medical home model holds promise for improved coordination of patient care needs and expectations.

Models that incorporate these principles are proposed to transform primary care. To make such models a reality, healthcare financing must be aligned with incentives that focus on care delivery that is safe, effective, and efficient. Obtaining funding to test innovative models and to evaluate resources that are necessary to ensure that the models work as designed is important to make them a reality. An example comes from the Louisiana Health Care Redesign Collaborative, which adopted the medical home as the cornerstone for post-Katrina New Orleans and submitted a proposal to the CMS for financing (Louisiana Health Care Quality Forum, 2008). Although they are based on primary care, these models have significant implications for re-visioning healthcare services and the roles of providers. They create an infrastructure for care that is coordinated through a primary care delivery system that connects tertiary services into a unified healthcare model. Healthcare providers in this new model deliver integrated care, which requires innovative and broader roles and functions.

Ambulatory Intensive-Care Units

Ambulatory intensive-care units (A-ICUs) are founded on the belief that individuals can be seen at the appropriate level of care and that decisions to change the level of care can be made in the patients' best interest rather than on financial incentives. Funded by a grant, the California HealthCare Foundation has tested the A-ICU model, which is designed to demonstrate significant cost savings in the care of high-risk, chronically ill individuals who incur the highest costs in the current system. A medical home provider links and coordinates appropriate care resources for patients to achieve efficiencies. The medical home provider has a continual relationship with the patient and oversees care across the continuum.

An A-ICU builds efficiency by moving the processes of care and organizational management to primary care. High-risk patients benefit from innovative, intensive primary care interventions to improve their health status and care management in a long-term relationship. Providers function not as gatekeepers but as partners with patients, engaging them to take responsibility for their own health in a system grounded in quality. The primary care team contracts with inpatient and specialty services based on demonstrated quality and efficiency indicators. Other providers must show worth and value to become ancillary to this process. Moving the locus of control from the insurer to the patient–provider relationship supports a more appropriate competitive process based on quality and efficiency rather than reimbursement regulations and rates.

Strategies for Leading Change

Key strategies for effective leadership in this transition involve adopting technology and change management. The Technology Informatics Guiding Education

Reform (TIGER) Initiative summary report notes that we must focus on "integrating informatics seamlessly into nursing, making it the stethoscope of the 21st century" (TIGER Initiative, 2007). Our ability to connect with patients is highly dependent on our adoption of technology. Cell phones, webinars for working with groups, online synchronous forms of communication, and decision support applications are tools we must incorporate into practice.

Echoing the TIGER report, we must become active players on all fronts related to the development and implementation of health information technology, enforcing the standard for evidence-based tools at the point of care for the use of both nurses and consumers. The TIGER report identified management and leadership as one of the key pillars for practice transformation in informatics and recommends leadership, direction, and support along with a shared mental model of the future (TIGER Initiative, 2007). These same principles serve us well in advocating for system redesign.

Today we are inundated with changes, and Ellis (2007) speaks to the acceleration of change. We are charged with managing these changes and their implications for stakeholders. Therefore, we must become students of change. In contrast to notions of rapid diffusion of innovations, Morrison (2000) describes the healthcare environment as one where healthcare providers experience rapid change; however, to those on the outside looking in, the pace is far from accelerated. While we are confronted with possibilities, we are also caught in this dilemma. We are charged with keeping the need for change and reevaluation at the forefront, and we are invited to create rather than react.

Traditional strategies for change management are based on planned change. Approaches to planned change apply to modifications in an existing structure that are reversible and do not require new learning. This type of change merely skims the surface compared with what is occurring and what needs to occur in health care. Consumers are calling for fundamental change in the healthcare system, and new models such as the A-ICU call nursing's attention to system's thinking and redesign of the work and how the workforce rethinks patient care delivery, teamwork, and care transitions.

To do this, we must also reconceptualize the tools and strategies we use to create change. This type of change, referred to as second-order change, occurs when there is a fundamental shift in an organization's basic structure. Frameworks for second-order change, although in need of further testing and research, may be more informative in guiding healthcare transformation. They call for new infrastructure that requires new learning. A new story is being told.

Changing Time, Location, and Relationship

The forces for change in health care are impacting the critical connection between nurses and patients. Patients no longer come to us as a captive audience. Historically, we have enjoyed a relationship with our patients based on the fact that they depend on us in the hospital at a time of acute vulnerability. Today, 56% of patients in hospitals stay for 4.5 or fewer hours. This has economic implications as well as implications for our survival.

If we want to maintain our signature relationship with patients, we must find ways to stay connected to them personally, but not necessarily in the place where we treat them. We must reimagine our definitions of how we serve patients and believe in them. The need to create work structures, employee work arrangements, and organizations that allow nurses to span episodes of care is critical.

New models, such as the advanced medical home and value-based competition, are built on concepts that have traditionally been in the nursing purview, such as compassionate, culturally sensitive, and coordinated care. These models may provide a venue to support our social contract with patients, but we must be involved in their evolution and testing. Research is needed to demonstrate qualitative and economic value and to evaluate designs that reinvent the role of nurses.

SUMMARY

We are in a new world of health care, and standard operating procedures (SOPs) may no longer serve the patient and the healthcare system. Understanding the organization through different lenses, such as CAS, may provide new tools for enhancing performance. Change, innovation, and infusion of evidence-based practice also contribute to greater efficacy and efficiency in leading. Being armed with an understanding of evidence-based practice and quality indicators improves one's success in creating a safe environment for patients, their families, and the workforce. Without transparent, authentic leadership, there is little hope for real change that can be sustained over time. The health of patients and families who are entrusted to our care depends on our courage to be great and to continually strive for excellence. It is the hope of these authors that increasing knowledge, skills, and abilities can serve this end.

REFLECTIVE QUESTIONS

1. Considering your own practice setting, discuss current trends in healthcare management and their impact on quality, safety, and value-added care (care delivery).
2. What innovative strategies do you envision leading in your own practice setting as you fast-forward to the future?
3. Describe major influences—such as the IOM, AHRQ, IHI, Magnet, Baldrige, and other major stakeholders—in healthcare systems.
4. Identify how ethics relates to managing healthcare services.

CASE STUDY 1-1   Who Speaks for the Patient?

Debbie R. Faulk and Arlene H. Morris

J. E. is the chief nursing officer (CNO) of a midsized regional hospital. One evening an older person was found unresponsive at a nearby long-term care facility, placed on ventilator support, and transferred to J. E.'s hospital. This person is awake and alert and has end-stage chronic obstructive pulmonary disease and severe rheumatoid arthritis with little likelihood of being weaned from the vent. Due to the patient's long-term chronic diseases and limited prognosis secondary to the illnesses, the lifetime Medicare reserve days are nearly exhausted.

(continues)

CASE STUDY 1-1   Who Speaks for the Patient? (Continued)

J. E. has been informed that the prior long-term care facility has no beds for readmission and that other hospitals or long-term care facilities in the geographic area are reluctant to accept transfer of this patient. Additionally, there is no family willing to care for the patient at home; the only living family members are two stepchildren who live in another state. They have requested that the patient be transferred to a facility that provides ventilator care. The physician assigned to provide care said, "The most humane plan of care is to take the patient off of the vent and allow a peaceful death through comfort care after extubation." It is anticipated that discontinuation of ventilator support will result in death, likely within a week.

J. E. believes there are only two options: extubation as suggested by the hospital physician or continuing care for the patient with the ventilator until death. The stepchildren call the case manager, who refers the call to J. E. The stepchildren are informed about the patient's status and the two options. J. E. told the stepchildren that the physicians are concerned the patient has no quality of life. Although J. E. requested consent to extubate, the stepchildren would not consent, stating they wanted to wait until December 26 to decide. When J. E. asked why they desired to wait and possibly prolong suffering, the stepchildren replied that they did not want to associate the memory of the patient's death with a holiday. The stepchildren asked how to get someone else appointed to make decisions. J. E. had been informed by the case manager that if a state agency appointed a legal guardian, the stepchildren could not have a say in funeral arrangements. J. E. relayed this information to the stepchildren, who were upset about no input regarding the funeral, but they asked no other questions.

The stepchildren later called back and consented over the phone to withdraw life support and requested to be informed when the patient died. J. E. is concerned about the phone consent and decided a consent form would be worded as follows: "We, _____ (name) and _____ (name), understand that if the ventilator is removed, death will likely occur soon, but this is in the best interest of _____ (name of patient)." This consent form was sent electronically to the stepchildren, who signed the form and returned it. J. E. then asked the case manager and the primary nurse to sign as witnesses on the form. However, the case manager said that the signing had not been witnessed and asked J. E. if a notary should have been involved and a hard copy of the form sent by mail. J. E. replied that electronic consent forms are part of the healthcare world as long as two people are present. The case manager and primary nurse expressed concern that the consent could have been coerced and actually provided for the physician to end the patient's life. J. E. asked another case manager and nurse to sign as witnesses for the consent form, and they agreed. However, the patient's case manager and other nurses on the patient's unit began discussing possible legal and ethical implications of these actions and asked if a line had been crossed.

Source: Morris & Faulk, 2012

Case Study Questions

1. What factors initially contributed to the development of this situation?
2. Do you believe there were other options than the two presented? Explain your thoughts.
3. Describe the ethical concerns for each of the following:
   The patient
   The family members
   The primary nurse
   The case manager
   J. E.
   The physician(s)
   The case manager and nurse who signed as witnesses
   The hospital as an organization
   The healthcare delivery system

> ## CASE STUDY 1-1   Who Speaks for the Patient? (Continued)
>
> **4.** Describe the legal implications for each of those listed in question 3.
> **5.** Who was the advocate for this patient?
> **6.** Was a consideration related to the patient's condition not discussed?
> **7.** What would you have done if you were J. E.?

REFERENCES

American Academy of Family Physicians, American Academy of Pediatrics, American College of Physicians, & American Osteopathic Association. (2007). Joint principles of the patient-centered medical home. Retrieved from http://www.acponline.org/acp_policy/policies/joint_principles_pcmh_2007.pdf

American Nurses Association. (2004). *Nursing: Scope & standards of practice.* Silver Spring, MD: nursesbooks.org.

Berry, M. J., & Edgman-Levitan, S. (2012). Shared decision making—the pinnacle of patient-centered care. *New England Journal of Medicine, 366,* 780–781.

Brody, J. E. (2008, January 22). A basic hospital to-do list saves lives. *New York Times.* Retrieved from http://www.nytimes.com/2008/01/22/health/22brod.html?pagewanted=print

Business Dictionary. (2015). Consumerism. Retrieved from http://www.business-dictionary.com/definition/consumerism.html

Chin, W. W., Hamermesh, R. G., Hickman, R. S., McNeil, B. J., & Newhouse, J. P. (2014). 5 Imperatives addressing healthcare's innovation challenge. *Forum on Healthcare Innovation.* Retrieved from http://www.hbs.edu/healthcare/Documents/Forum-on-Healthcare-Innovation-5-Imperatives.pdf

Coleman, E. A., Parry, C., Chalmers, S., & Min S. J. (2006). The care transitions interventions: Results of a randomized control trials. *Archives of Internal Medicine, 166,* 1822–1828.

Collins, J. C. (2001). *Good to great.* New York, NY: HarperCollins.

Collins, J. (2015). Level 5 leadership: The triumph of humility and fierce resolve. *Harvard Business Review.* Retrieved from https://hbr.org/2005/07/level-5-leadership-the-triumph-of-humility-and-fierce-resolve

Committee on Health, Education, Labor, and Pensions. (2014). Subcommittee hearing. More than 1,000 preventable deaths a day is too many: The need to improve patient safety. Retrieved from http://www.help.senate.gov/hearings/hearing/?id=478e8a35-5056-a032-52f8-a65f8bd0e5ef

Conway, P. (2013). U.S. efforts to reduce healthcare-associated infections. Retrieved from http://www.hhs.gov/asl/testify/2013/09/t20130924.html

Ellis, D. (2007). The acceleration of innovations. Retrieved from http://hfd.dmc.org/download/acceleration.pdf

Harvard-Partners Center for Genetics and Genomics. (2007). Improving health and accelerating personalized health care through health information technology and genomic information in population and community-based health care delivery systems. Retrieved from http://www.hpcgg.org/News/HPCGG_RFI _Response_1_0.pdf

Hussey, P. S., Mattke, S., Morse, L., & Ridgely, M. S. (2007). Chapter 5: Findings from the case studies. In *Evaluation of the use of AHRQ and other quality indicators*. Retrieved from http://www.ahrq.gov/about/evaluations/qualityindicators /qualindch5.htm

Institute for Healthcare Improvement. (2008). Patient safety and the reliability of healthcare systems. Retrieved from http://www.ihi.org/IHI/Topics/Patient Safety/MedicationSystems/Literature/Patientsafetyandthereliabilityofhealth caresystems.htm

James, J. T. (2013). A new, evidence-based estimate of patient harms associated with hospital care. *Journal of Patient Safety, 9*(3), 122–128. doi:10.1097/ PTS.0b013e3182948a69

Kouzes, J. M., & Posner, B. Z. (2003) *Encouraging the heart: A leaders' guide to rewarding and recognizing others.* San Francisco, CA: John Wiley & Sons, Inc.

Landrigan, C. P., Parry, G. J., Bones, C. B., Hackbarth, A. D., Goldmann, D. A., & Sharek P. J. (2010). Temporal trends in rates of patient harm resulting from medical care. *New England Journal of Medicine, 363*(22), 2124–2134.

Leapfrog Group. (2008). Leapfrog hospital survey and Leapfrog hospital rewards program. Retrieved from http://www.leapfroggroup.org/66445/hospital_contact

Leavitt, M. (2007). Remarks on personalized medicine coalition. Retrieved from http://www.hhs.gov/news/speech/2007/sp20070919a.html

Louisiana Health Care Quality Forum. (2008). The patient-centered medical home in Louisiana: Spring 2008 progress report. Retrieved from http://lhcqf .org/lapost-old/images/stories/PCMH%20in%20LA-Spring%202008%20 Progress%20Report.pdf

Maas, M., Johnson, M., & Moorehead, S. (1996). Classifying nursing-sensitive patient outcomes. *Journal of Nursing Scholarship, 28*, 295–301.

Morris, A., & Faulk, D. (2012). *Transformative learning in nursing. A guide for nurse educators.* New York, NY: Springer.

Morrison, I. (2000). *Health care in the new millennium: Vision, values and leadership.* Hoboken, NJ: Jossey-Bass.

National Quality Forum. (2008). Standardizing a patient safety taxonomy. Retrieved from http://www.qualityforum.org/Publications/2006/01/Standardizing_a _Patient_Safety_Taxonomy.aspx

Naylor, M. D., Brooten, D. A., Campbell, R. L., Maislin, G., McCauley, K. M., & Schwartz, J. S. (2004). Transitional care of older adults hospitalized with heart failure: A randomized, controlled trial. *Journal of the American Geriatric Society, 52*(5):675–684.

Needleman, J., Buerhaus, P. I., Mattke, S., Stewart, M., & Zelevinsky, K. (2002). Nurse-staffing levels and the quality of care in hospitals *New England Journal of Medicine, 346*(22), 1715–1722.

Pricewaterhouse Coopers Scientific Advancement. (2015). $232 billion personalized medicine market to grow 11 percent annually, says Pricewaterhouse-Coopers. Retrieved from http://www.prnewswire.com/news-releases/232 -billion-personalized-medicine-market-to-grow-11-percent-annually-says -pricewaterhousecoopers-78751072.html

Porter, M. E., & Teisberg, E. O. (2006). *Redefining health care: Creating value-based competition on results.* Cambridge, MA: Harvard Business School Press.

Porter, M. E., & Teisberg, E. O. (2007). How physicians can change the future of health care. *Journal of the American Medical Association, 297,* 1103–1111.

Porter-O'Grady, T., & Malloch, K. (2015). *Quantum leadership: A resource for healthcare innovation* (4th ed.). Burlington, MA: Jones & Bartlett Learning.

Rittenhouse, D. R., & Shortell, S. M. (2009). The patient-centered model home. Will it stand the test of health reform? *Journal of the American Medical Association, 301*(19), 2038–2040. doi:10.1001/jama.2009.691

Rock Island County. (n.d.). Health Department Maternal and Child Health: School Health LINK. Retrieved from http://www.rockislandcounty.org/HealthDept/SchoolHealthLINK.aspx

Schoen, C., How, I. W., Weinbaum, I., Craig, J. E., Jr., & Davis, K. (2006). Public views on shaping the future of the U.S. health system. Retrieved from http://hagel.senate.gov/index.cfm?FuseAction=News.HealthCareCommission

Stacey, R. (2010). *Complexity and organizational reality: Uncertainty and the need to rethink management after the collapse of investment capitalism* (2nd ed.). New York, NY: Routledge.

Stiefel, M., & Nolan, K. (2012). *A guide to measuring the triple aim: Population health, experience of care, and per capita cost* (IHI Innovation Series white paper). Cambridge, MA: Institute for Healthcare Improvement.

The Joint Commission. (2008). National patient safety goals. Retrieved from http://www.jointcommission.org/PatientSafety/NationalPatientSafetyGoals

TIGER Initiative. (2007). TIGER summary report. Retrieved from http://www.thetigerinitiative.org/

Vlasses, F. R., & Smeltzer, C. H. (2007). Toward a new future for healthcare and nursing practice. *Journal of Nursing Administration, 37*(9), 375–380.

SELECTED WEBSITES

Agency for Healthcare Research and Quality

www.ahrq.gov

The Agency for Healthcare Research and Quality funds, conducts, and disseminates research to improve the quality, safety, efficiency, and effectiveness of health care. The information gathered from this work and made available on the website assists all key stakeholders—patients, families, clinicians, leaders, purchasers, and policy makers—to make informed decisions about health care.

American Association of Critical-Care Nurses

www.aacn.org

The American Association of Critical-Care Nurses provides leadership and resources to their members to improve health care for critically ill patients and their families. The core concepts of patient- and family-centered health care are integrated throughout their practice guidelines.

American Hospital Association

www.aha.org

The American Hospital Association (AHA) is the premier membership organization for U.S. hospitals and provides leadership and advocacy for member hospitals to improve care for patients and their families. The IFCC (Institute for Patient- and Family-Centered Care) collaborated with the AHA to develop a tool kit called Strategies for Leadership: Patient- and Family-Centered Care, which is available for download at http://www.aha.org/advocacy-issues/quality/strategies-patientcentered.shtml.

Center for Health Design

www.healthdesign.org

The Center for Health Design is a nonprofit research and advocacy organization of healthcare and design professionals who are leading the effort to improve health quality through architecture and design.

Center for Medical Home Improvement

www.medicalhomeimprovement.org

A medical home is a community-based primary care setting that provides and coordinates high-quality, planned, patient- and family-centered health promotion, acute illness care, and chronic illness management throughout the continuum of care and across the life span.

Improvement Science Research Network

http://www.improvementscienceresearch.net/

The Improvement Science Research Network is the only improvement research network supported by the National Institutes of Health. The primary mission of the network is to accelerate interprofessional improvement of science in the context of systems across multiple hospital sites.

Institute for Healthcare Improvement

http://www.ihi.org/Pages/default.aspx

The Institute for Healthcare Improvement is an independent, not-for-profit organization based in Cambridge, Massachusetts. It focuses on inspiring and building the case for change; identifying and testing new models of care by partnering with both patients and healthcare professionals; and ensuring the broadest adoption of best practices and innovations.

CHAPTER 2

Leadership Theory and Application for Nurse Leaders

Linda Roussel, Patricia L. Thomas, and Carol Ratcliffe

LEARNING OBJECTIVES

1. Describe how leadership theory underpins healthcare management.
2. Discuss the guiding principles and competencies for nursing leadership practice.
3. Relate selected theories of leadership and management to organizational outcomes.
4. Discuss the role of nursing leadership in managing a clinical discipline.

AONE KEY COMPETENCIES

I. Communication and relationship building
II. Knowledge of the healthcare environment
III. Leadership
IV. Professionalism
V. Business skills

AONE KEY COMPETENCIES DISCUSSED IN THIS CHAPTER

III. Leadership
IV. Professionalism

III. Leadership
- Foundational thinking skills
- Personal journey disciplines
- Ability to use systems thinking
- Succession planning
- Change management

IV. Professionalism
- Personal and professional accountability
- Career planning
- Ethics
- Evidence-based clinical and management practices

- Advocacy for the clinical enterprise and for nursing practice
- Active membership in professional organizations

FUTURE OF NURSING: FOUR KEY MESSAGES

1. Nurses should practice to the full extent of their education and training.
2. Nurses should achieve higher levels of education and training through an improved education system that promotes seamless academic progression.
3. Nurses should be full partners with physicians and other health professionals in redesigning health care in the United States.
4. Effective workforce planning and policy making require better data collection and information infrastructure.

Introduction

Leadership counts, and leading like it matters is essential for inspiring and engaging our constituents, colleagues, and stakeholders. Without a spirited and deeply satisfied workforce, sustained safety and quality care are improbable. Gallup's *State of the American Workplace* report (2013) said a staggering 70% of Americans have negative feelings about their work. Some of the following findings were noted:

- Only 30% of employees are engaged and inspired at work.
- About 52% of employees are present but not engaged.
- A full 18% are actively disengaged or worse.
- As much as $550 billion in productivity is lost because of the 18% of actively disengaged employees.

This chapter focuses on leadership theories and models and their application to administrative practices. How leaders impact workforce and patient outcomes serves as the impetus for ongoing improvements and innovations.

WHAT DO LEADERS DO?

Kotter (2014) notes that management and leadership are different. Specifically, he notes the following:

- Management involves planning and budgeting. Leadership involves setting a direction.
- Management involves organizing and staffing. Leadership involves aligning people.
- Management provides control and solves problems. Leadership provides motivation and inspiration.

Gardner (1993) asserts that first-class managers are usually first-class leaders. Leaders and leader–managers distinguish themselves beyond run-of-the-mill managers in six respects:

- They think longer term—beyond the day's crises, beyond the quarterly report, beyond the horizon.

- They look beyond the unit they head and grasp its relationship to larger realities, such as the larger organization of which they are a part, conditions external to the organization, and global trends.
- They reach and influence constituents beyond their jurisdiction and beyond boundaries. Thomas Jefferson influenced people all over Europe. Gandhi influenced people all over the world. In an organization, leaders overflow bureaucratic boundaries, which is often a distinct advantage in a world that is too complex and tumultuous to be handled through channels. Their capacity to rise above jurisdictions may enable them to bind together the fragmented constituencies that must work together to solve a problem.
- They put heavy emphasis on the intangibles of vision, values, and motivation and intuitively understand the nonrational and unconscious elements in the leader–constituent interaction.
- They have the political skill to cope with the conflicting requirements of multiple constituencies.
- They think in terms of renewal. A routine manager tends to accept structures and processes as they exist. The leader or leader–manager seeks revisions of processes and structures that are required by a changing reality.

Good leaders, like good managers, provide visionary inspiration, motivation, and direction. Good managers, like good leaders, attract and inspire. People want to be led rather than managed. They want to pursue goals and values they consider worthwhile. Therefore they want leaders who respect the dignity, autonomy, and self-esteem of constituents (Morriss, Ely, & Frei, 2014).

The dynamic of complex relationship building in leading change necessitates various approaches to innovating health care. Dooley and Lichtenstein (2008) discuss methods for studying complex leadership interactions, centering on (1) micro, daily interactions using real-time experience, participant-observation actions; (2) meso interactions (days and weeks) involving social network analysis, where there is discovery of a set of agents and how they are connected and aligned over time; and (3) macro interactions (weeks, months, and longer) through event history analysis. The researchers describe agent-based modeling simulations, which are computer simulations using a set of explicit assumptions about how agents (leaders) are thought to operate and used as a means to study complexity leadership. Using a micro, meso, and macro interaction approach adds different lenses to social networks and interprofessional collaboration.

Effective nurse executives combine leadership and management and work to achieve these requisite goals. Leadership is a subsystem of a management system. It is included as an element of management science in management textbooks and other publications. In some sources, the term *leading* has replaced the term *directing* as a major function of management. In such a context, communication and motivation are elements of leadership (a concept that could be debated according to management theorists' philosophical bent) (Van Buren & Safferstone, 2014).

Management includes written plans, clear organizational charts, well-documented annual objectives, frequent reports, detailed and precise job descriptions, regular evaluations of performance against objectives, and the administrative ordering of theory. Nurse managers who are leaders can use these tools of management without making them a bureaucratic roadblock to autonomy, participatory management, maximum performance, and employee productivity.

LEADERSHIP VERSUS HEADSHIP

A job title does not make a person a leader, nor does it cause a person to exercise leadership behavior. This is as true of nurses as it is of personnel in industry or the military. It is a mistake to refer to the dean of a college, a professor of nursing, a nurse administrator, a supervisor, a nurse manager, or any nurse as a leader by virtue of position. That person is in a headship position rather than a leadership position; leadership is more a function of the group or situation than a quality that adheres to a person who is appointed to a formal position of headship. A person's behavior indicates whether that person occupies a functional leadership position. Leadership is an attempt to influence groups or individuals without the coercive form of power.

Avolio, Walumbwa, and Weber (2009) describe the concept of leadership as moving toward a more holistic approach and that more positive forms of leadership are being researched and integrated into the literature. How an individual develops leadership competencies and skills has always been essential to leadership development and has earned greater attention in healthcare innovation. Working in virtual teams across national and international boundaries is underscored as technology is embedded in our daily work, signifying how e-leadership will need to be included in leadership development. Impacting short- and long-term outcomes is critical, particularly as the return on investment becomes increasingly important to financial viability. Leadership and followership provide an important dynamic system as interprofessional collaboration and team building are identified as competencies in the education of healthcare professionals (Institute of Medicine [IOM], 2003). Distributed and shared leadership continue to be part of the leadership development conversation, as leadership is viewed as a complex and emergent dynamic in organizations.

When heads are elected by a group, they keep their positions only as long as they satisfy the members' needs for affiliating with the organization. They are responsible only to the group, whereas appointed heads are usually responsible to both the appointive authority and the group. Nurses who are elected to chair committees or who preside over professional organizations will not be reelected unless they satisfy the members' needs.

Appointed heads may lack the freedom to choose relationships with associates because their supervisors do not allow it. They have authority and power without being accepted by the group. If appointed nurse managers are allowed to and can exercise their leadership abilities, they can be accorded leadership status by the group. Nurse managers understand and motivate employees in order to be trusted by them.

Preparation of Nursing Leaders

Parks (2013) believes that leadership can be taught. Education begins in basic nursing education programs. To develop risk-taking behaviors and self-confidence, students should be encouraged to create new solutions and to disagree and debate, and they should be coached to make mistakes without fear of reprisal. Critical thinking and reflection are important to this process. Faculty should encourage and support students who exercise their leadership abilities in projects and organizations on campus and in the community.

Most nurses who graduate and enter the workforce are not ready to assume a leadership role. They require opportunities for self-discovery, self-reflection, and critical thinking to understand their strengths and build their skills. Skill building occurs through on-the-job training and coaching, along with support from peers and mentors who are effective leaders. Mentors must be dynamic, enthusiastic, and passionate about their work to positively influence those they mentor.

LEADERSHIP MATTERS

Hewertson (2015) shares eight insights that shape our understanding of leadership as being foundational to igniting those we work with. The insights include the following: leadership knowledge, though important, must be followed by action; leading people is messy; leadership is a discipline, not an accident; leadership and individual contributions require opposite skills sets and motivations. The other insights pertain to relationship-based leadership: in leadership it is all about relationships, soft skills are hard skills; although most change initiatives fail, they need not; and leaders create and destroy culture.

Hewertson (2015) also describes four core masteries that every leader needs to attain at a reasonable level of competency: personal mastery, interpersonal mastery, team mastery, and culture and systems mastery. A self-assessment of leadership style; knowing yourself and your emotional intelligence, preferences, life purpose, values, and vision; and how you influence others are the focus of personal mastery. Knowing how you communicate; deeply listening; providing critical and constructive feedback; and managing conflict are the skills of interpersonal mastery. How your team works; how members come together; how information is handed off; and group dynamics are skills of team mastery, along with decision making that works; delegation for development; and meetings that garner great results. Culture and systems mastery includes understanding the interaction of the organization's culture and systems dynamics. Doing a cultural assessment is important to understanding how culture facilitates or deters change initiatives (Hewertson, 2015).

Learning skills to lead and motivate interprofessional teams fosters collaboration and cooperation. An engaged workforce facilitates engaged patients through the patient experience and patient-centered care. Manary, Boulding, Staelin, and Glickman (2013) report on the patient experience and health outcomes. Their research notes that when studies are designed and administered appropriately, patient-experience surveys can provide robust measures of quality, as accessing patient experiences can be critical to continued quality improvement in healthcare redesign. The researchers report that while there are challenging methodologic issues related to measuring and interpreting patient experience, such as mode and timing of survey administration, and patients' prior experience, it is essential to find ways to capture this vital information. Capturing indicators of healthcare quality can serve to improve healthcare structures and processes (admission, discharge, and educating patient). The authors underscore the importance of focusing on how to improve the patient's care experience by emphasizing care coordination and patient engagement activities noted to be associated with both satisfaction and outcomes. Other important activities include evaluating the effects of new care-delivery models on patients' experiences and subsequent outcomes and developing appropriate measurement approaches that can provide timely and action-oriented information to enhance organizational change. These strategies can improve data collection methods and procedures and provide appropriate and accurate assessments of individual providers.

Stempniak (2014) describes patient engagement as a strategic imperative for hospital executives. Fully engaged patients can reduce costly readmissions and improve health literacy and patient satisfaction scores. Patients often come to a healthcare experience with past experience, expertise, and insights. This has been noted and addressed by the Centers for Medicare and Medicaid Services Stage 2 reimbursement, which is based on at least 5% of patients viewing, downloading, and transmitting their health information within 36 hours of discharge (Stempniak, 2014). Patients are consumers of health care, and engagement is an expectation for healthcare providers to meet regulatory mandates and standards of care. Leadership skills that provide innovative strategies for patient engagement are in demand. By creating a culture of engagement that inspires team members, the odds for patient engagement are increased.

ARCHETYPES OF LEADERSHIP

Kets de Vries (2013) describes his approach to leadership assessment that is based on observational studies of real leaders, primarily at the strategic apex of their organizations. His focus is helping leaders see and understand that their attitudes and interactions with people are the result of a complex confluence of their inner circles and may include their relationships with authority figures early in life, memorable life experiences, examples set by other executives, and formal leadership training. Kets de Vries posits that the complex confluences may play out over time, and often there are recurring patterns of behavior that influence an individual's effectiveness within an organization. The author considers these patterns to be leadership archetypes that reflect the various roles managers and executives assume in organizations. It is a lack of fit between a leader's archetype and the operational context that may result in team and organizational dysfunction and leadership failure. The eight archetypes are as follows:

- The strategist: Leadership is a game of chess. These managers often excel when dealing with developments in the organization's environment. They provide vision, strategic direction, and outside-the-box thinking to create new organizational forms and generate future growth.
- The change catalyst: Leadership is a turnaround activity. These leaders relish messy situations. They are exceptional at reengineering and creating new organizational blueprints.
- The transactor: Leadership is deal making. Leaders as transactors are great deal makers. Because they are skilled at identifying and tackling new opportunities, they thrive on negotiations.
- The builder: Leadership is an entrepreneurial activity. The leader as builder often dreams of creating something and has the talent and determination to make the dream come true.
- The innovator: Leadership is creative idea generation. Innovators focus on new, exciting, and creative ideas. They possess a great capacity to solve extremely difficult problems.

- The processor: Leadership is an exercise in efficiency. Leaders who are processors create organizations that run smoothly, like well-oiled machines. They are very effective at setting up structures and systems that are needed to support an organization's objectives.
- The coach: Leadership is a form of people development. Coaches know how to get the best out of people and create high-performance cultures.
- The communicator: Leadership is stage management. Leaders who are great influencers have a considerable impact on their surroundings.

Kets de Vries (2013) notes that determining which types of leaders are on the team can advance the group's effectiveness. It helps to recognize how you and your colleagues can individually make the best contributions, which will in turn create a culture of mutual support and trust, reduce team stress and conflict, and foster creative problem solving. This can also enhance searching for new talent for the team. What kinds of personalities and skills are missing? For example, if the team needs an executive with a strategic outlook and who had turnaround skills and experience, then a communicator and coach would be more effectively leveraged to resolve an operational crisis. Working with human resources to identify particular skill sets that are required on the executive management team could be expedited using an archetypes of leadership model, which provides a framework for enhancing team effectiveness.

TRANSFORMATIONAL LEADERSHIP

The healthcare system is immersed in tremendous change and chaos, and organizational situations and problems are increasingly complex. Healthcare organizations are restructuring and redesigning delivery models to meet the challenges of these changes. Health care is prohibitively expensive for many Americans. Hospitals and emergency rooms are financially burdened by uninsured people who may suffer from recurring and multiple chronic health issues, violence, drug overdose, and HIV infection. Many people, especially in rural areas and inner cities, do not have access to health care due to the downsizing of hospitals and a shortage of healthcare personnel. Leaders are tasked with keeping staff inspired and motivated in this chaotic, unstable environment. Effective leaders in this atmosphere of rapid change must acknowledge uncertainty, be flexible, and consider the values and needs of constituents.

Now more than ever, the need for transformational leadership is critical. Transformational leaders commit people to action, convert followers into leaders, and convert leaders into agents of change (Tuuk, 2011). The nucleus of leadership is power, as the basic energy to initiate and sustain action translating intention into reality. Transformational leaders do not use power to control and repress constituents. These leaders instead empower constituents to have a vision about the organization and trust the leaders so they work for goals that benefit the organization and themselves (Tuuk, 2012; Watkins, 2014).

Leadership is thus not so much the exercise of power itself as it is the empowerment of others. This does not mean that leaders must relinquish power, but rather that reciprocity, an exchange between leaders and constituents, exists. The goal is change in which the purpose of the leader and that of the constituent become enmeshed, creating a collective purpose. Empowered staff members become critical thinkers and are active in their roles within the organization. A creative and committed staff is the most important asset that administrators can develop.

Transformational leaders mobilize their staff by focusing on the welfare of the individual and humanizing the high-tech work environment. Experts favor a leadership style that empowers others and values collaboration instead of competition. People are empowered when they share in decision making and when they are rewarded for quality and excellence rather than punished and manipulated. When the environment is humanized, people are empowered, feel that they are part of the team, and believe they are contributing to the success of the organization. Leaders who share power motivate people to excel by inspiring them to be part of a vision rather than punishing them for mistakes. In nursing, empowerment can result in improved patient care, fewer staff sick days, and decreased attrition. Nurses who are transformational leaders have staff members with higher job satisfaction and who stay in the organization for longer periods. This can be accomplished through the establishment of a shared governance model that includes staff-led councils that are composed of, but are not limited to, nursing practice, staff development, research, quality, recruitment and retention, and unit-based councils.

Nurse executives who like to feel they are in charge may feel threatened by the concept of sharing power with staff members, so they need to be personally empowered to assist in the empowerment of others. They will have a sense of self-worth and self-respect, and confidence in their own abilities.

Transformational Leadership and Innovative Approaches

Transformational leadership and innovative approaches are needed for change in health care and are critical to successful organizational outcomes. Transformational leadership is central to safety in a variety of industries and to an organization's competitive cost position after a change initiative. Transformational leadership has been specifically identified by the Institute of Medicine (2001) in its work on medical error and patient safety. Changes in nursing leadership have been underscored in creating safe environments for patients and staff, particularly as the weakening of clinical leadership has been cited as a cause of organizational concerns and issues. The Institute of Medicine described outcomes of poor, problematic leadership (Buerhaus, Staiger, & Auerbach, 2000):

- Increased emphasis on production efficiency (bottom-line management)
- Weakened trust (reengineering initiatives, poor communication patterns)
- Poor change management (inadequate communication, insufficient worker training, lack of measurement and feedback, short-lived attention, limited worker involvement in developing change initiatives)
- Limited involvement in decision making pertaining to work design and work flow (hierarchical structures, limited voice on councils and committees)
- Limited knowledge management (process failures, limited second-order attention)

To address these challenges, the following recommendations were made for healthcare organizations by the Institute of Medicine, particularly related to acquiring nurse leaders for all levels of management (e.g., at the organization-wide and patient care unit levels). Nurse leaders are challenged to do the following (American Nurses Association [ANA], 2009):

- Participate in executive decisions within healthcare organizations.
- Represent nursing staff to organization management and facilitate their mutual trust.
- Achieve effective communication between nursing and other clinical leadership.
- Facilitate the input of direct-care nursing staff into operational decision making and work process and work flow designs.
- With organizational resources, support the acquisition, management, and dissemination to nursing staff of knowledge needed for quality clinical decision making and actions.

Although no one particular organizational structure was identified for the placement of nurse leadership, the focus of the recommendations was on well-prepared clinical nurse leaders at the most senior level of management. Magnet and Pathway to Excellence hospitals have found some positive outcomes related to staff and patient satisfaction that correlated with participatory and transformational leadership. Clearly, transformational leadership is called for to address these challenges, to improve quality outcomes for patients and staff, and to heighten overall organizational effectiveness (ANA, 2009).

Buffering

Nursing leaders can act as buffers or advocates for nurses. In doing so, they protect constituents from internal and external pressures of work. Nurse managers can reduce barriers to clinical nurses who are completing their clinical work. Buffering protects practicing clinical nurses from external health system factors, the healthcare organization, other supervisors and employees, top administrators, the medical staff, and themselves when their behavior jeopardizes their careers. Buffering is another facet of the theory of leadership related to management, and it requires leadership training (Zheng, Singh, & Mitchell, 2014).

Nurse managers can buffer, and therefore protect, nurse practitioners, extended-role nurses, staff nurses, and ancillary personnel. Professional nurses do not want to have additional responsibilities delegated to them if they are already under severe pressure and stress. The delegation of decision making is power; the delegation of work is drudgery. Professional nurses are there to motivate, inspire, and engage, not to dissatisfy.

Management writers say there is a difference between leaders and managers, but their textbooks and writings on the subject include leadership content. Professional nurses want to be led, mentored, and coached, not directed or controlled. Also, nurse managers can learn the concepts, principles, and laws that will assist them in becoming effective leader–managers.

Different situations require different leadership styles. The leader–manager assesses each situation and exercises the appropriate leadership style. Some employees want to be involved; others do not. There must be a fit between the leader and the constituents. The leader demonstrates this by changing the leadership style and training others until a transition is made. A flexible leadership style is necessary and vital. Participatory, transformational, innovative, and quantum leadership principles have received much attention. This is primarily due to the frenetic pace of health care and a focus on safe, quality care. Using leadership frameworks to guide practice may include authentic leadership, servant leadership, and lateral leadership (Avolio, Walumbwa, & Weber, 2009; Dinh et al., 2014; Johnson, 2014).

Competencies for Transformational Leaders

Bennis and Nanus (1985) believe the most important trait of successful leaders is having positive self-regard. Positive self-regard is not, however, self-centeredness or self-importance; rather, leaders with positive self-esteem recognize their strengths and do not emphasize their weaknesses. A leader who has positive self-regard seems to create in others a sense of confidence and high expectations. Techniques used to increase self-worth include visualization, affirmations, and letting go of the need to be perfect.

Through research and observations, Bennis (1991) defined four competencies for dynamic and effective transformational leadership: (1) management of attention, (2) management of meaning, (3) management of trust, and (4) management of self. The first competency, management of attention, is achieved by having a vision or a sense of outcomes or goals. Vision is the image of a realistic, attainable, credible, and attractive future state for an organization. Vision statements are written to define where the healthcare organization is headed and how it will serve society. They differ from mission and philosophy statements in that they are more futuristic and describe where energies are to be focused. The vision of nursing is supported by a nursing strategic plan that is integrated in and supports the overall organizational plan.

The second leadership competency is management of meaning. To inspire commitment, leaders must communicate their vision and create a culture that sustains the vision. A culture or social architecture, as described by Bennis and Nanus (1985), is "intangible, but it governs the way people act, the values and norms that are subtly transmitted to groups and individuals, and the construct of binding and bonding within a company" (p. 176). Barker (1991) believes that "social architecture provides meaning and shared experience of organizational events so that people know the expectations of how they are to act" (p. 207).

Nursing leaders transform the social architecture or culture of healthcare organizations by using group discussion, agreement, and consensus building, and they support individual creativity and innovation. To do this, Barker (1991) believes the nurse transformational leader will pay attention to the internal consistency of the vision, goals, and objectives; selection and placement of personnel; feedback; appraisal; rewards; support; and development. For example, rewards and appraisals must relate to goals, and the vision must be consistent with the goals and objectives. Most important, all elements must enhance the self-worth of individuals, allow creativity, and appeal to the values of nurses. For many nurse leaders, these are new skills that will take time and support from mentors to develop.

Because vision statements are a new concept to many, nursing leaders should provide opportunities for staff to openly explore feelings, criticize, and articulate negative reactions. Face-to-face meetings between nursing leaders and staff are desirable because in reactions involving trust and clarity, memoranda and suggestion boxes are not adequate substitutes for direct communication (Barker, 1991).

This can be achieved through nursing forums, rounding, huddles, or small group meetings.

The third competency is management of trust, which is associated with reliability. Nurses respect leaders whose judgment is sound and consistent and whose decisions are based on fairness, equity, and honesty. Staff can be heard to comment about leaders they trust with statements such as "I don't always agree with her decision, but I know she wants the best for the patients." Bennis (1991) believes that "people would much rather follow individuals they can count on, even when they disagree with their viewpoint, than people they agree with but who shift positions frequently" (p. 24).

The fourth competency is management of self, which is knowing one's skills and using them effectively. It is critical that nurses in leadership positions recognize when they lack management skills and take responsibility for their own continuing education. Incompetent leaders can demoralize a nursing unit and contribute to poor patient care. When leadership skills are mastered by nurse leaders, stress and burnout are reduced. Nurse leaders thus need to master the skills of leadership (Bennis, 1991).

Although effective leaders support shared power and decision making, they continue to accept responsibility for making decisions even when their decisions are not popular. Constituents like to have their wishes considered, but there are times when they want prompt and clear decisions from a leader. This is especially true in times of crisis.

Transformational leaders are flexible and able to adapt leadership styles to the chaos and rapid change that is occurring in the current healthcare environment.

Transformational Leader as Coach

Coaching and mentoring are important skill sets for transformational leaders. Coaching denotes a way of being with others that provides opportunities to facilitate growth and development. Coaching requires exquisite communication skills that model ways of interacting and networking with others, whereby those coached will find ready examples of best practices in working with others. Hill (2007) describes the predictable process of coaching, which includes the following:

- Observing
- Examining coach motives
- Creating a discussion plan for the coaching session
- Initiating
- Providing and eliciting feedback
- Having a follow-up meeting

As a coach, observing behaviors and responding with insights and strategies will go further than instructing others on what to do. This approach will afford greater opportunities for learning and advancing skills and opportunities. Porter-O'Grady and Malloch (2007) describe innovation coaching, stating the importance of creating the structure and content of the experience. Specifically, the following guidelines are given to facilitate this effort:

- Setting the bar high
- Being clear about who you are
- Treating transformation as a mission, not a job

BOX 2-1   Impediments to Effective Coaching

Use of power
- Inadequate power
- Autocratic application of power
- Lack of empowerment
- Nonstrategic use of power

Self-image
- Poor self-esteem
- Unclear role
- Psychological flaws

Knowledge
- Undeveloped knowledge
- Learning needs
- Inexperience
- Lack of personal technique

Problem solving
- Inadequate worldview
- Intolerance of diversity
- No clear process
- Situational solutions

- Exposing staff to different messages and different messengers
- Creating an egalitarian organizational structure
- Putting money where the ideas are
- Letting the talented experiment
- Allowing people to share in the fruits of their creativity

Box 2-1 illustrates impediments to effective coaching, and **Figure 2-1** illustrates a transformational model of coaching.

STRATEGIC LEADERSHIP

Schoemaker, Krupp, and Howland (2013) identified strategic leadership skills that are essential to leading. Their self-assessment tool for determining strategic leadership is available in the cited publication. It includes the following skills: anticipate, challenge, interpret, decide, align, and learn. Each skill includes methods to improve strategic leading; some examples are as follows:

- Anticipate: The actions include talking to customers, suppliers, and other partners to understand their challenges, and conducting market research and business simulations to understand competitors' perspectives, gauge their likely reaction to new initiatives or products, and predict potential disruptive offerings. Additional activities might include scenario planning to anticipate possible futures and prepare for the unexpected, and viewing trends and fast-growing rivals by examining strategies they have used that are surprising.
- Challenge: Leaders can improve by focusing on root causes, applying the five whys of Sakichi Toyoda, encouraging debate by creating safe-zone meetings that facilitate open dialogue and conflict, including naysayers in decision-making processes to discover challenges early, and capturing input from persons who are not directly affected by a decision who may have a good perspective on the repercussions.

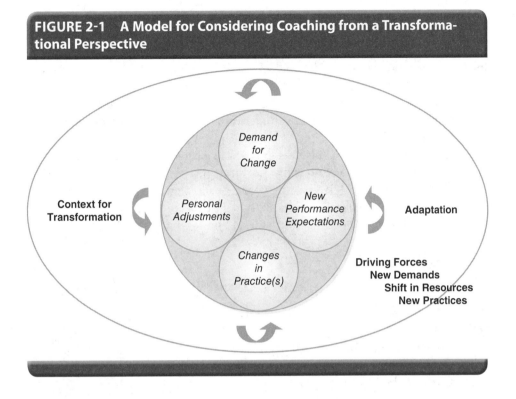

FIGURE 2-1   A Model for Considering Coaching from a Transformational Perspective

- Interpret: Strategies include listing three possible explanations for observations, inviting perspectives from diverse stakeholders, and supplementing observations with quantitative analysis. Additional strategies may include stepping away to get a fresh perspective, going for a walk, listening to unfamiliar music, looking at art, and other activities that promote open-mindedness.
- Decide: Leaders can reframe binary decisions by asking team members about other options for decision making, dividing decisions into chunks to understand component parts and reveal unintended consequences, and tailoring decision criteria to long-term versus short-term projects. Leaders can be transparent about decisions by letting others know if they are seeking divergent ideas and debate or if they are moving toward closure. It is also important to determine who needs to be directly involved and who can influence the success of the decision.
- Align: Leaders should communicate early and often to keep the two most common complaints in organizations from becoming a reality: no one ever asked me, and no one ever told me. Additional strategies include using structured and facilitated conversations to expose areas of misunderstanding or resistance and reaching out to resisters directly to understand their concerns and then address them.
- Learn: Useful strategies include creating a culture in which inquiry is valued and mistakes are considered learning opportunities, conducting learning audits to see where decisions and team interactions may have fallen short, and identifying initiatives that are not producing as anticipated and examining their root causes.

Organizational managers, including nurse executives, teach frontline managers the nature of leadership. They coach nurse managers in leadership skills and put managers in challenging scenarios to learn leadership. Critical reflection, debriefings, and innovative problem solving extend these lessons, which include starting up an operation, turning around a troubled division, moving from a staff position to a line position on an organizational chart, working under a wise mentor, serving on a high-level task force, and getting promoted to a more senior level of the organization.

Nurse executives and managers should be educated and socialized to coach their constituents on leadership skills and strategies. Constituents can be socialized to help managers with leadership. Leaders can listen and articulate, persuade and be persuaded, use collective wisdom to make decisions, and teach relationship building and upward communication skills (Galinsky & Kilduff, 2014).

Lateral Leadership

Johnson (2014) describes lateral leadership as involving a constellation of capabilities that includes the following:

- Networking
- Constructive persuasion and negotiation
- Consultation
- Coalition building

In networking, leaders cultivate broad networks of relationships with people inside and outside their companies whose support is needed to carry out initiatives. Johnson (2014) says if networking does not come naturally to a leader, it is important to connect with those who are portals to other people; that is, people who can connect the leader to bigger networks.

Constructive persuasion and negotiation is way to view those involved in projects and initiatives as peers, not targets. Developing constructive persuasion and negotiation abilities may be facilitated by taking courses and reading articles and textbooks to improve. These capabilities can also be enhanced by finding seasoned colleagues who can serve as confidantes and brainstorming partners.

Consultation is a useful skill in lateral leadership. It involves taking time to visit people whose buy-in is needed. Leaders should ask for others' opinions about initiatives they are championing and get their ideas and reactions. Lateral leaders will get better results if they commit to and advocate for the desired outcome, such as inviting peers to participate in defining the process for achieving specific outcomes.

Coalition building involves gathering influential people to form a single body of authority. By building coalitions, leaders ask the following questions: Who is most likely to be affected by the change? Whose blessing is needed, either in the form of political support or access to important resources or individuals? Whose buy-in is crucial to the success of the initiative?

There can be challenges to developing a lateral leadership style. Leaders may be too focused on their own functional silos that limit awareness of information and resources beyond one's internal group. They can combat functional focus by taking time to find out who makes things happen in the organization and asking the following questions:

- Who do people go to for advice and support?
- Who tends to set up roadblocks to changes and new ideas?

Informal contact and casual get-togethers can increase networking and reduce a functional focus. Additionally, by dedicating a specific amount of time each week to making contacts and getting support, lateral leadership skills can be sharpened.

LEADERSHIP AND JUST CULTURE

Creating a fair and just culture is an essential responsibility of nursing leadership. A fair and just culture is important to high-reliability organizations in facilitating safe patient care. Frankel, Leonard, and Denham (2006) describe three initiatives that are critical to the ethics of creating and maintaining a safe environment for patients and staff: (1) develop a fair and just culture; (2) intelligently engage by using frontline insights to directly influence operational decisions; and (3) provide systematic and reinforced training in teamwork and effective communication. Ethical decision making and actions underscore safe, high-quality care.

NURSING AND LEADERSHIP HEALTHCARE POLICY

Nursing is conspicuous in its absence from lists of national leaders. National consumers do not perceive nurse leaders as having power. The healthcare system has failed to recognize nurses as professionals who have knowledge that is useful in creating solutions to complex problems. The Institute of Medicine's (2011) report on the future of nursing further underscores the need for nurses to be at the table by being better educated and by being full partners with physicians and other healthcare professionals in redesigning health care in the United States.

Historically, nurses have avoided opportunities to obtain power and political muscle. The profession now understands that power and political savvy will help achieve the goals to improve health care and increase nurses' autonomy. Also, if the healthcare system is to be reformed, nurses must participate individually and collectively. Nurses need to find ways to influence healthcare policy making so their voices are heard. Milstead (2013) believes that nurses have the capacity for power to influence public policy and recommends the following steps to prepare:

- Organize.
- Do homework to understand the political process, interest groups, specific people, and events.
- Frame arguments to suit the target audience by appealing to cost containment, political support, fairness and justice, and other data that are relevant to particular concerns.
- Support and strengthen the position of converted policy makers.
- Concentrate energies.
- Stimulate public debate.
- Make the position of nurses visible in the mass media.
- Choose the most effective strategy as the main one.

- Act in a timely fashion.
- Maintain activity.
- Keep the organizational format decentralized.
- Obtain and develop the best research data to support each position.
- Learn from experience.
- Never give up without trying.

Nurses in leadership positions are most influential in organizational, systems, national, and international changes that impact global policy initiatives.

FUTURE DIRECTION: QUANTUM LEADERSHIP

Porter-O'Grady and Malloch (2015) describe quantum leadership as new leadership for a new age. From a conceptual perspective, quantum theory considers the whole, integration, synthesis, relatedness, and team action. **Box 2-2** compares the Newtonian and the quantum perspectives. According to Porter-O'Grady and Malloch (2015), quantum theory has informed leaders that change is not an occurrence or an event; it is a dynamic that is essential to the universe. Quantum leadership incorporates transformation, a dynamic flow that integrates transitions from work, rules, scripts, chaos, and loss. Adaptation considers driving forces from sociopolitical, economic, and technical perspectives. The term *chaos*, as used in quantum leadership, refers to the transitional period focused on relational and whole systems thinking, as compared with separate components and linear thinking (**Figure 2-2** and **Figure 2-3**).

Porter-O'Grady and Malloch (2015) further describe seven imperatives for the new age (**Box 2-3**).

INNOVATIVE LEADERSHIP

Porter-O'Grady and Malloch (2007) describe concepts of innovative leadership in preparing organizational systems for change. They outline stages of innovation adoption that include knowledge, persuasion, decision, implementation, and confirmation. Individuals are also identified and include innovators, adopters, early majority, late majority, and laggards. Concepts include design thinking, thinking inside the box, disruptive innovation, and scenario planning.

Design thinking involves integrating work from art, craft, science, and business. Understanding consumers and the market is essential to designing programs

---

BOX 2-2   Newtonian Characteristics

- Vertical orientation
- Hierarchical structures
- Focus on control
- Process-driven action
- Reductionistic scientific processes
- Top-down decision making
- Mechanistic models of design

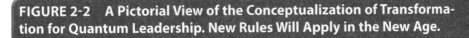

FIGURE 2-2   A Pictorial View of the Conceptualization of Transformation for Quantum Leadership. New Rules Will Apply in the New Age.

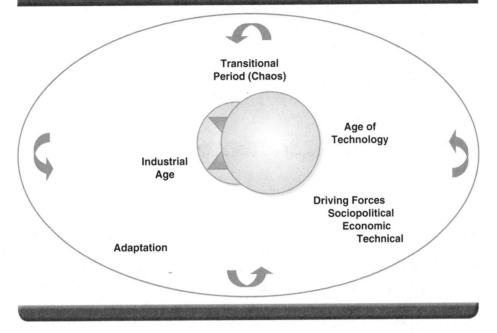

FIGURE 2-3   A Pictorial View of the Conceptualization of Transformation for Quantum Leadership. New Rules Will Apply in the New Age.

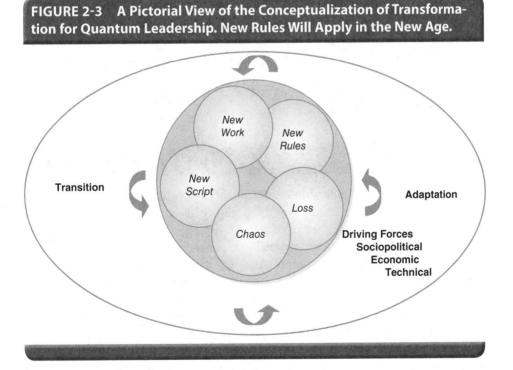

BOX 2-3   Seven New Age Imperatives

1. Open access to health information
2. Medicine and nursing based on genomics
3. Mass-customized diagnosis and treatment
4. User-specific insurance programs
5. Integration of allopathic and alternative therapies
6. Payment incentives tied to outcomes (quality)
7. Focused service settings for specific populations

---

that are sensitive to the needs of patients. Thinking inside the box considers that those closest to the work and those who are familiar with the existing challenge have the greatest insights into the processes. As innovation leaders become knowledgeable about processes by thinking inside and outside the box, positive deviants become evident. Positive deviants increase the knowledge pool by offering different perspectives that may, on the surface, be divergent to the status quo. Disruptive innovation defines a performance trajectory by introducing new dimensions of performance compared with existing innovations. New markets are created by bringing new features to nonconsumers or offering more convenient or lower prices to consumers. Scenario planning allows for a dry run and creating what-if scenarios for new ideas. Scenario planning provides an opportunity to capture essential elements for evaluating healthcare situations. The information garnered from this type of strategy provides invaluable information that teams can use to confront uncertainty and deal with serious problems that may seem outrageous from a traditional thinking perspective. "The purpose is to move out of traditional thinking patterns and develop creative solutions not previously considered" (Porter-O'Grady & Malloch, 2015, p. 113).

SUMMARY

The theory of nursing leadership is part of the theory of nursing management. Leadership is a process of influencing a group to set and achieve goals. Bennis and Nanus (1985) define a theory of leadership they call transformational. This leadership style involves change in which the purposes of the leader and follower become intertwined. Effective leaders create a vision for the organization and then develop a commitment to the vision. Bennis and Nanus (1985) believe the wise use of power is the energy needed to develop commitment and to sustain action.

Nurse managers should learn to practice leadership behaviors that stimulate motivation within their constituents, practicing professional nurses, and other nursing personnel. These behaviors include promotion of autonomy, decision making, and participatory management by professional nurses. They are facilitated by effective nurse manager–leaders. Strategic and lateral leadership also provide frameworks for contextual thinking about leading.

Quantum leadership offers a new-age perspective as one transforms and redesigns the workplace into a culture of greater safety and quality.

REFLECTIVE QUESTIONS

1. Reflect on how you lead and follow and describe how leadership theory underpins how you manage.
2. Describe the guiding principles and competencies that frame your leadership style and the perceptions of those you lead.
3. Consider leadership theory as a lens through which you view your leadership practice. Does this relate to selected theories of leadership and management, as well as organizational outcomes, within your healthcare system?
4. How do you view the role of nursing leadership in managing a clinical discipline?

CASE STUDY 2-1   Is a Leader Only a Leader When Paid?

Arlene H. Morris and Debbie R. Faulk

S. M., a midlevel administrator in a medical home, has been quite active in the state nurses' association since moving to the state 10 years ago. S. M. was recently elected to the office of president-elect (a 2-year term followed by 2 years in the president role). Although S. M. perceives election as an honor and an expression of other members' confidence in her leadership abilities, she wondered what preparation would be needed and how much time would be involved in this professional volunteer service. Additionally, it was a surprise when the higher-level administrators did not look favorably on her election. In fact, a few asked S. M. to describe how the state nurses' association was or was not functioning as a labor union and how the officer role would influence her role as midlevel administrator.

Although she was surprised at the administration's response, S. M. met with her supervisor to discuss the mission and vision of the state nurses' association, focusing on promoting excellence in nursing practice across all settings of care and advocating both for nurses within the healthcare delivery system and for quality and safe health care for the state population. The chief executive officer (CEO) later met with S. M. and asked her to specify what the role would entail and how it would impact her work role. S. M. thought of a past state association president who encouraged her to run for office and who was a role model and mentor for her. The past president often spoke of transformational leadership theory, and from what S. M. had encountered, it was the best example of this theory in action.

S. M. responded to the CEO by relaying her hopes of developing her own leadership skills and influencing the quality and safety of nursing in the healthcare delivery system within the state and across the nation. The CEO emphasized that the volunteer activities must not interfere with S. M.'s job responsibilities in any way. S. M. left the meeting puzzled and discouraged, wondering why the CEO did not see her election as a way for S. M. to increase her leadership competencies and a wonderful opportunity to advance professional nursing practice within the state.

(continues)

CASE STUDY 2-1   Is a Leader Only a Leader When Paid? (Continued)

Case Study Questions

1. What are the intended purposes and benefits of membership in a state nurses' association?
2. What are similarities and differences between state nurses' associations and state or national nursing specialty organizations?
3. What theory (or theories) of leadership would be helpful for S. M. as she assumes a leadership role in a voluntary professional membership association?
4. In the role of advocate for the thousands of licensed nurses within S. M.'s state, what issues should S. M. anticipate, and how will they most effectively be addressed?
5. How could S. M. pursue interaction with current state nurses' association leaders to ensure adequate succession planning for her benefit and for the benefit of the association?
6. Describe how S. M.'s leadership role in the state nurses' association would potentially benefit her performance in her midlevel management role.
7. What business skills, management abilities to work with state nursing association employees and volunteers, and knowledge of the healthcare delivery system are needed? How can S. M. develop the necessary knowledge, skills, and abilities?

CASE STUDY 2-2   Managing Conflict

Sergül Duygulu

Sevda has worked for 6 years at a private hospital with a capacity of 20 beds. She recently earned her bachelor's degree in nursing and is now working as a clinic nurse in orthopedics and traumatology at the hospital. As a student, Sevda wanted to change several unfavorable conditions in patient care after she graduated. Her belief that nothing could be done about system failures had solidified after spending so many years working at the hospital. On the other hand, Sevda is experiencing family burdens, including caring for her husband, who is unemployed, and her 3-year-old daughter, which led Sevda to continue working at the same hospital. She goes to work every day with the hope that she can at least make a difference in the lives of her patients.

There are eight nurses and a unit charge nurse in the orthopedics and traumatology department where Sevda works. Four of them have bachelor's degrees in nursing, and four of them are graduates of vocational schools. The hospital management is forced to hire vocational graduates because of a high turnover rate. Three nurses work the day shift, two nurses work the evening shift, and one nurse works the night shift. Although there is an effort to provide service in accordance with predefined standards, it is known that there are often patient care mistakes. However, the measures taken to reduce the mistakes have been limited. People have been held responsible, and the necessary warnings have been made.

Sevda is working with another nurse on the evening shift. She is more senior than the other nurse, who is a vocational school graduate and has recently completed her first year in the profession. After they take over from the day shift nurses, Sevda and her colleague divide the patients and start to provide care. Two of the patients under Sevda's care require careful attention because they have recently come out of surgery. Midway through the shift, one patient's fever has gone up, and the other has started to bleed. Sevda asks the other nurse to help her by checking the vital signs of her other patients, but the nurse says she is too busy with her own patients.

CASE STUDY 2-2   Managing Conflict (Continued)

Sevda was barely able to finish her work as her shift drew to a close. She remembered that the daughter of one of the other nurse's patients asked Sevda to give pain medication to her mother. Because Sevda was busy with her postsurgical patients, she told the daughter that the other nurse was assigned to her mother, and that she should be available soon. At the end of the shift, Sevda and her colleague handed off their patients to the night nurse and went home.

The next morning, when the unit charge nurse visited patient rooms, the daughter who asked Sevda for her mother's pain medication complained, saying that neither of the evening nurses stopped by her mother's room, and her mother did not get her pain medication until the night nurse gave it to her. The unit charge nurse, who believes that patient satisfaction is essential, apologized and said she would take care of the situation. She reviewed the records from the evening shift and found a note saying the evening nurse visited the patient three times to take her vital signs and twice to give medication. The unit charge nurse called Sevda and the other evening nurse and asked them to come to a meeting that afternoon.

In the meeting, the unit charge nurse asked Sevda and her colleague to explain what happened. Sevda said the woman was not her patient; she cared for 10 patients, two of whom were in critical condition. She explained that the daughter who complained had asked her for pain medication, and she told the daughter that the other nurse should come by. Sevda said she did not know anything else about the situation. Sevda's colleague said the patient and her daughter were lying. She said she went to the patient's room at least five times, as noted in the hospital record.

The unit charge nurse did not know what to do, so she referred the issue to the nursing services director, who requested the videotape from the camera that records patient room entrances. The tape showed that no nurse had entered the patient's room except when the patient was handed off between shifts.

The nursing services director called Sevda to her office. She told Sevda that, as an experienced nurse, she should manage the evening shift better. She told Sevda that if another such mistake is made, her employment will be terminated. Sevda loses her motivation and begins to think that she should take the necessary steps to find a job in another hospital.

The nursing services director told the other nurse that her employment was terminated. The nurse responded by saying that many nurses make the same mistake, but the director said her conduct is unacceptable. She stands by her decision to terminate the nurse so the other nurses will see the outcome of such behavior.

Now that one evening nurse has been terminated, only one nurse will work that shift.

Case Study Questions

1. Describe the issues that complicate the case. How are these issues interrelated?
2. What possible system problems occurred in this situation?
3. If you were Sevda, how would you have handled the situation?
4. How do you assess the leadership behaviors of Sevda, the unit charge nurse, and the nursing services director in handling this situation?
5. Who are the power holders in this case, what power sources did they use, and how did they use that power to manage the situation?
6. How did the players' actions impact the resolution of the problem?
7. Do you think the problem was solved?
8. How do you assess this case in terms of effective leadership?
9. If you were the unit charge nurse or the nursing services director, how would you have handled the situation?

REFERENCES

American Nurses Association. (2009). *Scope and standards for nurse administrators* (2nd ed.). Washington, DC: Author.

Avolio, B., Walumbwa, F., & Weber, T. J. (2009). Leadership: Current theories, research, and future direction. *Management Department Faculty Publications.* Paper 37. Retrieved from http://digitalcommons.unl.edu/managementfacpub/37

Barker, A. M. (1991). An emerging leadership paradigm. *Nursing and Health Care, 12,* 204–207.

Bennis, W. (1991). Learning some basic truisms about leadership. *Phi Kappa Phi Journal, 71,* 12–15.

Bennis, W., & Nanus, B. (1985). *Leaders: The strategies for taking charge.* New York, NY: Harper Row.

Buerhaus, P., Staiger, D., & Auerbach, D. (2000). Implications of an aging registered nurse workforce. *Journal of the American Medical Association, 283,* 2948–2954.

Dinh, J. E., Lord, R. G., Gardner, W. L., Meuser, J. D., Liden, R. C., & Hu, J. (2014). Leadership theory and research in the new millennium: Current theoretical trends and changing perspectives. *The Leadership Quarterly, 25*(1), 36–62.

Dooley, K. J., & Lichtenstein, B. (2008). Research methods for studying the dynamics of leadership. In M. Uhl-Bien & R. Marion (Eds.), *Complexity leadership: Part I: Conceptual foundations* (pp. 269–290). Charlotte, NC: Information Age Publishing, Inc.

Frankel, A. S., Leonard, M. W., & Denham, C. R. (2006). Fair and just culture, team behavior, and leadership engagement: The tools to achieve high reliability. *Health Services Research, 41*(4), 1690–1709.

Galinsky, A. D., & Kilduff, G. J. (2013). Be seen as a leader: A simple exercise can boost your status and influence. *Harvard Business Review, 91,* 127–30.

Gallup. (2013). *State of the American workplace.* Retrieved from http://www.gallup.com/services/178514/state-american-workplace.aspx

Gardner, J. W. (1993). *On leadership.* New York, NY: The Free Press.

Hewertson, R. B. (2015). *Lead like it matters, because it does.* New York, NY: McGraw-Hill Education.

Hill, L. A. (2014). Becoming the boss. *Harvard Business Review OnPoint, Seize Your Leadership Moment,* 34–43.

Institute of Medicine. (2001). *Crossing the quality chasm: A new health system for the 21st century.* Washington, DC: National Academies Press.

Institute of Medicine. (2011). *The future of nursing: Leading change, advancing health.* Washington, DC: National Academies Press.

Johnson, L. K. (2014, Fall). Exerting influence without authority. *Harvard Business Review OnPoint, Seize Your Leadership Moment,* 31–32.

Kets de Vries, M. F. R. (2013, December 18). The eight archetypes of leadership. Retrieved from https://hbr.org/2013/12/the-eight-archetypes-of-leadership

Kotter, J. P. (2014, Fall). What leaders really do. *Harvard Business Review OnPoint. Seize Your Leadership Moment,* 52–62.

Manary, M. P., Boulding, W., Staelin, R., & Glickman, S. W., (2013). The patient experience and health outcomes. *New England Journal of Medicine, 368,* 201–203.

Milstead, J. (2013). *Health policy and politics, a nurse's guide* (4th ed.). Burlington, MA: Jones & Bartlett Learning.

Morriss, A., Ely, R. J., & Frei, F. (2014, Fall). Stop holding yourself back. *Harvard Business Review OnPoint*. Retrieved from http://www.neccf.org/whitepapers/HBR_Managing_Yoursellf.pdf

Parks, S. D. (2013). *Leadership can be taught*. Benton, MA: Harvard Business Press.

Porter-O'Grady, T., & Malloch, K. (2007). *Quantum leadership: A resource for healthcare innovation* (2nd ed.). Sudbury, MA: Jones and Bartlett Publishers.

Porter-O'Grady, T., & Malloch, K. (2010). *Innovation leadership: Creating the landscape of health care*. Sudbury, MA: Jones and Bartlett Publishers.

Porter-O'Grady, T., & Malloch, K. (2015). *Quantum leadership: A resource for healthcare innovation* (4th ed.). Burlington, MA: Jones & Bartlett Learning.

Schoemaker, P. J., Krupp, S., & Howland, S. (2013). Strategic leadership: The essential skills. *Harvard Business Review OnPoint*. Retrieved from: http://www.harvardbusiness.org/sites/default/files/HBR_Strategic_Leadership.pdf

Stempniak, M. (2014). Your not-so-secret weapon to transform care. Retrieved from http://www.hhnmag.com/display/HHN-news-article.dhtml?dcrPath=/templatedata/HF_Common/NewsArticle/data/HHN/Magazine/2014/Feb/fea-patient-engagement

Tuuk, E. (2012). Transformational leadership in the coming decade: A response to three major workplace trends. Retrieved from http://www.cornellhrreview.org/transformational-leadership-in-the-coming-decade-a-response-to-three-major-workplace-trends/

Van Buren, M., & Safferstone, T. (2014, Fall). The quick wins paradox. *Harvard Business Review OnPoint*. Retrieved from http://www.executiveboard.com/exbd-resources/pdf/leadership-transition/The%20Quick%20Wins%20Paradox.pdf

Watkins, M. D. (2014). How managers become leaders. *Harvard Business Review OnPoint*. Retrieved from http://www.harvardbusiness.org/sites/default/files/HBR_How_Managers_Become_Leaders.pdf

Zheng, W., Singh, N., & Mitchell, W. (2014). Buffering and enabling: The impact of interlocking political ties on firm survival and sales growth. *Strategic Management Journal*. doi:10.1002/smj.2301

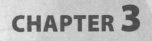

CHAPTER 3

Professional Practice: A Prototype Linking Nursing in Interprofessional Teams

Gay Landstrom and Donald D. Bignotti

LEARNING OBJECTIVES

1. Develop processes to lead and manage nursing and interprofessional teams.
2. Apply principles of management to reach desired organizational outcomes and a shared vision.
3. Design models that strengthen synergistic nursing and interprofessional effectiveness.

AONE KEY COMPETENCIES

I. Communication and relationship building
II. Knowledge of the healthcare environment
III. Leadership
IV. Professionalism
V. Business skills

AONE KEY COMPETENCIES DISCUSSED IN THIS CHAPTER:

I. Communication and relationship building
II. Knowledge of the healthcare environment
III. Leadership
IV. Professionalism

I. Communication and relationship building
- Effective communication
- Relationship management
- Influence of behaviors
- Ability to work with diversity
- Shared decision making
- Community involvement
- Medical staff relationships
- Academic relationships

II. Knowledge of the healthcare environment
- Clinical practice knowledge
- Patient care delivery models and work design knowledge
- Healthcare economics knowledge
- Healthcare policy knowledge
- Understanding of governance
- Understanding of evidence-based practice
- Outcomes measurement
- Knowledge of, and dedication to, patient safety
- Understanding of utilization and case management
- Knowledge of quality improvement and metrics
- Knowledge of risk management

III. Leadership
- Foundational thinking skills
- Personal journey disciplines
- Ability to use systems thinking
- Succession planning
- Change management

IV. Professionalism
- Personal and professional accountability
- Career planning
- Ethics
- Evidence-based clinical and management practices
- Advocacy for the clinical enterprise and for nursing practice
- Active membership in professional organizations

FUTURE OF NURSING: FOUR KEY MESSAGES

1. Nurses should practice to the full extent of their education and training.
2. Nurses should achieve higher levels of education and training through an improved education system that promotes seamless academic progression.
3. Nurses should be full partners with physicians and other health professionals in redesigning health care in the United States.
4. Effective workforce planning and policy making require better data collection and information infrastructure.

Introduction

There are a number of irrefutable changes facing health care in the United States over the next decade. The United States will likely surpass the point where 20% of the nation's gross domestic product is related to healthcare spending. As a society, we must decide whether we can afford to continue down this path or if we will find a way to improve the health of our population while reducing the per capita cost and improving the experience of those entering the healthcare arena. If we do not address these issues successfully, many believe there will be a tremendous negative impact on the standard of living in the United States.

What are the key drivers for the next decade? We know that within the United States we have an aging population to care for. Data from the U.S. Census Bureau clearly show a near doubling of the U.S. population aged 75 years and older, and aged 85 years and older, between 2010 and 2050 (Ortman, Velkoff, & Hogan, 2014). Other data show that historically there is a direct relationship between per capita spending on personal health care and age. Data from the Centers for Medicare and Medicaid Services (CMS) clearly show the cost per capita basis rises dramatically at about age 75 years and definitely jumps at age 85 years.

This is not the only phenomenon impacting the increase in per capita cost in the United States. Data from the Centers for Disease Control and Prevention reveal that in 1990, no state had an obesity rate as high as 15%. The data reveal that by 2010, no state had an obesity rate under 20%, and a large number of states had surpassed a 30% obesity rate. Data from the Congressional Budget Office demonstrate the relationship between body weight and per capita healthcare cost (Congressional Budget Office, 2010; Volsky, 2010). The data reveal a dramatic change in both the proportion of obesity and its relationship to healthcare expenditures over a 20-year period, between 1987 and 2007, and reflect the change from being underweight to being overweight as the driver of cost.

It should not be surprising that the combination of an aging population, obesity, and progress in treating chronic diseases should lead to an increase in the average number of chronic conditions experienced by our population. In fact, data from CMS show that the percentage of Medicare fee-for-service beneficiaries having four or more chronic conditions exceeded 34% in 2008 (Centers for Medicare and Medicaid Services, 2011). With the increase in the number of chronic conditions comes an increase in cost, reflected by the percentage of spending for Medicare. In 2008, the 34% of the population with four or more chronic diseases was responsible for 72% of Medicare spending, according to CMS (2011).

While utilization, as reflected by increased chronic diseases per capita and increased healthcare spending per capita, continues to climb at an alarming rate, we find ourselves in a growing misdistribution and shortage of clinicians in key areas. Data from the Association of American Medical Colleges project that the shortage of primary care physicians may be as high as 91,500 physicians by 2020 (Association of American Medical Colleges [AAMC], 2010). We already know there are tremendous shortages of primary care physicians and OB/GYN positions in parts of the country (Cunningham, 2011; Richards, Albright, & Rayburn, 2011). We continue to face a shortage of nurses that is greater than the shortage of physicians by at least a factor of 10. Similarly, according to the American Association of Colleges of Nursing (AACN), there is a substantial nursing misdistribution within the United States (American Association of Colleges of Nursing [AACN], 2014b). As the population ages, the current workforce continues to age in place. In 1985, physicians aged 65 years and older represented 9.4% of the physician workforce. By 2011, physicians aged 65 years and older grew to represent 15.1% of the physician workforce (AAMC, 2011). Similarly, the age distribution of nurses reveals progression from 1980 through 2020 (AACN, 2014b; Buerhaus, 2008).

In addition to aging, we are now realizing the impacts of burnout on the healthcare workforce. As it relates to physicians, reports indicate that nearly half of physicians struggle with burnout, which impacts their ability to relate to patients and focus on work in a way that avoids medical error (Shanafelt et al., 2012). Similar burnout rates are reported for registered nurses (Erickson & Grove, 2007; Todaro-Franceschi, 2013).

Yet clearly clinicians are not the only ones within the healthcare system to experience substantial stress. Patients are experiencing economic stress as they navigate the healthcare system. In addition to the personal stress of illness, substantial economic stress results. Himmelstein, Thorne, Warren, and Woolhandler (2009) studied bankruptcies that were filed in 2007 in the United States. They found that 62% of all bankruptcies filed that year related to medical expenses. Of those who filed for bankruptcy that year, nearly 80% had health insurance. Himmelstein and colleagues (2009) said the findings of this study show that middle-class families "frequently collapse under the strain of the health care system that treats physical wounds but inflicts fiscal ones" (p. 746).

Where do these revelations lead us? We have evidence that the U.S. population will continue to utilize healthcare resources at an ever-increasing pace. We have clear evidence that there is an existing misdistribution and shortage of clinical professionals. We have a system to pay for health care that puts the middle class at risk for bankruptcy and arguably prevents the poorest and most vulnerable from being able to access health care where and how they need it. We have a growing distance between what the United States and other countries, with whom we compete economically on a global scale, pay for health care (Kaiser Family Foundation, 2011). The authors believe that to meet this challenge, clinical professionals must come to the table with a different mind-set and a different skill set if we are to avert potential healthcare shortages or prevent the cost of caring for the current population to be borne by many future generations. In this chapter we share some thoughts and insight about how we can manage this Herculean task. It not us, who? If not now, when?

THE CALL FOR A DIFFERENT APPROACH

No. individual discipline—medicine, nursing, pharmacy, social work, physical therapy, or others—can meet the needs of U.S. citizens alone. Many of the structures and processes we currently enjoy were created within disciplinary silos. But our current system is fragmented, contains costly redundancies, and is not achieving necessary outcomes. We have to create a different health system that absorbs fewer resources and yields better outcomes. We have to find a way to fully leverage the strengths and perspective of each discipline and cocreate the future system. The best system will be created by consumers, nursing, medicine, dieticians, physical and occupational therapists, pharmacy, mental health clinicians, community agents, and the faith community all coming together to develop a shared vision, required outcomes, and the processes and structures necessary to achieve these outcomes. It is through shared perspectives, knowledge, and experience that we will find the best answers to the challenges we face as a nation.

For nursing to participate fully in this interprofessional effort, individual nurses need to first fully understand their own practice. What do nurses uniquely bring to the table in helping the population maintain health or in helping those patients with illness regain health or find optimal functioning with their disease? Too often nurses have a hard time defining for others what nursing is and what the discipline brings to patient care (Parse, 2013). Competencies of nursing, such as skill in modifying the patient's environment to maintain or regain a state of health, are just not salient to many nurses today. When joining an interprofessional team, nurses can be reticent contributors, unsure about what they can uniquely bring to the planning of patient care. Without clarity about nursing's contributions, nurses will not be good partners in creating the health system of the future (Engel & Prentice, 2013; Haskins, 2008).

Nurses also need to have clarity about their accountability to the public. Nurses are issued a license by their state governmental agency. This license gives the nurse a right to care for people, have access to sensitive patient information, perform critical assessments and treatments, have the privilege of teaching patients and families, and make decisions about the right course of nursing interventions to bring about a return to a level of health. In return, nurses accept accountability to always do what is in the best interest of the patient, maintain currency in the best nursing practice, protect patient rights and personal information, advocate for patients, families, and communities, and practice with the highest ethical behavior (American Nurses Association [ANA], 2010a, 2010b).

The Institute of Medicine (IOM) report *The Future of Nursing: Leading Change, Advancing Health* (2010) also provided clear guidance that nurses need to expand their knowledge and skills through formal education and practice to the full extent of their license. Then nurses need to be willing to engage and collaborate with physicians and other healthcare professionals in redesigning health care in the United States. For those positioned to affect the nursing educational system, they have the additional responsibility of advocating for seamless academic progression and improved data collection structures to create more effective workforce planning and public health policy. Now is not the time for nurses to be hesitant or wait for someone else to come forward to do the job.

Personal Accountability for Competency

Nurses and other members of the healthcare team need to bring their very best selves to the collaborative effort to be good partners in creating the health system of the future. Team members need to learn skills beyond expert knowledge of their own discipline. It is essential for team members to understanding the complex nature of systems, particularly the healthcare system that currently exists in the United States. And they need an understanding of the outcomes and resource consumption that will be required of systems in the future. Team members will need to be critical thinkers who are able to evaluate ideas and reflect on them in light of the required outcomes, constrained resources, and available assets.

There is a set of skills that are perhaps even more important. These include listening skills, emotional intelligence, change leadership, and personal journey disciplines. Exquisite listening skills will be required of each team member. Each member will bring a unique set of knowledge, skills, and experiences to the table. There will be differences in language that must be understood through listening and clarification. Some team members may be called on to serve as translators, verbalizing what they understand and helping other teammates comprehend meanings. Through listening, clarifying, and translating for others, members of the collaborative team will be able to share their perspectives and ideas and pool them with the perspectives and ideas of their teammates, and thus create the broadest set of options for consideration in designing the health system (Bridges, Davidson, Odegard, Maki, and Tomkowiak, 2011; Interprofessional Education Collaborative Expert Panel, 2011).

Emotional intelligence is a set of skills that are purported to contribute to accurate assessment and expression of emotion in oneself and in others (Salovey & Mayer, 1989). Goleman (2006) went on to explain that without emotional intelligence, humans cannot be fully successful in relationships, work, and even physical well-being. Goleman explains that emotional literacy can be enhanced, yielding the ideal combination of both mental and emotional intelligence. Members of the collaborative healthcare team need to individually develop their emotional intelligence to accurately assess and express emotion as a component of idea exchange and understanding, and emotional intelligence skills in interpersonal negotiations.

Change leadership is a hot topic in health care. Healthcare leaders, including those engaged in designing the health system of the future, need a solid understanding of change and the skills to plan for change, communicate to people about the needed change and the steps that will need to be taken, and ultimately lead people through change. If change is to be successful and sustainable over time, it needs to be understood on multiple levels. In his model of change, Kotter (2002) describes the need to create urgency or a compelling case for not staying in the present state. Without a compelling reason to change, people will not expend the energy to leave their current behaviors and thinking. Schein (2004) describes change on four organizational levels. For change to be successful, leaders need to not only address technical and process changes but also deal with what people need to know and the skills they need to possess, and they need to address the beliefs, attitudes, and behaviors of those going through the desired change. Change can be sustained only if the effort reaches into this last cultural level and takes hold. The healthcare team members need to recognize that resistance can be a positive sign of initial engagement that needs to be embraced and nurtured, rather than avoided or fought. Without basic change leadership knowledge and skills, the collaborative team members will be limited in their ability to plan for the implementation of change and sustain it.

In an arena like health care, which is complex and rapidly changing, keeping up on what one needs to know about external influences, changing clinical knowledge, and personal growth requires more than traditional learning. Personal journey disciplines are key practices that help individuals learn from every experience, every encounter, and every potential source of learning. These disciplines are not a book that can be read or a lecture that can be attended. Personal journey disciplines involve practices such as action learning and reflective practice (American Organization of Nurse Executives, 2005).

Professional Accountability

Members of the collaborative team, including nurses, need to fully understand what professional accountability requires of them. Guanci (2007) notes that a combination of various tenets makes up a profession. These include (1) a well-defined body of knowledge, (2) depth of education, (3) control over practice and the practice environment, (4) self-regulation, (5) use of evidence-based practice and nursing research, (6) peer review, (7) the ability to practice autonomously, (8) affiliation with professional organizations, (9) a system of values, and (10) the development of a unique relationship with patients. We will take a closer look at just a few of these.

Values guide the creation of any organization or structure. Outcomes that are the target of the initial design express the values of the individuals or sponsoring body that forms an organization. These values may be implicit or explicit, but they are always there. Ethics is closely related to a system of values. Ethical behavior and ethical practice, both of which serve to help protect the public, are absolutely essential. Ethics are used to guide how the work of the organization or system is accomplished, and each professional needs to understand his or her discipline's standards of ethical behavior (ANA, 2009, 2010a, 2010b; Engel & Prentice, 2013).

Professional practice is based on the best evidence. In creating the health system of the future, the best evidence will be required, both for clinical practice in each of the involved disciplines and for leadership. Too often, evidence-based practice is applied only to the clinical realm. Leadership and management require the use of the best knowledge available, and old methods that no longer serve to accomplish the desired outcomes should be discarded. In designing health care for the future, the best clinical and leadership evidence needs to be used. Borrowing from Sackett and his colleagues (2000), this evidence needs to include not only the best research evidence, but also the experience of expert clinicians and the values and priorities of the people that will be served. Yet how do we manage the explosion of information and evidence? Clinical professionals across disciplines will need to employ a different approach if we are to effectively cope with the amount of information that appears annually in an increasing number of publications. Clinical leaders will need to develop new systems through which information on the best evidence can be supplied to clinicians in the trenches where and when it is most needed. Expecting that clinicians will continue to personally read all the available literature, make critical decisions on the value of the literature, and implement that knowledge effectively and rapidly may be unrealistic. In the future—perhaps already—individual clinicians will need to trust teams of subject matter experts who will review evidence and particular topics and put together recommendations and supportive rationales that they will be able to access, accept, and follow.

INTERPROFESSIONAL COLLABORATION

The authors perceive that, in this context, interprofessional teams will work in collaboration to review evidence and deliver recommendations for team-based approaches to deliver the highest quality, lowest cost, evidence-based care that also maximizes the patient experience. As such, we see that the leadership challenge is in the willingness, and ability, to work in teams representing different disciplines and potentially different cultures. In fact, the historically different cultures that impact how clinical professionals train, work, think, and behave should not be underestimated as a potential impediment to future interprofessional collaboration. We believe that when open discussion among clinical professionals in interprofessional teams occurs to address cultural differences and to create similar mental models of the future of healthcare design, the stage will be set for effective collaboration leading to rule clarification, professional respect, and trust. These elements are essential to the effectiveness of both clinical leaders and clinical professionals at the bedside.

Communication, Relationship-Building Competence, and the Care of a Partnership

Many books have been written about the need for clear communication within teams and building foundational relationships. Teams also need to have a common purpose. This provides motivation for expending energy to form relationships. We all know that some relationships give us energy and stoke our creativity, while others seem to drain us of those things. Members of the best interprofessional teams bring their best selves to the work, but they don't focus on recognition. Instead, team members take deliberate steps to understand other members. They commend input that is offered by another. They use "we" language and focus on the goals of the team. They draw attention to the perspectives and contributions of others. Taking team relationships a step further, collaborative relationships are careful to set aside personal interests and focus on cooperative efforts with no sense of vanquishing or beating others (World Health Organization, 2010). Power and authority are shared in collaboration, and efforts are focused on understanding the unique contributions of collaborators (Kagan, 2004). As discussed earlier, there are multiple disciplines in health care, with unique education and differing perspectives and areas of focus. Team members must understand and respect one another's unique contributions to the common purpose and goals.

It is important to note that collaborators within healthcare design teams are likely to include nontraditional participants. Competitors might have to collaborate to serve a population. A single former competitor might be a competitor in one situation and serve as a collaborator and full member of the team for a different service. New collaborators are emerging as drugstores, grocery stores, and others enter the urgent care and health maintenance arena. Still other collaborative partners are likely to be insurance companies who are funding the care of patients by clinicians. Teams will have to collaborate not only across disciplines but also across entirely different organizations with differing objectives and experiences. All stakeholders need to be at the table to design systems that meet the needs of a given population.

Relationships require care, attention, and feeding. Collaborators can begin to misunderstand motives and misinterpret behaviors if ongoing communication and relationship building are not embedded in the process. Time must be set aside not only for planning itself but also for team members to continually communicate, seek clarity, and ensure that the relationship is strong and functional.

Best Management Science of Interprofessional Teams

Interprofessional teams need to base their design work on the best evidence from clinical and leadership literature, expert opinions, and patient values and preferences. This evidence needs to be drawn from multiple disciplines and vetted by team members. The days of nurses working on teams but focusing most of their efforts on isolating nursing and creating protective walls to guard nursing are long past. This isolationist behavior was in response to perceived threats, but it was counterproductive and sometimes led to nurses' voices not being heard. Nurses need to be strong and know their assets, but these qualities need to be in service of better caring for the population.

INTERPROFESSIONAL PRACTICE PARTNERSHIPS

Several landmark reports have catapulted interprofessional learning and partnerships to the forefront. While patients, lawyers, and each discipline recognized the strengths and shortcomings of their work, prior to 2000 relatively little effort was put forward to address common concerns around patient safety and quality of care.

The first report was the IOM's *To Err Is Human: Building a Safer Health System* (1999), followed by the IOM Committee on Quality of Health Care in America report *Crossing the Quality Chasm: A New Health System for the 21st Century* (2001), which recognized that healthcare professionals working in interprofessional teams can communicate and address the complex needs of patients and families most effectively. This was followed by an IOM report on interprofessional education, *Health Professions Education: A Bridge to Quality* (2003), which was recently updated in *Interprofessional Education for Collaboration: Learning How to Improve Health from Interprofessional Models across the Continuum of Education to Practice* (2013). Last, the *Future of Nursing: Leading Change, Advancing Health* (Institute of Medicine, 2010) report stressed the need for nurses to become equal partners in health policy, decision making, and practice. Common to each of these reports is the recognition that collaboration, effective communication, shared learning, and building teams are neither intuitive nor commonplace, yet they are essential in the provision of high-quality, safe patient care.

The AACN has established two notable partnerships in support of interprofessional team development and collaboration. First were formal academic–practice partnerships, established in 2003, to support the transition of nurse graduates, irrespective of educational program, in becoming practice organization leaders. The task force members, comprising nurse leaders spanning practice and academe, joined together to establish parameters and criteria in support of effective and meaningful transitions from the school setting to practice. The task force generated a white paper that became the foundation to a decade of long work to bridge the worlds of practice and academe for effective entry into the profession. The white paper was the impetus for several academic–practice collaborations regarding professional development, interprofessional learning, and curricular expectations for bachelor's, master's, and doctoral education of nurses (AACN, 2003).

Most recently, the AACN joined the American Association of Colleges of Osteopathic Medicine, the American Association of Colleges of Pharmacy, the American Dental Education Association, the Association of American Medical Colleges, and the Association of Schools and Programs of Public Health to establish an expert panel that generated *Core Competencies for Interprofessional Collaborative Practice* (Interprofessional Education Collaborative Expert Panel, 2011) as a product of the Interprofessional Education Collaborative. Inspired by a shared vision of interprofessional practice forming the foundation for safe, high-quality, accessible, patient-centered care, a commitment to develop interprofessional competencies with health profession students was seen as key to preparing the future workforce. While each profession builds from distinct disciplinary learning, each member of the collaborative agreed that the need to move beyond discipline-specific education by engaging students in interactions with other disciplines would be fundamental to interprofessional learning, team building, and ultimately becoming an effective team member in the workplace (Interprofessional Education Collaborative Expert Panel, 2011).

The AACN and the American Organization of Nurse Executives (AONE) joined together to form a task force on academic–practice partnerships to initiate a national dialogue, recognizing that although nurse leaders who are responsible for education and operations would need to partner, this would be insufficient. As such, they established an expectation that academic–practice partnerships should include other health disciplines, leverage evidence and best practices, and make recommendations based on definitions, expectations, qualities, and products of academic–practice partnerships (AACN, 2015). As an outcome of this work, eight guiding principles for academic–practice partnerships were established (AACN, 2012), and a tool kit that supports ongoing education was created (AACN, 2014a).

Practice leaders also stepped forward to create expectations and structures for interprofessional collaboration and learning within the practice environment. Supported by the Agency for Healthcare Research and Quality and based on work developed in the U.S. Department of Defense, Team Strategies and Tools to Enhance Performance and Patient Safety (TeamSTEPPS) established a teamwork system to improve safety that is predicated on improved communication and teamwork skills within practice organizations across the continuum of care (Agency for Healthcare Research and Quality, 2011). TeamSTEPPS is an evidence-based, systematic approach to improve and sustain a culture of safety by providing an interdisciplinary curriculum, readiness assessments, and consultations to organizations that commit to implementation. Shared learning within and among disciplines is emphasized and supported by leadership engagement, coaching, feedback, and skill building across disciplines throughout the organization.

As the nation moves into an era of population health, accountable care, and healthcare reform, additional partnerships will enter the landscape. They will include community partners that are not commonly considered members of a healthcare team, such as business entities, wellness disciplines, health educators, navigators, technology-based industry members, and policy makers. Their shared goal will be to improve the health of our country through innovative practice models that embrace partnering to improve care outcomes.

SUMMARY

The United States is headed in the wrong direction in terms of the costs of health care, health-harming personal behaviors, and outcomes. Change is not just inevitable, it is essential to future success. We have to turn around the current trends and create a health system that will yield a higher degree of health at a lower cost.

The solution will come through the collaboration of interprofessional teams that will include nurses, physicians, other clinical disciplines, patients, insurers, and many new providers of urgent care and health maintenance. Nurses need to prepare themselves educationally and mentally to participate as members of these teams and work to design the health system of the future. They need to understand their own practice and unique contributions. Additionally, nurses must be prepared to fulfill their contract to serve the public good and behave with the highest degree of ethical behavior and integrity. They need to gain knowledge of the best available evidence and hone their skills in relationship building, teamwork, change leadership, and how to best participate as a full collaborative member of an inter-professional team. As nurses bring their best selves to this work, they will cast a strong leadership shadow and positively contribute to the work of the whole team.

The United States needs courageous nurses to prepare for and take their seat at the redesign table. When nurses, physicians, and members of the healthcare team come to the table fully prepared, the design of the new health system will take off.

REFLECTIVE QUESTIONS

1. Describe an experience you have had working with an interprofessional team. What frameworks (lens) did you use to understand and work with processes in managing the team's goals?
2. Considering your work with an interprofessional team, how would an emotionally intelligent leader use specific skills to impact positive outcomes?
3. How would you design models that strengthen synergistic nursing and interprofessional effectiveness?
4. Supported by the Agency for Healthcare Research and Quality and based on work developed in the U.S. Department of Defense, TeamSTEPPS provides an evidence-based teamwork system to improve safety that is predicated on improved communication and teamwork skills within practice organizations across the continuum of care. Describe two strategies from this evidence-based practice that could improve hand-off communication in your practice.

CASE STUDY 3-1   Academic–Clinical Partnership and Team Cohesion

Lori Lioce and Kristen Herrin

Natalie Busby was recently hired as a department nurse manager by a regional not-for-profit healthcare system. She has master's degree preparation in nursing administration. Natalie served as a nurse manager at a small private hospital for 2 years after graduation.

Natalie just completed new employee orientation. Last week she had her first meeting with the chief nursing officer, who addressed department goals. During the meeting, Natalie became aware of several concerns in the department. Historically, the department had run smoothly and efficiently and was one of the premier departments within the organization. During the past 6 months, some of the nurses began requesting transfers to other departments, and some left to seek employment outside the organization. The chief nursing officer is concerned and would like Natalie to make this her first priority as the new department head.

In Natalie's first department manager meeting, the unit nurse managers voiced concerns about the increase in the number of nursing students on the floor at one time and nursing instructors sitting in the break room while relying on floor nurses to guide the students' clinical experience. Additionally, some nurses are refusing to take students or are calling in sick when students are expected on the floor, resulting in short staffing and incivility among staff members.

(continues)

CASE STUDY 3-1   Academic–Clinical Partnership and Team Cohesion (Continued)

The department has 152 full- and part-time employees, consisting of 88 RNs, 40 LPNs, and 24 nursing assistants. Each unit has a staffing mix of 22 RNs, 10 LPNs, and 6 nursing assistants. In the past, the staff has worked well together. The recent increase in turnover has resulted in additional stress among the staff, creating a negative and distrusting culture. The unit nurse managers said that because many seasoned nurses are leaving and new nurses are coming on board, the staff feels overburdened with training new nurses and dealing with nursing students. In addition, the staff feels like the patients may not be getting the proper care.

Case Study Questions

1. What additional coaching would be beneficial for Natalie?
2. How should Natalie address the nurse managers' concerns?
3. What strategies can Natalie employ internally with the following groups:
   - Nurse managers
   - Staff nurses (LPNs and RNs)
   - Nursing assistants
4. What strategies can Natalie employ externally with the following groups:
   - Schools of nursing
   - Nursing instructors
5. Which leadership style or styles should Natalie use to create a positive work environment?
6. What change theory or theories could be used in this situation?
7. Why is there a culture of incivility? How can this be addressed? How can Natalie involve staff to change the culture?
8. Natalie asks for current patient outcome data for her department. The Catheter Associated Urinary Tract Infection (CAUTI) rates are reported as the second highest in the hospital. How can Natalie use this data when working with her team? What strategies would be effective in improving patient outcomes?

REFERENCES

Agency for Healthcare Research and Quality. (2011). TeamSTEPPS: Strategies and tools to enhance performance and patient safety. Retrieved from http://teamstepps .ahrq.gov

American Association of Colleges of Nursing. (2003). Building capacity through university hospital and university school of nursing partnerships. Retrieved from http://www.aacn.nche.edu/publications/white-papers/building-capacity

American Association of Colleges of Nursing. (2012). AACN-AONE task force on academic–practice partnership: Guiding principles. Retrieved from http://www .aacn.nche.edu/leading-initiatives/academic-practice-partnerships/Guiding Principles.pdf

American Association of Colleges of Nursing. (2014a). Academic–practice partnerships tool kit. Retrieved from http://www.aacn.nche.edu/leading-initiatives /academic-practice-partnerships/tool-kit

American Association of Colleges of Nursing. (2014b). Nursing shortage fact sheet. Retrieved from http://www.aacn.nche.edu/media-relations/NrsgShort ageFS.pdf

American Association of Colleges of Nursing. (2015). AACN-AONE academic–practice partnerships steering committee. Retrieved from https://www.aacn.nche.edu/about-aacn/committees-task-force/aacn-aone-task-force-on-academic-practice-partnerships

American Nurses Association. (2009). *Scope and standards for nurse administrators* (3rd ed.). Silver Spring, MD: Author.

American Nurses Association. (2010a). *Guide to code of ethics for nurses: Interpretation and application.* Silver Spring, MD: Author.

American Nurses Association. (2010b). *Scope and standards of practice* (2nd ed.). Silver Spring, MD: Author.

American Organization of Nurse Executives. (2005). Nurse executive competencies. Retrieved from http://www.aone.org/resources/leadership%20tools/nursecomp.shtml

Association of American Medical Colleges. (2010). The impact of health care reform on the future supply and demand for physicians updated projections through 2025. Retrieved from https://www.aamc.org/download/158076/data/updated_projections_through_2025.pdf

Association of American Medical Colleges. (2011). *2011 state physician workforce data book.* Retrieved from https://www.aamc.org/download/263512/data/statedata2011.pdf

Bridges, D., Davidson, R., Odegard, P., Maki, I., and Tomkowiak, J. (2011). Interprofessional collaboration: Three best practice models for interprofessional education. Retrieved from: http://www.ncbi.nlm.nih.gov/pmc/articles/PMC3081249/.

Buerhaus, P. (2008). Current and future state of the US nursing workforce. *Journal of the American Medical Association, 300*(20), 2422–2423.

Centers for Medicare and Medicaid Services. (2011). *Chronic conditions among Medicare beneficiaries.* Retrieved from http://www.cms.gov/Research-Statistics-Data-and-Systems/Statistics-Trends-and-Reports/Chronic-Conditions/Downloads/2011Chartbook.pdf

Congressional Budget Office. (2010). How does obesity in adults affect spending on healthcare? Retrieved from http://www.cbo.gov/publication/21772

Creating Minds. (2015). Practical tools and wise quotes on all matters creative. Retrieved from http://creatingminds.org/quotes/thinking.htm

Cunningham, P. (2011). State variation in primary care physician supply: Implications for health reform Medicaid expansions (HSC Research Brief No. 19). Retrieved from http://www.hschange.com/CONTENT/1192/?PRINT=1

Engel, J., & Prentice, D. (2013). The ethics of interprofessional collaboration. *Nursing Ethics, 20*(4), 426–435.

Erickson, R., & Grove, W. (2007). Why emotions matter: Age, agitation, and burnout among registered nurses. *Online Journal of Issues in Nursing, 13*(1). Retrieved from http://www.nursingworld.org/MainMenuCategories/ANAMarketplace/ANAPeriodicals/OJIN/TableofContents/vol132008/No1Jan08/ArticlePreviousTopic/WhyEmotionsMatterAgeAgitationandBurnoutAmongRegisteredNurses.html. doi:10.3912/OJIN.Vol13No01PPT01

Goleman, D. (2006). *Emotional intelligence.* New York, NY: Bantam Books.

Guanci, G. (2007). *Feel the pull: Creating a culture of nursing excellence.* Minneapolis, MN: Creative Health Care Management.

Haskins, A. (2008). *An exploration of satisfaction, psychological stress, and readiness for interprofessional learning in medical, nursing, allied health, and social work students in an interprofessional health course* (Doctoral dissertation). University of North Dakota, Grand Forks.

Himmelstein, D., Thorne, D., Warren, E., & Woolhandler, S. (2009). Medical bankruptcy in the United States, 2007: Results of a national study. Retrieved from http://www.amjmed.com/article/S0002-9343%2809%2900404-5/pdf

Institute of Medicine. (1999). *To err is human: Building a safer health system*. Washington, DC: National Academies Press.

Institute of Medicine. (2001). *Crossing the quality chasm: A new health system for the 21st century*. Washington, DC: National Academies Press.

Institute of Medicine. (2003). *Health professions education: A bridge to quality*. Washington, DC: National Academies Press.

Institute of Medicine. (2010). *The future of nursing: Leading change, advancing health*. Washington, DC: National Academies Press.

Institute of Medicine. (2013). *Interprofessional Education for Collaboration: Learning how to improve health from interprofessional models across the continuum of education to practice*. Retrieved from http://iom.edu/Reports/2013/Interprofessional-Education-for-Collaboration.aspx

Interprofessional Education Collaborative Expert Panel. (2011). *Core competencies for interprofessional collaborative practice: Report of an expert panel*. Washington, DC: Author.

Kagan, R. (2004). *Of paradise and power: America and Europe in the new world order*. New York, NY: Vintage Books.

Kaiser Family Foundation. (2011). Snapshots: Health care spending in the United States and selected OECD countries. Retrieved from http://kff.org/health-costs/issue-brief/snapshots-health-care-spending-in-the-united-states-selected-oecd-countries/

Kotter, J. (2002). *The heart of change*. Boston, MA: Harvard Business School.

Ortman, J. M., Velkoff, V. A., & Hogan, H. (2014). An aging nation: The older population in the United States. Retrieved from www.census.gov/prod/2014pubs/p25-1140.pdf

Parse, R. (2013). What we've got here is a failure to communicate. *Nursing Science Quarterly, 26*(1), 5–6.

Richards, M., Albright, B., & Rayburn, W. (2011). Measuring the obstetrician workforce: Access to maternity centers using geographical information systems (GIS) mapping. Retrieved from https://www.aamc.org/download/185474/data/2011_pwc_rayburn.pdf

Sackett, D. L., Straus, S. E., Richardson, W. S., Rosenberg, W., & Haynes, R. B. (2000). *Evidence-based medicine: How to practice and teach EBM* (2nd ed.). Edinburgh, Scotland: Churchill Livingstone.

Salovey, P., & Mayer, J. (1989). Emotional intelligence. *Imagination, Cognition and Personality, 9*(3), 185–211.

Schein, E. H. (2004). *Organizational culture and leadership* (3rd ed.). San Francisco, CA: Jossey-Bass.

Shanafelt, T., Boone, S., Litjen, T., Dyrbye, L., Sotile, W., Satele, D., . . . Oreskovich, M. (2012). Burnout and satisfaction with work-life balance among US physicians relative to the general US population. *Archives of Internal Medicine, 172*(18), 1377–1385. doi:10.1001/archinternmed.2012.3199

Todaro-Franceschi, V. (2013). *Compassion fatigue and burnout in nursing: Enhancing professional quality of life.* New York, NY: Springer.

Volsky, I. (2010). How much does obesity contribute to health spending? Retrieved from http://thinkprogress.org/health/2010/09/08/171640/obesity-spending-cbo/

World Health Organization. (2010). *Framework for action for interprofessional education and collaborative practice.* Geneva, Switzerland: Author.

CHAPTER 4

Professional Development: An Imperative for Leadership in Nursing and Healthcare Organizations

Patricia L. Thomas, Micki McMillan, Patricia A. Barlow, and Lesa Becker

LEARNING OBJECTIVES

1. Identify the elements of an executive coaching relationship.
2. Draw distinctions between coaching for performance management and executive coaching for transformative leadership practice.
3. Integrate professional responsibility and power, authenticity, integrity, and emotional intelligence into leadership practice.
4. Analyze organizational challenges that promote and inhibit authentic nursing leadership.

AONE KEY COMPETENCIES

I. Communication and relationship building
II. Knowledge of the healthcare environment
III. Leadership
IV. Professionalism
V. Business skills

AONE KEY COMPETENCIES DISCUSSED IN THIS CHAPTER:

I. Communication and relationship building
III. Leadership
IV. Professionalism

I. **Communication and relationship building**
  - Effective communication
  - Relationship management
  - Influence of behaviors
  - Ability to work with diversity
  - Shared decision making
  - Community involvement
  - Medical staff relationships
  - Academic relationships

III. Leadership

- Foundational thinking skills
- Personal journey disciplines
- Ability to use systems thinking
- Succession planning
- Change management

IV. Professionalism

- Personal and professional accountability
- Career planning
- Ethics
- Evidence-based clinical and management practices
- Advocacy for the clinical enterprise and for nursing practice
- Active membership in professional organizations

FUTURE OF NURSING: FOUR KEY MESSAGES

1. Nurses should practice to the full extent of their education and training.
2. Nurses should achieve higher levels of education and training through an improved education system that promotes seamless academic progression.
3. Nurses should be full partners with physicians and other health professionals in redesigning health care in the United States.
4. Effective workforce planning and policy making require better data collection and information infrastructure.

Introduction

In this time of unprecedented change in health care, professional growth and development have taken on new meaning. It will not be sufficient to find a mentor or read on your own as a means to keep pace with industry changes, much less develop leadership ability (Benner, Sutphen, Leonard, & Day, 2010). The imperative for nurses to develop their leadership presence and visibility has been emphasized as a goal for the nursing profession in two of the four recommendations in *The Future of Nursing: Leading Change, Advancing Health* (Institute of Medicine [IOM], 2010). To develop this report, in 2008 the Robert Wood Johnson Foundation and the Institute of Medicine (IOM) launched a 2-year study to assess the nursing profession, recognizing that redesign of the healthcare delivery system would require nurses' active, visible engagement and influence, given their numbers and proximity to patients. The intent of the report was to transform the nursing profession through an action-oriented blueprint to meet the healthcare needs of the 21st century.

Foundational to meeting these expectations is a reconceptualization of the role of nurses within the context of the entire workforce and development of innovative solutions to address societal needs in a rapidly changing delivery system. New competencies for nurse leaders were anticipated in recognition of a gap between current and future states. Powerful, competent, and confident nurse leaders who can interact with a variety of stakeholders in health care, business, government, and the insurance industry will be needed. Thus, the need for professional development of nurses and learning new skills was catapulted into the healthcare reform dialogue.

Significant emphasis has been placed on the need for nurses to position themselves as equal partners with other health professionals to lead the improvement and redesign of the healthcare system in a variety of environments, including hospitals, schools, homes, retail health clinics, long-term care facilities, battlefields, and community and public health centers. As such, nurses will be positioned to bridge the gap between coverage and access, to coordinate increasingly complex care for a wide range of patients, and to innovate new care delivery systems across the care continuum to satisfy unmet patient needs in our current delivery system (IOM, 2010).

The IOM report identified that historic restrictions on the scope of practice, policy- and reimbursement-related limitations, and professional tensions have undermined the nursing profession's ability to provide and improve both general and advanced care. In light of this, they call upon all nurse leaders to develop a leadership presence to influence decisions and policy making from the bedside to the boardroom and in education and research (Khoury, Blizzard, Wright-Moore, & Hassmiller, 2011). The need to examine professional development, leverage existing effective strategies, and nurture transformational development opportunities will be essential. Many of our current professional development strategies based on formal education have been moderately effective. The radical change before us dictates the need for dynamic, responsive, innovative strategies for professional development within organizations and universities. The models for this development may reside outside the healthcare industry (Benner et al., 2010).

EXPECTATIONS FOR NURSE LEADER PROFESSIONAL DEVELOPMENT

Professional development is multifaceted, spanning formal education and ongoing development within roles. Leadership competence will become part of expected practice for all nurses, not just those holding formal leadership positions (Benner et al., 2010). In light of this, educational institutions will need to incorporate leadership development into all nursing curricula. Additionally, those in nursing operations will need to embed leadership development into career planning and provide opportunities to learn and lead simultaneously.

Organizations have invested heavily in leadership and nurse leader development, recognizing that the work of the organization resides in the effectiveness of its leaders (Locke, 2008; Taft, 2011). Taft (2011) identified strong, effective executive leaders in nursing as a scarce commodity, emphasizing that organizations often experience inconsistent leadership performance within the ranks even with highly effective executive leaders in place. Recently organizations have acknowledged that while clinical indicators and outcomes of care may be strong, patient satisfaction, physician satisfaction, employee engagement, and retention are heavily influenced by the effectiveness of nurse leaders to support staff through planned and unplanned change (Bamford, Wong, & Laschinger, 2013; Karsten,

Baggot, Brown, & Cahill, 2010). Given this, efforts directed toward nurse leader development are worthy of time, attention, and resources.

The American Organization of Nurse Executives (AONE), which represents nurse leaders across practice and academe, set research and education priorities to address critical issues facing the profession. Recognizing the changing role of nurse leaders, AONE recommends five areas for nurse leader competence: communication and relationship building, knowledge of the healthcare environment, leadership skills, professionalism, and business skills (American Organization of Nurse Executives [AONE], 2011). They also called for bachelor's and master's degrees as the minimal educational preparation of nurse leaders and doctoral degrees for those in executive positions. Their guiding principles for nurses entering the profession recognize dimensions of development in clinical reasoning, technical skills acquisition, shaping emotional intelligence, socialization, professional engagement, and ongoing continuing education. These guidelines, when effectively implemented, will define the model that ensures the success of nurses as they transition into professional roles, creating a bond between the nurse and the organization in a professional culture to sustain the discipline (AONE, 2010). This chapter will highlight the elements of professional development and the transformation anticipated in how we support nurses in developing a strong, authentic, sustainable presence to lead in a 21st-century healthcare system.

SYSTEMS THINKING AS A FRAMEWORK

Systems thinking, introduced by Senge in *The Fifth Discipline* (1990), identifies that learning organizations understand how things work by appreciating that in a system, activity in one area influences elements of the whole. Systems thinking becomes a lens for seeing wholes and provides a structure to see interrelationships and patterns among objects rather than separate objects or static snapshots of situations.

In organizations, systems consist of people, structures, and processes that work together to make an organization healthy or unhealthy. The illusion of the world created by separate, unrelated forces needs to be eliminated so learning organizations can be built. This allows organizations to move past survival learning into creative, generative learning (Senge, 1990).

Senge identifies five disciplines that must be embraced to become a learning organization (Senge, 1990; Senge, Kleiner, Roberts, Ross, & Smith, 1994):

1. Personal mastery is defined as the discipline of continually clarifying and deepening our personal vision, focusing our energies, developing patience, and seeing reality objectively.
2. Mental models are deeply ingrained assumptions, generalizations, or pictures of images that influence how we understand the world and how we take action.
3. Building shared vision is the practice of creating a shared picture of the future that fosters genuine commitment and engagement rather than compliance.
4. Team learning starts with dialogue and the capacity of the team to suspend assumptions and think together.
5. Systems thinking integrates all the previous disciplines.

As a guide to professional development, systems theory and organizational learning provide a way to view our work through a generative, integrated lens rather than a static experience that has a start and an end.

QUALITIES AND CHARACTERISTICS OF EFFECTIVE LEADERS

It is generally agreed that nurse leaders face uncertainty, turbulence, unprecedented change, and ambiguity in their daily work (AONE, 2011; IOM, 2010). This is instructive as we consider ways to support and develop leaders to succeed in executing their leadership role. Whether leading clinically at the bedside, in the boardroom, or in midlevel management, the literature is rich with studies that examine qualities, attributes, and characteristics of leaders who thrive in their roles despite ambiguity (Thompson, Wolf, & Sabatine, 2012; Westphal, 2012).

Nurse leaders face enormous challenges. In the coming years they will be called upon to manage costs within new reimbursement structures, work in newly designed care delivery systems, and deal with workforce turnover, shortages, and retirements of proficient and knowledgeable clinicians. They will also be faced with rapidly changing technological applications, the need to develop new knowledge for the discipline, and the responsibility to educate and mentor a new generation of nurses. As the care delivery system and models change, nurse leaders will be called upon to supervise an evolving, diverse workforce of new unlicensed personnel who have entered the landscape in response to care coordination, navigation, and the drive toward health promotion and public health (Manix, Wilkes, & Daly, 2013; Westphal, 2012). Although this future is daunting, there are great opportunities for nurse leaders to move into positions of greater responsibility and visibility as they are given new opportunities for personal and professional growth to develop their leadership role (Khoury et al., 2011; Shanta & Connelly, 2013; Thompson et al., 2012; Weinstock, 2011).

Nurse leaders are central to daily operational leadership and strategic visions within organizations. For this reason, many nurses aspire to executive leadership positions. Nurses are often promoted or asked to serve in interim positions based on their clinical accomplishments, education, or credentials. Johnson, Billingsley, Crichlow, and Ferrell (2011) found that 79% of healthcare organizations do not include succession planning in their strategic plan; without a plan, organizations promote nurses irrespective of their interest or potential to fill an executive role (Manix et al., 2013; Taft, 2011; Thompson et al., 2012).

Ongoing, deliberate skills development coupled with support is essential across a nurse's career trajectory. Those who aspire to nurse executive roles need to be intentional in their career development, but they often fail because they lack knowledge, support, and guidance. Leadership competencies, strengths, and opportunities for growth need to be identified through a variety of assessment mechanisms, mentorship, and 360-degree reviews. Underlying formal assessments, self-awareness, and reflection are vital to inform a systematic plan. Failure to support the transition into an executive role can lead to negative outcomes for patient care, the nursing workforce, and the organization. For the nurse leader, ineffective or difficult executive transition leads to disillusionment; for the organization, it results in the loss of a promising leadership candidate (Akerjordet & Severinsson, 2008; Koloroutis, 2008; Manix et al., 2013; Thompson et al., 2012; Westphal, 2012).

With any role change, a range of dynamic shifts that impact our internal and external lives occurs. The opportunity and anticipated challenges can be exciting and fulfilling, while at the same time distressing, because they deconstruct how we have known ourselves in the world (Richez, 2014). As leaders are promoted and move into a new space in the organizational hierarchy, the new job boundaries can create feelings of separation and loneliness. Additionally, if a leader has been promoted from a position with a close peer group, the familiar support systems have been eliminated. New questions arise about where to go with questions, whose input can be trusted, and with whom it is safe to express uncertainty and doubt (Coetzee & Harry, 2014; Weinstock, 2011).

Once, the ability to lead and manage change was viewed as a major skill of successful leaders. However, recent studies highlight that developing higher levels of emotional intelligence, mindfulness, and resilience are qualities of effective and successful leaders (Akerjordet & Severinsson, 2008). Understanding these concepts provides a springboard for nurse leader professional development. Support in many forms, including leadership coaching, mentoring, leadership development, and self-directed learning, can be a tremendous catalyst for new leaders to find integration, realignment, and new solid ground following role transition or promotion (Coetzee & Harry, 2014; Koloroutis, 2008; Weinstock, 2011; Westphal, 2012).

EMOTIONAL INTELLIGENCE

Mayer and Salovey (1997) defined emotional intelligence as "the ability to perceive, appraise and express emotion, access and process emotional information, generate feelings, understand emotional knowledge and regulate emotions for emotional and intellectual growth" (p. 10). As such, emotional intelligence supports us in recognizing our feelings and motivates us toward managing them in ourselves and others (Bulmer-Smith, Profetto-McGrath, & Cummings, 2009; Hay Group, 2014; Taft, 2011). Emotional intelligence frames a sense of clarity, meaning, and purpose within role functions as part of the social context. By developing skills and competence in emotional intelligence, leaders can support and build a sense of connectedness that many people desire (Bamford et al., 2013). Emotional intelligence provides a venue to understand and appreciate the interrelatedness of leadership, organizational culture, and achievement of organizational goals.

The nursing literature shows widespread support for the idea that emotional intelligence is central to nursing practice (Akerjordet & Severinsson, 2008; Bulmer-Smith et al., 2009; Taft, 2011). Emotional intelligence includes capabilities that are distinct from but complementary to intelligence or the purely cognitive capacities measured by intelligence quotient. Emotional competencies are defined as "learned capabilities based on emotional intelligence that contribute to effective performance at work" (Côté, Lopes, Salovey, & Miners, 2010). From extensive research conducted by Goleman and colleagues, emotional competence has been found to matter twice as much as intelligence quotient and technical skill combined in producing superior managerial job performance (Goleman, 1995; Hay Group, 2014).

Emotional intelligence develops in humans as a result of genetics and socialization. Individuals born with average emotional intelligence might become exceptionally emotionally competent in adulthood if their parents tune into their feelings, leadership was practiced in college, and experience with emotionally competent managers occurred in early work experiences. Similarly, it is possible to have experiences that erode emotional intelligence. Individuals born with high natural emotional intelligence could become limited in emotional competencies if they are raised in a home where a parent suffered with addiction, if they were bullied as a young child, or if they had a boss early in their career who was abusive (Taft, 2011).

Emotional competencies can be learned and developed (Akerjordet & Severinsson, 2008; Murphy, 2012; Taft, 2011). Emotional self-awareness, accurate self-assessment, self-confidence, emotional self-control, and empathy are core emotional competencies; therefore, they are the most important. To develop emotional competencies, a person's strengths and weaknesses need to be evaluated, followed by nurturing ideal behaviors to address targeted weaknesses. To grow emotional competencies, an honest appraisal of motivation and willingness to practice and enact new behaviors is required (Bulmer-Smith et al., 2009; Kupperschmidt, Kientz, Ward, & Reinholz, 2010; Taft, 2011). While it is relatively new to health care and nursing, executive coaching offers a platform for this development.

Emotional Intelligence and Nursing Leadership

The nursing profession requires a high degree of emotional labor. Nurses are expected to regulate their own emotions and recognize the expression of emotions for the sake of their patients. Nurses are expected to display caring, understanding, and compassion toward patients while regulating their own feelings (Adams & Iseler, 2014; Bulmer-Smith et al., 2009; Kooker, Shoultz, & Codier, 2007). For new nurses, the emotional burden in the transition from school to work is enormous. The role of the nurse leader is important in establishing a work environment that helps nurses cope with concurrently managing their emotions and the emotion of others.

The concept of emotional intelligence is important when considering skills and competencies needed for effective, responsive, and adaptable leadership during times of change and uncertainty (Bulmer-Smith et al., 2009; Taft, 2011). The ability to connect with followers, communicate a sense of purpose in work, and establish influential relationships with others resides in the ability to create a social context of shared goals and common interests. Leaders with emotional intelligence are prepared to use their social prowess as a tool to promote and support change, which is congruent with behaviors and traits of transformational leaders (Akerjordet & Severinsson, 2008; Bamford et al., 2013; Murphy, 2012).

The need for emotionally intelligent nurse leaders is well represented in research literature that pertains to recruitment and retention, staffing, turnover, nurse satisfaction, healthy work environments, shared leadership and decision making, staff empowerment, nurses leaving the profession, burnout and resilience, and improving trust and communication (Akerjordet & Severinsson, 2008; Bamford et al., 2013; Bulmer-Smith et al., 2009; Kravits et al., 2010). Additionally, the American Nurses Association's (2009) scope and standards for nurse administrators highlights nurse leaders' responsibilities for ensuring patient and nurse satisfaction; considering ethics in actions and decision making; demonstrating trustworthiness and integrity; facilitating difficult conversations; facilitating interpersonal, interdisciplinary, and inter- and intraorganizational communication; teambuilding;

leading performance improvement; creating environments of practice and practice innovation; managing change; empowering others; and motivating others to learn and excel. The standards reflect the values and priorities of the profession, direct the leadership of professional nursing practice, and identify areas in which nurse leaders are accountable (American Nurses Association, 2009; Taft, 2011). The parallels among competence in emotional intelligence, the American Nurses Association's scope and standards, and research that is supportive of this work are noteworthy.

Emotionally intelligent nurse leadership is characterized by self-awareness and supervisory skills that emphasize empowerment and a climate characterized by resilience, innovation, and change (Akerjordet & Severinsson, 2008; Bulmer-Smith et al., 2009; Kooker et al., 2007; Murphy, 2012). The role of nurse leaders is evolving from a top-down orientation to a participatory, team-based interdisciplinary approach and is challenging historic supervisory strategies that guided individual performance. Nurse leaders are faced with developing new ways to optimize working relationships and team effectiveness without the structures of clear hierarchy or authority to guide the work. This means that greater trust will need to be placed in others since direct contact and supervision of work will be unlikely given the fluid nature of teams in matrix organizations or where work crosses multiple care settings (Bamford et al., 2013). Emotionally intelligent, transformational leaders inspire followers to achieve high performance by articulating a vision and tapping the passions and emotion to mobilize the team and guide it toward a desired outcome (Akerjordet & Severinsson, 2008).

Emotional intelligence may provide access to one's own resources and is characterized by self-awareness, self-motivation to carry out tasks, creativity, and the desire to perform well (Akerjordet & Severinsson, 2008; Goleman, 1995; Schneider, Lyons, & Khazon, 2013). In addition, emotional intelligence supports nurse leaders in generating healthy work environments and subjective well-being and quality of life for followers because it incorporates an emotional understanding of the complex situations that are inherent in working with people (Adams & Iseler, 2014; Bamford et al., 2013; Kooker et al., 2007; Murphy, 2014). It appears that emotional intelligence may allow nurse leaders to develop buffers, such as a healthier mood, more adaptive ways of interpreting the world, and better social support (Akerjordet & Severinsson, 2008).

Emotional intelligence is not a panacea, but it offers nurse leaders a framework for thinking and being. It honors the intelligence of feelings, a social context, and a process for evaluating and continuously improving leadership. As emotional intelligence competencies grow, it generates social capital and improves qualities of the individual and the organization. Clinical efficiency, professional readiness, and personal and organizational commitment may be promoted by emotional intelligence as nurse leaders create situations for interdisciplinary teamwork and team-based caring (Adams & Iseler, 2014; Akerjordet & Severinsson, 2008; Montes-Berges & Augusto-Landa, 2007).

BURNOUT AND RESILIENCE

Burnout, stress, low job satisfaction, and disengagement are common occupational pitfalls for those who have difficulty finding meaning in their work. This is experienced by clinicians and leaders alike. Historically, burnout was viewed as a problem for an individual. In organizations where burnout rates are high, turnover, an inability to achieve clinical and organizational goals, and a loss of competitive advantage are commonly experienced. Today there is recognition that organizations have some responsibility in mediating burnout, and leaders are tasked to create healthy work environments (Buchda et al., 2012; Kravits et al., 2010; Larrabee et al., 2010). This means nurse leaders need to recognize factors that contribute to and behaviors that are indicative of workplace stress so interventions directed toward minimizing deleterious effects can be implemented.

Nurses are challenged to develop coping skills to protect them from burnout in the work environment (Anewalt, 2009; Kupperschmidt et al., 2010). Like others in caring professions, nurses experience compassion fatigue and compassion stress that encompasses cognitive, emotional, behavioral, spiritual, interpersonal, and physical aspects of being. Compassion stress, which leads to compassion fatigue, is the compulsive demand for action to relieve the discomfort of others. Symptoms may include diminished concentration, powerlessness, anxiety, sleep disturbances, nightmares, anger, loss of purpose, decreased libido, headache, dizziness, and rapid heartbeat, although many other symptoms have been identified (Lombardo & Eyre, 2011; Rivers, Pesata, Beasley, & Dietrich, 2010).

Burnout has been described as a syndrome of emotional exhaustion, depersonalization, and reduced personal achievement caused by prolonged exposure and engagement in emotionally taxing situations (Kearney, Weininger, Vachon, Harrison, & Mount, 2009; Lombardo & Eyre, 2011). Nurses describe how pressures to perform, technology, workload, and systems issues can create barriers that prevent them from providing humane care. The environment detracts them from caring for others and themselves. This contributes to burnout, dissatisfaction, and compassion fatigue, so it is incumbent on leaders to address these concerns to preserve the spirit and core values of the profession (Larrabee et al., 2010). Resilience has been identified as the capacity for coping successfully and functioning competently despite chronic stress and adversity. The good news is that resilience can be learned, and mindfulness has been identified as one method to build resilience.

Resilience

The development of resilience in individuals and organizations is viewed by many as a potential answer to the stress associated with contemporary lifestyles and workplaces (Lombardo & Eyre, 2011). Presently, definitions of resilience vary but include the following: an innate developmental process; a process or outcome; a deficit or measure of well-being; and a process that emphasizes benefits for individuals and workplaces (Grafton, Gillespie, & Henderson, 2010; Kabat-Zinn, 1994; Rivers et al., 2010). Building a strong and resilient workforce, however, has been explicitly linked to the development of mindfulness (Grafton et al., 2010; Thompson, Arnkoff, & Glass, 2011).

Anewalt (2009) coined the phrase *dual awareness* for a skill to be developed as part of resilience. Dual awareness is the ability to focus on the needs of others while being mindful of our personal reactions and responses to suffering. Caregivers who use self-care without self-awareness are often overwhelmed, and a recommendation to mitigate this is dual awareness. As an observer and participant, the sense of being weighed down by emotion is buoyed and supports coping and resilience (Anewalt, 2009; Kearney et al., 2009).

Grafton and colleagues (2010) say that inquiry into resilience has come in three waves. The first wave focused on resilience as a set of characteristics like hardiness, coping, self-efficacy, optimism, and adaptability. The second wave shifted focus to view resilience as a dynamic process in which adversity meets adaptation through learning and gained experiences. The most recent wave views resilience in terms of innate energy or a motivating life force within an individual that enables him or her to cope with adversity, learn from experience, and engage in cognitive transformations (Grafton et al., 2010). This wave of resilience lends itself to applications of self-care practices and mindfulness meditation. Mindfulness practices are a systematic approach to developing new kinds of control and wisdom in our lives, based on our inner capacities for relaxation, paying attention, awareness, and insight. Therefore, mindfulness is self-care practice that is integral to the development of cyclical resilience (Aikens et al., 2014; Grafton et al., 2010; Keng, Smoski, & Robins, 2011). While nurse leaders are charged to generate resilience in followers, these practices and interventions are also necessary skills for effective nurse leaders.

MINDFULNESS

As demands on healthcare providers escalate, the interest in the applications of mindfulness training grows. External stressors are a part of life that cannot be changed. Despite this, opportunity rests in how we cope with stress and how we respond. In terms of nurse leader development and coaching, mindfulness serves as a foundational practice to enhance awareness to promote transformational learning. In turn, mindfulness enhances presence, promotes engagement, provides insights for innovative solutions to long-standing problems, supports leaders in behaviors that demonstrate authenticity, and serves as a practice that supports the development of emotional intelligence (Bamford et al., 2013; Kupperschmidt et al., 2010; Schutte & Malouff, 2011).

Research suggests that mindfulness can serve as a viable tool for the promotion of self-care and well-being (Aikens et al., 2014; Irving, Dobkin, & Park, 2009; Keng et al., 2011; Schutte & Malouff, 2011). Mindfulness has been described as the miracle by which we can master and restore ourselves. It has been theoretically and empirically associated with psychological well-being and has been promoted for many centuries as a part of Buddhist and other spiritual traditions. The application of mindfulness in Western medicine started in the 1970s and includes practices such as yoga and meditation (Keng et al., 2011).

A commonly cited definition comes from Kabat-Zinn (1994), who describes mindfulness as awareness that arises through "paying attention in a particular way, on purpose, in the present moment, and nonjudgmentally" (p. 4). When we are mindful, we learn to observe the steady stream of internal and external stimuli as they arise, we suspend judgment, and we become aware of our thought patterns.

Mindfulness has been conceptualized as having two components: regulation of attention and adoption of openness toward experiences framed by curiosity and acceptance. Acceptance in this context is not passivity or resignation but rather the ability to experience situations fully without excessive preoccupation or suppression (Keng et al., 2011). Awareness and nonjudgmental acceptance of moment-to-moment experiences are viewed as potentially effective antidotes for distress, such as anxiety, worry, fear, and anger. Trait mindfulness has been associated with higher levels of life satisfaction, agreeableness, conscientiousness, vitality, self-esteem, empathy, sense of autonomy, competence, and optimism (Keng et al., 2011; Schutte & Malouff, 2011). In a 2014 study, Aikens and colleagues demonstrated statistically significant improvements in stress and vigor that were further improved 6 months following mindfulness interventions.

In light of this, and given the complexity of nursing leadership, building mindfulness as a tool offers many benefits in executing the role of nurse executives. Mindful practices cultivate habits of mind through attentive observation, critical curiosity, a beginner's way of thinking, and presence (Irving et al., 2009; Schutte & Malouff, 2011). This work has been incorporated into medical schools as a tool to prevent compassion fatigue and burnout because individuals who are self-aware are more likely to engage in self-care activities and to manage stress effectively (Dobkin & Hutchinson, 2013; Irving et al., 2009; Schutte & Malouff, 2011). Likewise, mindfulness is a tool that supports being fully present with a client, developing keen observation skills, and listening more attentively.

Mind–Body Stress Reduction Programs

Mind–body stress reduction programs have become more popular and are gaining attention in organizations and educational institutions because of their impact on reducing stress, anxiety, and depression (Aikens et al., 2014). The goal of mind–body stress reduction programs is to increase awareness of the present moment by activating a unique, individualized way of coping with stress. Concepts of mindfulness are learned through lectures, self-exploration, and activities such as breathing, yoga, body scanning, and slow walking, which aim to help bring awareness of the present moment to cultivate mindfulness (Aikens et al., 2014; Blue Mesa Group, n.d.; Flugel-Colle et al., 2010).

Mindfulness-based stress reduction, a psychoeducational program developed by Kabat-Zinn and colleagues at the University of Massachusetts Medical Center, has demonstrated positive results on self-reported measures of psychological symptoms experienced by medical students and nurses. Mindfulness-based stress reduction decreased anxiety, depression, and burnout, and it increased empathy, relaxation, life satisfaction, and spirituality. Spanning 8 weeks, the program consists of 2.5 hours of class weekly, a day of silence, and various types of meditation practices applied in class and at home to routine aspects of daily life, such as eating, driving, walking, washing dishes, and interacting with others (Irving et al., 2009). Evidence suggests that mindfulness-based stress reduction improves health, enhances a sense of coherence between experiences, and lowers stress and anxiety, all of which could benefit nurse leaders and their organizations.

LEARNING ORGANIZATIONS AND PROFESSIONAL DEVELOPMENT

The success of healthcare organizations has been tied to an investment in human capital. Recognizing that organizational goals are achieved by the strength of the workforce, employee engagement has become a top organizational priority. Successful organizations are the by-product of leaders sharing a clear and compelling vision coupled with equipping the workforce with resources and tools to achieve results. Leaders who fail to recognize the link between an engaged workforce and organizational outcomes place their organizations at risk (Koloroutis, 2008; Locke, 2008; McCabe & Mackenzie, 2009; Westphal, 2012).

Education and training alone will not produce results organizations need to remain competitive. Unprecedented change is before us, and the very skills that made us successful today will not serve us well in future organizations. Change will come at a speed not previously experienced in health care, and a clear answer about what needs to be done for success will be generated as the new care delivery system is built. In light of this, developmental coaching has been identified as an intervention to bridge learning and practice. Used with individuals, teams, and organizations, coaching achieves demonstrable results, contributes to organizational success, and improves the bottom line (Joo, Sushko, & McLean, 2012; Locke, 2008; Narayanasamy & Penney, 2014; Serio, 2014).

COACHING

As the need for strong, positive, responsive nursing leaders increases, challenges for our current nurse leaders are magnified. With greater visibility, authority, and spans of control, nurse leaders will likely face new trials for which they have not been prepared (Serio, 2014; Weinstock, 2011; Westphal, 2012). Coaching, whether labeled executive coaching, leadership coaching, or developmental coaching, is an intervention for nurse executives and managers and is a tool to leverage strengths, gifts, and talents within an organization. Coaching provides support needed to excel in current roles, access self-awareness, and improve relationships, which ultimately brings greater effectiveness to the individual and the organization (Blue Mesa Group, n.d.; Boyatzis, Smith, & Beveridge, 2012; Joo et al., 2012; Karsten et al., 2010; Kempster & Iszatt-White, 2013; Koloroutis, 2008; Locke, 2008; Serio, 2014).

Nurse leaders make a significant difference in how nurses perceive and perform their jobs. Repeatedly, effective behaviors and practices of nurse leaders have been found to influence work environments, resulting in greater levels of nurse job satisfaction and organizational commitment (Koloroutis, 2008; Murphy, 2012; Narayanasamy & Penney, 2014). Nurse executives in any healthcare setting establish standards, provide resources, buffer staff nurses from the effects of ongoing uncertainties in the healthcare industry, lead with high expectations, and negotiate with other professional groups for control over nursing practice. Additionally, top-level emotionally intelligent nursing leadership is necessary to support the effective selection and development of nurse middle managers. In turn, nurse executives need support from their executive colleagues to create work environments that enable professional practice by nurses (Taft, 2011).

An underlying assumption in many organizations is that talented, high-potential people will be effective and successful in roles of greater responsibility. In fact, the challenges of leadership are so different from those of an individual contributor that, without proper leadership skill training, newly promoted leaders struggle to be effective in these roles (Cox, Bachkirova, & Clutterbuck, 2014; Serio, 2014).

Although organizational processes allow for performance feedback to leaders, feedback typically occurs annually at a performance evaluation and is not an effective means to shape and develop leadership skills in real time. That lack of real-time feedback leaves room for ineffective habits to take hold, ignores developmental opportunities, and allows escalating conflicts to arise. Coaching offers a vehicle to provide meaningful, ongoing, timely feedback to prevent ineffective patterns from derailing a promising leadership career (Koloroutis, 2008; Serio, 2014).

In the literature, coaching is described as one-on-one interactions to identify development opportunities, receive feedback on strengths, explore areas for improvement, and obtain support and guidance to modify individual behaviors that can contribute to the organization by more effective enactment of a leader's role in the organization (Boyatzis et al., 2012; Joo et al., 2012; Karsten et al., 2010; Kempster & Iszatt-White, 2013; McDermott & Levenson, 2007). Effective coaching bridges the hard stuff (organizational strategies, financial expectations, and customer loyalty) and the soft stuff (effective communication, emotional and social intelligence, mindfulness, and personal mastery).

The International Coach Federation's (ICF) definition of coaching is as follows:

> Coaching is partnering with individuals in a thought-provoking and creative process that inspires them to maximize their personal and professional potential. Professional coaches provide an ongoing partnership designed to help clients produce fulfilling results in their personal and professional lives. Coaches help people improve their performance and enhance the quality of their lives. Coaches are trained to listen, to observe and to customize their approach to individual needs. The coach's job is to provide support to enhance the skills, resources, and creativity that the client already has. (International Coach Federation [ICF], Code of Ethics, paragraph 1, 2014 and ICF Michigan, What is Coaching?, 2014.)

Leadership coaching is described in many ways, but it typically involves establishing a relationship between the coach and the individual being coached, an agreed-upon plan, a widening of the leaders' self-awareness, progress tracking and monitoring, and attainment of desired outcomes (Blue Mesa Group, n.d.; Kowalski, 2007; Smith-Glasgow, Weinstock, Lachman, Dunphy-Suplee, & Dreber, 2009; Weinstock, 2011). Through coaching, leaders develop the capacity to do something in the future that they cannot do today.

Common areas of focus for leaders in coaching relationships include time management, delegation, managing others, strategic planning, and aligning values with organizational actions. With coaching, leaders develop greater self-awareness, understand their knowledge gaps, and learn new behaviors that enable them to fulfill their true potential. While the research on coaching in health care has been sparse, there is growing evidence that physicians, nurses, and educators value coaching to learn leadership competencies (Blue Mesa Group, n.d.; Koloroutis, 2008; McNally & Lukens, 2006; Weinstock, 2011).

Coaching and Learning

Foundational to coaching is the belief that we all can learn. When faced with challenges, we make choices about how to react or respond, and when we are successful, we want to repeat the behavior in similar situations. Likewise, if we have made choices that do not lead to success, different choices and options are available, but we may not readily identify them (Blue Mesa Group, n.d.). With any job change or promotion, we experience modifications in our work tasks, a new leadership hierarchy, different productivity expectations, and changes in our relationships with others (Narayanasamy & Penney, 2014; Serio, 2014; Westphal, 2012). Since success as an individual in a clinical role serves as the basis for promotions in health care, many nurses are surprised by the maze of emotions they experience at the time of role transition.

When a deliberate leadership development process using coaching is put in place, leaders have a learning experience that combines leadership theory with the opportunity to practice new skills in a safe setting. This practice enables leaders to develop confidence to employ new skills and behaviors to gain the competencies necessary to function at a higher level (Joo et al., 2012; Kempster & Iszatt-White, 2013; Narayanasamy & Penney, 2014; Serio, 2014).

In any organization it is rare to find a setting where practicing on the job and getting it wrong is acceptable. After formal education and technical training are complete, leaders are expected to show up every day and lead well. Often, this implied expectation puts pressure on leaders without corresponding developmental support. Individuals often describe this as being thrown in the deep end of the pool and being expected to swim. This can result in isolation and loneliness that are self-reinforcing. The quandary plays itself out in a variety of ways, but leaders often report feeling like impostors who have been promoted but lack skills to perform effectively in their new position (Blue Mesa Group, n.d.). Coaching helps us identify options and practice strategies that are aligned to behavior change to address these perceptions and optimize the likelihood of success.

In light of the evolving healthcare delivery system, role changes and transitions are commonplace for nurses. With each shift, change, or promotion an array of emotions are experienced both personally and professionally. They range from accomplishment, fulfillment, and satisfaction to uncertainty and upheaval in how we see ourselves in the world (Richez, 2014; Weinstock, 2011). Leaders who are not properly prepared for new roles frequently reference a general sense of being overwhelmed (Blue Mesa Group, n.d.; Koloroutis, 2008). They are caught in the perceived need to get things done themselves (based on previous role expectations), and they get lost in detail. Many lack the knowledge and confidence to use the very skills that got them the promotion. Rather than taking the appropriate leadership role, they try to complete the work of their subordinates and their own work (Blue Mesa Group, n.d.). In the end, they cannot see the forest for the trees. Coaching helps leaders learn practical new skills for their executive or leader role and moves them from feeling incompetent and isolated to fully confident so they can join other leaders within the organization.

Since coaching is about learning, it addresses developmental leadership gaps that have gone unrecognized or unattended by current feedback mechanisms in organizations (Kempster & Iszatt-White, 2013). At its core, coaching is about creating a space for exploring patterns in thought and action that have prevented optimal performance. With coaching guidance, mindfulness practices create greater awareness and allow realizations to unfold about how situations might be handled differently to result in desired outcomes (Blue Mesa Group, n.d.; Cox et al., 2014; Serio, 2014). As a proactive process, coaching helps leaders define their learning gap and a desired future state. Through thoughtful questions, the coach guides the leader to self-selected actions for accountability. This process helps leaders "get unstuck from their dilemmas and assist(s) them to transfer their learning into results for the organization" (O'Neil, 2000, p. 6).

What Coaches Do

Separating what a coach does from who they are is virtually impossible. Effective coaches walk the talk. Through their own example, they inspire the actions of others and earn their trust and respect. A coach's greatest influence, far greater in proportion to their spoken word, comes from authenticity, the demonstration of personal excellence, and credibility. This paves the way for sustainable progress and continued learning for the individuals they coach (Blue Mesa Group, n.d.).

Coming from a place of service, humility, and clarity, coaches know themselves and are committed to a journey of lifelong learning. At their best, coaches are change agents and role models who practice mindfulness strategies, full listening, and the openness they share with their clients as part of how they show up in the world. They support others in learning and embrace the wisdom each of us has but need support to access (Blue Mesa Group, n.d.). Coaches are masters in applied learning that has both immediate and sustainable results. Central to this is the ability to explore the gap between the current situation and what is desired to establish development goals, cocreate learner commitments and actions for behavior change, and define the next steps and accountability for the person being coached. As such, they are dedicated to creating a safe space to enable growth, learning, the development of confidence, and flexibility to support the resilience and adaptation needed in constantly changing environments (Blue Mesa Group, n.d.; Kempster & Iszatt-White, 2013; Locke, 2008; Serio, 2014).

Coaching competencies fall largely into the domain of interpersonal skills and emotional intelligence. Grounded in a profound curiosity, coaches ask thought-provoking questions, listen fully and actively, and share observations without generating defensiveness (Blue Mesa Group, n.d.; Boyatzis et al., 2012; Joo et al., 2012; Kowalski & Casper, 2007). Although technical competence enhances a coach's credibility with the learner, it is the coach's ability to form respectful, honest, collaborative relationships that builds trust and receptivity that are vital to the learning process.

Coaching mirrors elements of Kolb's model of experiential learning. The model's use of experience to test one's thinking and its use of feedback and reflection are noteworthy (Kolb, 1984). Inquiry is the instrument of learning in this model, and it is used to stimulate the learner's ability to apply lessons from current or previous experiences to a future situation. This methodology leads to deeper learning and development of critical thinking skills. As transformative lessons are integrated into routine practice, the learner's level of performance begins to rise. Fundamentally, this is where the results of coaching are seen.

Three distinctions exhibited by coaches strongly influence learning outcomes. First is the coach's ability to maintain objectivity and concentrate on facts, not assumptions, beliefs, or personal interpretations of the development opportunity. Second is the coach's ability to hear beyond the spoken word and offer observations as a helpful way to support the leader in reframing a situation to see a pattern or situation differently (Blue Mesa Group, 2013, n.d.). Last is the development of a trusting, respectful alliance with the learner so feedback leads to an identified action rather than a directive for change. Preserving the autonomy and self-esteem of the learner boosts learning. Conceivably the greatest attribute of a coach is the ability to use oneself as an instrument of change. As transformative lessons are integrated into routine practice, the learner's level of performance begins to rise

(Blue Mesa Group, n.d.; Kempster & Iszatt-White, 2013; Locke, 2008; Narayana-samy & Penney, 2014).

Distinctions between Performance Management and Coaching

Although coaching has been popular for workforce development in other indus-tries, health care has been slow to adopt it (Narayanasamy & Penney, 2014; Serio, 2014). This can, in part, be explained by the confusion and misuse of the term *coaching* as it relates to managing poor performance. Confusion about what coach-ing is, and what it is not, has contributed to the perception that the process should be avoided (Batson & Yoder, 2011). The benefits of developmental coaching will be realized only when it is consistently and clearly defined in terms of both purpose and process.

Feldman and Lankau (2005) discuss the overlap and differences between executive coaching and other helping relationships like career coaching, therapy, or mentoring. The distinction in the literature between coaching and mentoring or therapy emphasizes that executive coaching focuses on the development of a person in his or her current role. The focus is on future behavior changes to bring greater effectiveness rather than the history or the why behind issues that are explored in therapy or the direction and guidance that is offered by mentors (Blue Mesa Group, n.d.; Karsten et al., 2010).

One widely held myth that has impeded the acceptance of coaching is that the process is offered only to individuals with performance problems (Batson & Yoder, 2011; Locke, 2008). Leadership or developmental coaching is commonly confused with performance management, which is as a function of supervisors in the evalu-ation of job performance. Performance management upholds acceptable levels of performance based on practice standards to ensure competence in performing a job. The appraisal or performance period typically spans a year and often includes identifying opportunities for development. In and of itself, performance manage-ment is not a learning activity but rather a summary of past performance com-pared to job duties. As a point of contrast, leadership or developmental coaching focuses on performance enhancement to move solid performers to exceptional sta-tus through focused guidance. Ultimately, the definitive outcome of developmental coaching is performance excellence and enhancement (Batson & Yoder, 2011; Blue Mesa Group, n.d.; Boyatzis et al., 2012; Joo et al., 2012; Locke, 2008).

It is also important to distinguish coaching from performance counseling. Coaching is future oriented and aimed toward growth. Performance counseling is discipline oriented and intended for remediation of a past behavior, action, or outcome. Counseling can result in the development of an improvement plan that defines clear expectations for behavioral change and what the consequences will be if the undesirable performance continues. In coaching, the developmental plan is proactive and expands current potential. In essence, leadership and developmental coaching promote learning and growth, not compliance (Blue Mesa Group, n.d.; Cox et al., 2014; Locke, 2008).

Who Benefits from Coaching?

Coaching has emerged as a cornerstone of learning organizations in which the development of people is a high priority. Karsten and colleagues (2010) provide evidence that coaching leads to higher engagement among leaders, enhances communication skills, and improves decision-making skills, motivation, retention, and improved outcomes; these factors demonstrate a significant return on investment. Although coaching is commonly used to develop the skills of high-potential, emerging leaders and executives who have a strong intrinsic drive to learn and make an organizational impact, there is growing evidence that all new managers could benefit from developmental coaching. Likewise, the coaching of teams and groups is gaining popularity as organizations embrace shared learning to promote the achievement of organizational goals (Boyatzis et al., 2012; Joo et al., 2012; Narayanasamy & Penney, 2014).

Middle managers can make or break the care delivery process, given their position between executive leaders and those providing care. Faced with pressures and expectations from those in positions both above and below them in the hierarchy, nurse managers face different expectations about what their work should be focused on. They move from highly effective individual performers to novice leaders who are responsible for the performance and development of others, which has a steep learning curve. Given that organizational objectives are achieved through people, frontline managers are in a critical and pivotal position to accomplish organizational goals. The literature suggests that midlevel nursing leaders need support to be more fully engaged and effective in their work (Akerjordet & Severinsson, 2008; Karsten et al., 2010; Serio, 2014). Through coaching, frontline managers are given support to develop self-awareness and self-regulated positive behaviors and to expand their spheres of influence to motivate and develop their staff (Bamford et al., 2013; McNally & Lukens, 2006; Serio, 2014). The investment in coaching is therefore viewed as wise and worthwhile.

Return on Investment in Coaching

Many executives inquire about the return on investment (ROI) of coaching. In the past decade, several studies have highlighted elements of workforce engagement and organizational performance to showcase the impact coaching has had in organizations. The most frequently cited study about coaching was performed by the ICF in 2009. It reported a 700% ROI for companies and 344% return for individual coaches (ix).

Anderson (2014) published an ROI case study for coaching across several industries. In the case study, the experience of MetrixGlobal is highlighted, which in 2001 published the results of coaching in a Fortune 500 company with participants from the United States and Mexico. The results were positive, with 77% of the 30 respondents indicating that coaching had a significant or a very significant impact on at least one of nine business measures. Other results, besides ROI, were increases in employee satisfaction and productivity. A 529% ROI was produced by the coaching process, excluding benefits from employee retention. These outcomes demonstrate why, despite minimal empirical evidence, executive coaching has become widely utilized in recent years. In the healthcare sector, McNally and Lukens (2006) demonstrated positive coaching outcomes with nurse leaders who reported increased competence and confidence in their leadership abilities resulting in an ROI related to turnover.

In 2013, ICF and PricewaterhouseCoopers conducted an international study of leadership coaching across industries to provide businesses, coaches, stakeholders, and the general public with information and insights about the status, value, effectiveness, and impact of professional coaching within organizations. The key messages highlight variability in how and where coaches are used, whether coaches are internal or external to the organization, and whether coaches' reputations are significant when leaders make decisions about engaging a coach. Most organizations reported positive impacts in employee engagement, reduced turnover, improved teamwork, and leadership development. Although some organizations utilize 360-degree reviews and employee surveys to measure coaching effectiveness, formally assessing and quantifying ROI remain a challenge (Pricewaterhouse-Coopers, 2013). Participants across various industries view coaching as positive and valuable. The development of an acceptable quantification and evaluation method to measure ROI is needed.

In 2012, the *Measuring the Success of Coaching* study offered a detailed, step-by-step description of how to accurately assess the ROI of coaching (Phillips, Phillips, & Edwards). The steps include evaluation planning and data collection, isolation of coaching effects, data conversion, and reporting results. In addition to the process used to establish the ROI, six case studies are provided. One case study looks at a manufacturer of high-quality plastics and the effect coaching had on employee work engagement. Overall, the company reported a 300% ROI. Employee engagement was measured at 45-day intervals for 6 months following the coaching intervention in both the control and intervention groups. At every measurement point, the group that received coaching had higher engagement scores (Phillips et al., 2012).

Anecdotal reporting of coaching ROI is common. Many organizations and leaders are passionate and emphatic when offering qualitative analyses regarding the benefit of coaching. As a demonstration of this, Banner Health received the ICF Prism Award based on their success and commitment to coaching within their organization. Banner Health explained: "For us, leadership is a direct connection to patient care and excellent clinical results. Equipping Banner leaders with coaching competency is one important way we do so. Banner's community of internal coaches grows in a very intentional pay-it-forward way. As we train internal coaches, they engage in coaching and the community grows" (Banner Health, 2012, para. 5).

What is clear in examining ROI in coaching is that an acceptable, quantifiable, and consistent methodology is needed. While improvements in leadership, organizational culture, and performance indicators are offered, the methods by which these results are derived are fluid. Future evaluative research methodology is warranted as coaching becomes more widely utilized by organizations and nurse leaders.

SUMMARY

Each of us has observed leaders and made determinations about their proficiency. Leadership is enacted through individual choices, behaviors, and actions. This chapter was devoted to gaining awareness of leadership development with an eye to the future, recognizing that traditional professional development programs will not be sufficient in this era of healthcare reform. Central to success is the ability to learn, modulate our emotions, and be resilient, which are cornerstones developed through coaching. Evidence has been presented to demonstrate that emotionally competent organizational leadership raises the level of performance for everyone, places nurses as equal partners in the executive suite, and improves staff engagement and work environments to achieve desired organizational outcomes.

REFLECTIVE QUESTIONS

1. What are the elements of an executive coaching relationship and their impact on employee performance, including team collaboration?
2. Describe the distinctions between coaching for performance management and executive coaching for transformative leadership practice.
3. How would you integrate professional responsibility and power, authenticity, integrity, and emotional intelligence into leadership practice?
4. Analyze organizational challenges that promote and inhibit authentic nursing leadership.

CASE STUDY 4-1   Chief Nursing Officer Development: Transformational Coaching

Micki McMillan, Patricia A. Barlow, Gay Landstrom, and Patricia L. Thomas

In response to a 30% chief nursing officer (CNO) turnover in 2 years, the senior vice president of Patient Care Services and Chief Nursing Officers in a national health system engaged Blue Mesa Group (BMG) to create a CNO development program. The program consisted of three phases: (1) assessment of each CNO's current situation, (2) classroom training, and (3) leadership coaching.

Assessment Phase

This phase established a solid base for classroom training and follow-up leadership coaching. The biggest portion of the assessment was to gather key stakeholder feedback from the chief executive officers, chief financial officers, chief operating officers, and chief human resources officers who were supervisors and peers of the CNOs. Other stakeholder feedback included a sample of direct reports to each CNO. This feedback was assembled and presented privately to each CNO during the classroom training phase. It included real examples that helped the CNO understand his or her strengths and shortcomings. It highlighted how many CNOs function at a detailed, operational level rather than a strategic, leading level in their organizations. Because the feedback was specific to the individual CNO, it made the CNOs aware of the importance of working at the right level. Each CNO grasped how working at the wrong level was a recipe for failure. Many left inspired and confident to step into a new leadership approach.

Classroom Training

The classroom training was designed after BMG understood the challenges presented in the assessment phase. BMG designed a program that included leadership skill building and social and emotional intelligence. The culmination of the training was a C-suite simulation that represented real cases that were common to most CNOs. This simulation allowed the CNOs to practice the newly developed skills in real time. It also enabled them to perceive the implications of leading at the wrong level.

(continues)

CASE STUDY 4-1   Chief Nursing Officer Development: Transformational Coaching (Continued)

The final activity in the classroom training was to develop an individualized coaching and learning plan that would be the foundation for leadership coaching. These plans were reviewed and approved by the senior vice president and CNO as part of the program closing exercise. The CNOs committed to sharing these plans with their chief executive officers when they returned to their hospitals.

Leadership Coaching

Each CNO had a leadership coach who supported him or her in executing the coaching and learning plan. This coaching was intended to inspire the leaders to continuously practice their newly developed skills and implement them in daily practice. Most CNOs had up to 8 hours of coaching over a 2-month period.

Six months after the program concluded, a follow-up survey was conducted with the same stakeholders who provided preprogram input. **Table 4-1** shows the percentages of responses that were rated good, significant, or excellent.

After the program, the stakeholders provided the following feedback:

- "D is becoming more comfortable in her role"
- "More visibility; more association with CMO and President"
- "Doesn't jump into an 'ugly story' so quickly"
- "Nice focus on communication"
- "Proactive managing up"
- "Performance management and focus of her management team on results"
- "Noticed that she has been very reflective and open to renewed ideas and approach"
- "Doing a nice job in developing team and delegating tasks/responsibilities"
- "I see her more comfortable in her leadership role than a year ago"
- "Much more willing to speak up; highly accountable in her words and actions"
- "P. is making herself a more integrated member of the team"
- "She has worked to listen and seek to understand and be more accepting and respectful of her peers. She is working better with all members of the senior leadership team"
- "She is more inclusive and able to discuss openly without fears—I would say she has made a good improvement overall"

In the 3 years after implementation of the BMG program, there was less than 5% turnover in the health system's CNOs.

As healthcare systems grapple with significant change, retention of talented nursing leaders will be essential to the stability and success of organizations. Executive coaching offers a venue to support nurse leaders as they develop to their full potential, benefitting the individual CNO, those they lead, and the C-suite.

Case Study Questions

1. Consider your organization and the leaders who are at risk for turnover. What category of nurse leaders is at risk for turnover? Why?
2. What elements of executive and developmental coaching might mitigate the turnover?
3. How would you make the business cases to engage executive coaches? What research or evidence might be drawn upon to make the case?

TABLE 4-1　Percentage of Responses That Were Rated Good, Significant, or Excellent

Stakeholder feedback	Good to excellent improvement
1. More strategic thinking and planning	87.1%
2. Improved listening skills	83.6%
3. Clear communications	79.0%
4. More collaboration with others	78.7%
5. Stronger voice at the leadership table	77.6%
6. Less silo behavior	75.8%
7. Increased delegation to direct reports	69.3%

CASE STUDY 4-2　Group Executive Coaching for Directors of Nursing and Service Line Administrators

Micki McMillan, Patricia A. Barlow, Patricia L. Thomas, Lesa Becker, and Abigail Veliquette

During the year of consolidation of two large national healthcare systems, an executive coaching program for directors of nursing and service line administrators was developed. The impetus for this program came from a request of CNOs who recognized that these nurse leaders had limited opportunity for professional development to guide them through the magnitude of change they were experiencing. Additionally, most experienced a larger span of control and increased performance pressures from internal and external stakeholders. Many of the CNOs had received executive coaching and believed it would benefit the nurse leaders and organizations.

Research has demonstrated the pivotal role that frontline, midlevel leaders have in organization performance, particularly in clinical indicators, safety metrics, staff retention, turnover, and satisfaction. Organizations across the country have identified that traditional leadership development programs are only marginally successful, and the sustainability of initial improvements is rare.

Building on the success with the healthcare system CNOs, BMG was invited back to deliver their Envision Excellence in Nursing Leadership Program to 31 nurse leaders who reported to the CNOs. The participants included nursing directors and service line administrators from multiple functional areas in hospitals from various geographic locations. The program included a one-on-one review of individual assessments, a 2-day onsite workshop, and 8 hours of telephonic executive group coaching in the 3 months following the onsite education.

The goals of the Envision Excellence program were for participants to understand attributes of effective leadership, including leading at the right level; to explore self-assessment and peer feedback for insights about their leadership strengths; to examine cultural competence and the neuroscience of behavior change; and to identify future development opportunities and construct an individual leadership development action plan.

The group underwent several leadership assessments to assist participants in identifying strengths and opportunities for development to inform their individual learning action plans. Each participant received 360-degree feedback from five key stakeholders and also took the California Psychological Inventory (CPI 260). The CPI 260 measures 18 leadership competencies in the areas of self-management,

(continues)

CASE STUDY 4-2   Group Executive Coaching for Directors of Nursing and Service Line Administrators (Continued)

organizational capabilities, team building and teamwork, problem solving, and sustaining a vision. According to an Aberdeen Group research brief (2013), assessments can help organizations and individuals understand capability gaps.

Based on the themes from the 360-degree feedback, the categories most frequently noted by peers and supervisors for development were leadership and communication. Additionally, collaboration and delegation were two of the most frequently noted individual areas for improvement in stakeholder feedback. Findings from the CPI 260 preassessment identified the collective strengths of these leaders as responsibility and accountability, comfort with organizational structures, interpersonal skills, and resilience. The leadership characteristic that showed the group's greatest developmental opportunity was managing change. Based on these themes, BMG tailored the didactic content to address these areas.

The didactic portion of the program included content delivered by master coaches on skillful communication, listening, advocacy and inquiry, social and emotional intelligence and management, reflection, trust building, mental models and ladder of inference, management commitments, and managing time. Each participant also met individually with an executive coach twice during the 2-day workshop for input about their assessments and what they were learning so their individualized learning and action plan could be completed before leaving the onsite training.

The didactic portion of the program was followed by 8 hours of group coaching spread over 3 months. Participants were placed into groups of five. They had various levels of leadership experience and were from diverse geographic locations. The goal of the group coaching process was to reinforce the content provided in the 2-day onsite sessions, to provide one-on-one coaching, and to build a community of practice among nursing leaders.

Themes from the evaluation and feedback of the group coaching program identified that participants found the experience to be valuable. They indicated that the most valuable parts of the program were as follows:

- The ability to network and collaborate with their peers from across the national healthcare system
- Value in learning from more experienced leaders in similar roles
- The simulation exercise that required them to role-play C-suite roles to understand the responsibilities and expectations of those in the C-suite
- Content on intentional listening, being comfortable with silence, being rigorous with time management, and understanding advocacy versus inquiry

After participating in the Envision Excellence program, there was an 11% increase in the number of leadership characteristics tested as a strength on the postimplementation CPI 260, which was taken 2 months after completion of the program. In addition, there was a 20% reduction in the number of leadership characteristics tested as a developmental opportunity. The top five group strengths following the Envision Excellence program were responsibility and accountability, interpersonal skills, self-confidence, influence, and (tied) working through and with others and resilience.

Case Study Questions

1. What are the advantages of group or team coaching? Are there any disadvantages?
2. Consider the tools used in your organization to assess leadership competencies. If you were asked by a colleague why coaching needs to be added to the leadership development strategy, what would your answer be? What gap does coaching fill?
3. As you consider nurse leaders you know and admire, which of their qualities or characteristics inspire you?

REFERENCES

Aberdeen Group. (2013). Take charge of your organization's future with talent lifecycle assessments. Retrieved from http://aberdeen.com/Aberdeen-Library /8697/RB-talent-lifecycle-assessments.aspx

Adams, K., & Iseler, J. (2014). The relationship of bedside nurses' emotional intelligence with quality of care. *Journal of Nursing Care Quality*, *29*(2), 174–181.

Aikens, K., Astin, J., Pelletier, K., Levanovich, K., Baase, C., Park, Y., & Bodnar, C. (2014). Mindfulness goes to work: Impact of an online workplace intervention. *Journal of Occupational and Environmental Medicine*, *56*(7), 721–731.

Akerjordet, K., & Severinsson, E. (2008). Emotionally intelligent nurse leadership: A literature review study. *Journal of Nursing Management*, *16*, 565–577.

American Nurses Association. (2009). *Nursing administration: Scope and standards of practice*. Silver Spring, MD.

American Organization of Nurse Executives. (2010). *AONE guiding principles for the newly licensed nurse's transition into practice*. Retrieved from http://www .aone.org/resources/PDFs/AONE_GP_Newly_Licensed_Nurses.pdf

American Organization of Nurse Executives. (2011). Nurse executive competencies. Retrieved from http://www.aone.org/resources/leadership%20tools /nursecomp.shtml

Anderson, M. (2014). Leadership coaching return on investment (ROI). Retrieved from http://www.findyourcoach.com/roi-study.htm

Anewalt, P. (2009). Fired up or burned out? Understanding the importance of professional boundaries in home health care hospice. *Home Healthcare Nurse*, *27*(10), 591–597.

Bamford, M., Wong, C., & Laschinger, H. (2013). The influence of authentic leadership and areas of worklife on work engagement of registered nurses. *Journal of Nursing Management*, *21*, 529–540.

Banner Health. (2012). Banner Health earns award for coaching excellence. Retrieved from http://www.bannerhealth.com/About+Us/News+Center /Press+Releases/Press+Archive/2012/Banner+Health+earns+award+for +coaching+excellence.htm

Batson, V., & Yoder, L. (2011). Managerial coaching: Concept analysis. *Journal of Advanced Nursing*, *68*(7), 1658–1669.

Benner, P., Sutphen, M., Leonard, V., & Day, L. (2010). *Educating nurses: A call for radical change*. San Francisco, CA: Jossey-Bass.

Blue Mesa Group. (n.d.). Transformational Coaching Program. Unpublished course guide for TCP Leadership for coaching program.

Boyatzis, R., Smith, M., & Beveridge, A. (2012). Coaching with compassion: Inspiring health, well-being, and development in organizations. *Journal of Applied Behavioral Science*, *49*(2), 153–178.

Bulmer-Smith, K., Profetto-McGrath, J., & Cummings, G. (2009). Emotional intelligence and nursing: An integrative literature review. *International Journal of Nursing Studies*, *46*(12), 1624–1636.

Coetzee, M., & Harry, N. (2014). Emotional intelligence as a predictor of employees' career adaptability. *Journal of Vocational Behavior*, *84*, 90–97.

Côté, S., Lopes, P., Salovey, P., & Miners, C. (2010). Emotional intelligence and leadership emergence in small groups. *The Leadership Quarterly*, *21*, 496–508.

Cox, E., Bachkirova, T., & Clutterbuck, D. (2014). Traditions and coaching genres: Mapping the territory. *Advances in Developing Human Resources, 16*(2), 139–160.

Dobkin, P., & Hutchinson, T. (2013). Teaching mindfulness in medical school: Where are we now and where are we going? *Medical Education, 47*(8), 768–779.

Feldman, D., & Lankau, M. (2005). Executive coaching: A review and agenda for future research. *Journal of Management, 31*, 829–848.

Flugel-Colle, K., Vincent, A., Cha, S., Loehrer, L., Bauer, B., & Wahner-Roedler, D. (2010). Measurement of quality of life and participant experience with the mindfulness-based stress reduction program. *Complementary Therapies in Clinical Practice, 16*(2010), 36–40.

Goleman, D. (1995). *Emotional intelligence: Why it can matter more than IQ.* New York, NY: Bantam.

Grafton, E., Gillespie, B., & Henderson, S. (2010). Resilience: The power within. *Oncology Nursing Forum, 37*(6), 698–705.

Hay Group. (2014). Emotional intelligence training. Retrieved from http://www .haygroup.com/leadershipandtalentondemand/your-challenges/emotional -intelligence/index.aspx

Institute of Medicine. (2010). *The future of nursing: Leading change, advancing health.* Retrieved from http://www.iom.edu/Reports/2010/The-Future-of-Nursing -Leading-Change-Advancing-Health.aspx

International Coach Federation Michigan Charter Chapter. (2014). What is Coaching? Retrieved from http://icfmichigan.org/about-icf-michigan/what -is-coaching/

International Coach Federation. (n.d.). Code of Ethics: Part 1 Definition of Coaching. Retrieved from http://coachfederation.org/Ethics/

Irving, J., Dobkin, P., & Park, J. (2009). Cultivating mindfulness in health care professionals: A review of empirical studies of mindfulness-based stress reduction (MBSR). *Complementary Therapies in Clinical Practice, 15*, 61–66.

Johnson, J., Billingsley, M., Crichlow, T., & Ferrell, E. (2011). Professional development for nurses: Mentoring along the U-shaped curve. *Nursing Administration Quarterly, 35*(2), 119–125.

Joo, B., Sushko, J., & McLean, G. (2012). Multiple faces of coaching: Manager-as-coach, executive coaching, and formal mentoring. *Organization Development Journal, 31*(1), 19–37.

Kabat-Zinn, J. (1994). *Wherever you go there you are: Mindfulness meditation in everyday life.* New York, NY: Hyperion.

Karsten, M., Baggot, D., Brown, A., & Cahill, M. (2010). Professional coaching as an effective strategy to retaining frontline managers. *Journal of Nursing Administration, 40*(3), 140–144.

Kearney, M., Weininger, R., Vachon, M., Harrison, R., & Mount, B. (2009). Self-care of physicians caring for patients at the end of life. *Journal of the American Medical Association, 301*(11), 1155–1165.

Kempster, S., & Iszatt-White, M. (2013). Towards co-constructed coaching: Exploring the integration of coaching and co-constructed autoethnography in leadership development. *Management Learning, 44*, 319–336.

Keng, S., Smoski, M., & Robins, C. (2011). Effects of mindfulness on psychological health: A review of empirical studies. *Clinical Psychology Review, 31*, 1041–1056.

Khoury, C., Blizzard, R., Wright-Moore, L. & Hassmiller, S. (2011). Nursing leadership from bedside to boardroom: A Gallup national survey of opinion leaders. *Journal of Nursing Administration, 41*(7/8), 299–306.

Kolb, D. A. (1984). *Experiential learning: Experience as the source of learning and development*. Englewood Cliffs, NJ: Prentice Hall.

Koloroutis, M. (2008). Telephone coaching for clinical nurse managers. *Creative Nursing, (14)*3, 122–127.

Kooker, B., Shoultz, J., & Codier, E. (2007). Identifying emotional intelligence in professional nursing practice. *Journal of Professional Nursing, 23*(1), 30–36.

Kowalski, K., & Casper, C. (2007). The coaching process: An effective tool for professional development. *Nursing Administration Quarterly, 31*(2), 171–179.

Kravits, K., McAllister-Black, R., Grant, M., & Kirk, C. (2010). Self-care strategies for nurses: A psycho-educational intervention for stress reduction and the prevention of burnout. *Applied Nursing Research, 23*, 130–138.

Kupperschmidt, B., Kientz, E., Ward, J., & Reinholz, B. (2010). A healthy work environment: It begins with you. *Online Journal of Issues in Nursing, 15*(1), Manuscript 3.

Larrabee, J. H., Wu, Y., Persily, C. A., Simoni, P. S., Johnston, P. A., & Marcischak, T. L. (2010). Influence of stress resiliency on RN job satisfaction and intent to stay. *Western Journal of Nursing Research, 32*, 81–102.

Locke, A. (2008). Developmental coaching: Bridge to organizational success. *Creative Nursing, 14*(3), 102–109.

Lombardo, B., & Eyre, C. (2011). Compassion fatigue: A nurse's primer. *Online Journal of Issues in Nursing, 16*(1). Retrieved from http://www.nursingworld.org/MainMenuCategories/ANAMarketplace/ANAPeriodicals/OJIN/TableofContents/Vol-16-2011/No1-Jan-2011/Compassion-Fatigue-A-Nurses-Primer.html

Mayer, J., & Salovey, P. (1997). What is emotional intelligence? In P. Salovey & D. Sluyter (Eds.), *Emotional development and emotional intelligence: Educational implications* (pp. 1–31). New York, NY: Basic Books.

Manix, J., Wilkes, L., & Daly, J. (2013). Attributes of clinical leadership in contemporary nursing: An integrative review. *Contemporary Nurse Leaders: A Journal for the Australian Nursing Profession, 45*(1), 10–21.

McCabe, K., & Mackenzie, E. (2009). The role of mindfulness in healthcare reform: A policy paper. *Explore, 5*(6), 313–323.

McDermott, M., & Levenson, A. (2007). What coaching can and cannot do for your organization. *Human Resource Planning, 30*(2), 30–37.

McNally, K., & Lukens, R. (2006). Leadership development: An external-internal coaching partnership. *Journal of Nursing Administration, 36*(3), 155–161.

Montes-Berges, B., & Augusto-Landa, J. (2007). Emotional intelligence and affective intensity as life satisfaction and psychological well-being predictors of nursing professionals. *Journal of Professional Nursing, 23*(1), 30–36.

Murphy, L. (2012). Authentic leadership: Becoming and remaining an authentic nurse leader. *Journal of Nursing Administration, 42*(11), 507–512.

Narayanasamy, A., & Penney, V. (2014). Coaching to promote professional development in nursing practice. *British Journal of Nursing, 23*(11), 568–573.

O'Neil, B. (2000). *Executive coaching with backbone and heart: A systems approach to engaging leaders with their challenges*. San Francisco, CA: Jossey-Bass.

Phillips, P., Phillips, J., & Edwards, L. (2012). *Measuring the success of coaching: A step by step guide for measuring impact and ROI.* Danvers, MA: ASTD Press.

Pipe, T., Buchda, V., Launder, S., Hudak, B., Hulvey, L., Karns, K., & Pendergast, D. (2012). Building personal and professional resources of resilience and agility in the healthcare workplace. *Stress and Health, 28,* 11–22.

PricewaterhouseCoopers. (2013). *Executive summary: 2013 ICF organizational coaching study.* Retrieved from http://icf.files.cms-plus.com/FileDownloads/2013OrgCoachingStudy.pdf

Richez, M. (2014). Resilience-building strategies for nurses in transition. *Journal of Continuing Education in Nursing, 45*(2), 54–55.

Rivers, R., Pesata, V., Beasley, M., & Dietrich, M. (2010). Transformational leadership: Creating a prosperity-planning coaching model for RN retention. *Nurse Leader, 9*(5), 48–51.

Schneider, R., Lyons, J., & Khazon, S. (2013). Emotional intelligence and resilience. *Personality and Individual Differences, 55,* 909–914.

Schutte, N., & Malouff, J. (2011). Emotional intelligence mediates the relationship between mindfulness and subjective well-being. *Personality and Individual Differences, 50,* 1116–1119.

Senge, P. (1990). *The fifth discipline: The art and practice of the learning organization.* New York, NY: Currency-Doubleday.

Senge, P., Kleiner, A., Roberts, C., Ross, R., & Smith, B. (1994). *The fifth discipline fieldbook: Strategies and tools for building a learning organization.* New York, NY: Currency Doubleday.

Serio, I. (2014). Using coaching to create empowered nursing leadership to change lives. *Journal of Continuing Education in Nursing, 45*(1), 12–13.

Shanta, L., & Connolly, M., (2013). Using King's interacting systems theory to link emotional intelligence and nursing practice. *Journal of Professional Nursing, 29*(3), 174–180.

Smith-Glasgow, M., Weinstock, B., Lachman, V., Dunphy-Suplee, P., & Dreher, H. (2009). The benefits of leadership program and executive coaching for new nurse academic administrators: One college's experience. *Journal of Professional Nursing, 25*(4), 204–210.

Taft, S. (2011). Emotionally intelligent leadership in nursing and healthcare organizations. In L. Roussel (Ed.), *Management and leadership for nurse administrators* (6th ed., pp. 59–85). Burlington, MA: Jones & Bartlett Learning.

Thompson, R., Arnkoff, D., & Glass, C. (2011). Conceptualizing mindfulness and acceptance as components of psychological resilience to trauma. *Trauma, Violence, Abuse, 12*(4), 220–335.

Thompson, R., Wolf, D., & Sabatine, J. (2012). Mentoring and coaching: A model guiding professional nurses to executive success. *Journal of Nursing Administration, 42*(11), 536–541.

Weinstock, B. (2011). The hidden challenges in role transitions and how leadership coaching can help new leaders find solid ground. *Holistic Nursing Practice, 25*(4), 211–214.

Westphal, J. (2012). Characteristics of nurse leaders in hospitals in the USA from 1992 to 2008. *Journal of Nursing Management, 20,* 928–937.

CHAPTER 5

Transformational Leadership in an Era of Healthcare Reform

Lisa Mestas, Rita Stockman, Patricia L. Thomas, and Linda Roussel

LEARNING OBJECTIVES

1. Describe attributes of transformational leadership that promote contemporary care models.
2. Envision how nurse leaders position the discipline for success.
3. Acknowledge contributions of all team members in achieving organizational imperatives.

AONE KEY COMPETENCIES

I. Communication and relationship building
II. Knowledge of the healthcare environment
III. Leadership
IV. Professionalism
V. Business skills

AONE KEY COMPETENCIES DISCUSSED IN THIS CHAPTER

I. Communication and relationship building
II. Knowledge of the healthcare environment
III. Leadership
IV. Professionalism

I. **Communication and relationship building**
   - Effective communication
   - Relationship management
   - Influence of behaviors
   - Ability to work with diversity
   - Shared decision making
   - Community involvement
   - Medical staff relationships
   - Academic relationships

II. **Knowledge of the healthcare environment**
  - Clinical practice knowledge
  - Patient care delivery models and work design knowledge
  - Healthcare economics knowledge
  - Healthcare policy knowledge
  - Understanding of governance
  - Understanding of evidence-based practice
  - Outcomes measurement
  - Knowledge of, and dedication to, patient safety
  - Understanding of utilization and case management
  - Knowledge of quality improvement and metrics
  - Knowledge of risk management

III. **Leadership**
  - Foundational thinking skills
  - Personal journey disciplines
  - Ability to use systems thinking
  - Succession planning
  - Change management

IV. **Professionalism**
  - Personal and professional accountability
  - Career planning
  - Ethics
  - Evidence-based clinical and management practices
  - Advocacy for the clinical enterprise and for nursing practice
  - Active membership in professional organizations

FUTURE OF NURSING: FOUR KEY MESSAGES

1. Nurses should practice to the full extent of their education and training.
2. Nurses should achieve higher levels of education and training through an improved education system that promotes seamless academic progression.
3. Nurses should be full partners with physicians and other health professionals in redesigning health care in the United States.
4. Effective workforce planning and policy making require better data collection and information infrastructure.

Introduction

Nurse administrators utilize many leadership styles, such as situational, motivational, transformational, and servant leadership, to drive change and sustain success. Today's healthcare environment requires transformational leaders to inspire necessary culture shifts within healthcare systems as they move forward. In 2010, the Affordable Care Act (ACA) was passed by Congress with the intent of creating a more affordable, accessible healthcare system while improving patient safety and quality (American Nurses Association [ANA], 2014; Centers for Medicare and Medicaid Services, 2010). Escalating costs to provide care, the aging of the baby boomer generation, and an economic downturn culminated in a crisis in 2008. Healthcare costs in the United States represented 18% of the gross domestic product in 2009. The situation was deemed unsustainable, and observers noted that if the trend was not curtailed, it would debilitate an already struggling American economy (Executive Office of the President Council of Economic Advisers, 2009). In spite of the United States spending the most dollars on health care worldwide, a 2009 World Health Organization report ranked the country's healthcare system 37th in quality and cost (Murray, Phil, & Frenk, 2010). The U.S. healthcare system was the most expensive and performed poorly compared to other industrialized nations in measures of quality, efficiency, and effectiveness (Commonwealth Fund, 2014).

The technological revolution has resulted in a society that is highly informed and expects superior results, exceptional customer service, and instant gratification. Patients no longer allow physicians to make healthcare decisions independently; they expect to partner with the healthcare team. Quality scores are posted publically and are tied to reimbursement. Savvy customers are willing to travel outside their hometowns and around the globe for world-class care (Plonien & Baldwin, 2014).

Other forces affecting the current state of health care in the United States are an aging population and epidemic levels of obesity compounded with poor-quality food sources, limited accessibility, and compartmentalized care delivery models that lead to failures. Since January 2011, 10 thousand baby boomers have become eligible for Social Security each day (Kessler, 2014). Medicaid and Medicare face increasing financial struggles as costs and demands continue to grow. According to Nix (2012), Medicaid is consuming larger portions of state budgets, and Medicare's long-term unfunded obligations are estimated as high as $36.9 trillion. Since 2008, Medicare has been running deficits in the Hospital Insurance Trust Fund. It is anticipated that with the flood of new baby boomer enrollees, Medicare costs will continue to soar. Technological advances have increased the life span of adults, adding significant costs to the healthcare system. In 1958, the average American worker spent about $1,080 per year on health care compared to about $8,950 today (Health Management Academy, 2013).

In spite of the ACA being signed into law, many uninsured people have found healthcare premiums to be unaffordable. Medicaid enrollment has increased, but those who access the exchanges find that high-deductible plans that reduce monthly premiums are still out of reach, and the imposed penalties are less than the cost of insurance. Some uninsured people have decided to pay for health care out of pocket because the expense is less than paying either a premium or the penalty (Gorman & Appleby, 2014). Uninsured individuals who do not qualify for Medicaid and who cannot pay for insurance are often turned away by providers, which results in undiagnosed and untreated pathologies and increased hospitalizations (Johnson & Johnson, 2010). A radical and innovative approach to the design of new care delivery models will be essential if we are to meet the varied and complex health needs of the country. Unraveling the current disease-focused approach to care and the payment systems for these services will require an unwavering commitment to health promotion, establishing competencies and role functions of all engaged in care delivery, and an inspiring vision to bring care providers together to achieve the desired outcomes. This shift will demand the best of interdisciplinary teams that are led by those who recognize each of us will need to learn new ways to interact with patients as consumers. An evidence-based model called Team Strategies and Tools to Enhance Performance and Patient Safety (TeamSTEPPS) is one strategy to improve team communication and effectiveness.

TEAMSTEPPS

A recent emphasis has been placed on the impact of teams in providing care, recognizing that each team member provides a unique perspective that collectively maximizes interprofessional collaboration. The Agency for Healthcare Research and Quality created the TeamSTEPPS curriculum (2008) in collaboration with the U.S. Department of Defense Patient Safety Program. The curriculum defines teamwork as a "set of interrelated knowledge, skills, and abilities (KSAs) that facilities co-coordinated, adaptive performance, supporting one's teammates, objectives and missions" (Agency for Healthcare Research and Quality [AHRQ], 2008, p. 1).

The TeamSTEPPS core program is based on 20 years of research and experience from the application of team science and principles in team building. The aim of TeamSTEPPS is to improve patient safety through the coordination and collaboration of interdisciplinary members. It is an evidence-based system to facilitate communication and teamwork skills among healthcare professionals. TeamSTEPPS provides useful tools and a training curriculum that is readily available through online resources. The program emphasizes role clarity, responsibilities of team members, language to be used for handoffs, dealing with conflict to improve information sharing, and reducing barriers to quality and safety.

TeamSTEPPS has a three-phase process aimed at creating and sustaining a culture of safety with a pretraining assessment for site readiness, training for onsite trainers and healthcare staff, and implementation and sustainment. The AHRQ describes the three phases as follows:

> The three phases of TeamSTEPPS are based on lessons learned, existing master trainer or change agent experience, the literature of quality and patient safety, and culture change. A successful TeamSTEPPS initiative necessitates a thorough assessment of the organization and its processes and a carefully developed implementation and sustainment plan.

> **Phase 1: Assess the Need**
> The goal of Phase 1 is to determine an organization's readiness for undertaking a TeamSTEPPS-based initiative. Such practice is typically referred to as a training needs analysis, which is a necessary first step to implementing a teamwork initiative.

> **Phase 2: Planning, Training, and Implementation**
> Phase 2 is the planning and execution segment of the TeamSTEPPS initiative. Because TeamSTEPPS was designed to be tailored to the organization, options in this phase include implementation of all tools and strategies in the entire organization, a phased-in approach that targets specific units or departments or a selection of individual tools that are introduced at specific intervals (called a *dosing strategy*). As long as the primary learning objectives are maintained, the TeamSTEPPS materials are adaptable.

Phase 3: Sustainment
The goal of Phase 3 is to sustain and spread improvements in teamwork performance, clinical processes, and outcomes resulting from the TeamSTEPPS initiative. The key objective is to ensure that opportunities exist to implement the tools and strategies that are being taught, practice and receive feedback on skills, and provide continual reinforcement of the TeamSTEPPS principles on the unit or within the department. As an effective, evidence-based practice, TeamSTEPPS provides a multifaceted approach to improving team communication, patient handoffs, and safety, which can reduce the chaos and disorder of the complexity in health care. (AHRQ, 2008, About TeamSTEPPS section)

TeamSTEPPS 2.0 Core Curriculum is an iteration of the original work done on improvement interprofessional communication. It is meant to help teams tailor a plan to train staff on teambuilding skills facilitating improvement work in the organization. The Core Curriculum starts with the initial concept development, implementation, spread of the evidence-based strategies, and sustainment of positive outcomes.

The TeamSTEPPS curriculum is a user-friendly, comprehensive multimedia kit that contains basic modules in text and presentation format, a pocket guide that corresponds to the essentials version of the course, video vignettes to reinforce key concepts, and workshop materials, including a supporting CD and DVD on change management, coaching, and implementation (AHRQ, 2008, p. 1).

There are specific tools within the TeamSTEPPS model. One communication tool identifies the situation, background, assessment, and recommendations (SBAR). It is a situational briefing model that was developed to bridge differences in individual communication styles and perceived authority or power gradients of the people involved. The tool can reduce dependency on memory and uses prompts on an SBAR reporting document to help develop what information needs to be communicated. TeamSTEPPS integrates situational monitoring as the process of actively scanning and assessing elements of the situation in which the patient care team is functioning (AHRQ, 2008). Situational monitoring involves actively and systematically scanning the whole patient care environment. It includes problem recognition and promotes flexibility and adaptability, serving to keep the environment safer. A more focused form of situational monitoring is situation awareness, which is knowing what conditions affect the work.

Complex Care Delivery System

Attention is now being paid to the complex care delivery system in the United States and the care being provided across the continuum. Historically, high-acuity care was provided only within the confines of acute care hospitals. This has shifted so that higher-acuity care is now being offered in long-term care facilities, in long-term acute care hospitals, and in patients' homes (Mor, Caswell, Littlehale, Niemi, & Fogel, 2009). Nurse leaders are now expected to provide supervision and oversight to clinical care and quality outcomes across settings in healthcare systems.

As healthcare reform evolves and more care is provided in a variety of sites within a community, the need for transformational leadership requires the recognition that all members of a team—nurses, physicians, physical and occupational therapists, pharmacists, social workers, health coaches, assistants, and payer care coordinators and navigators—will require different leadership skills. Likewise, expectations surrounding patient safety, which are highlighted in The Joint Commission National Patient Safety Goals, emphasize care across the continuum and the contributions of interdisciplinary team members to affect outcomes (The Joint Commission, 2015).

In terms of safety, the link between how teams function and how each of us perceives the quality and safety of care calls for leaders to engage staff in conversation and a disciplined approach to improvement work. Systems theory acknowledges that a change in one element of care influences other elements, and impacts the entire system (AHRQ, 2008).

With the need to manage care coordination and care across the system, emerging themes in population health management and transitions in care have generated a paradigm shift. A recognition of care fragmentation, managing disease rather than wellness (Schultz, Pineda, Lonhart, Davies, & McDonald, 2013), and cost, efficiency, and effectiveness on the national stage have changed the conversations among providers, patients as consumers, employers, regulators, and healthcare policy makers (Dahl, Reisetter, & Zismann, 2014).

POPULATION HEALTH

Managing care across the continuum in this era of healthcare reform is focused on population health, recognizing that the current disease-focused, episodic, fee-for-service delivery model is costly and not effective in managing the overall health and well-being of individuals. The goal of population health is to keep people healthy, minimize high-cost interventions in emergency rooms or hospitals, and judiciously use imaging tests and procedures. In this model, individuals interface with providers throughout a disease trajectory and are offered tools and information that promote health (Felt-Lisk & Higgins, 2011; Institute for Health Technology Transformation, 2012). This not only offers care in a lower-cost setting, it also redefines health care as a service based on concern about individuals when they are sick and when they are taking steps to maintain their health for an overall sense of well-being.

Although population health does not ignore high-risk ill individuals, it distributes resources toward prevention and health promotion, particularly for those with chronic illness, recognizing that some risk factors are modifiable. Medical care is one of many factors that influence outcomes. Public health intervention, sociodemographic status, genetics, and individual behaviors are also important determinants of health (Institute for Health Technology Transformation, 2012; Kindig & Stoddart, 2003).

Population health improvement has been defined by the Care Continuum Alliance as having three components: (1) primary care providers taking leadership roles that are central to care delivery; (2) patients becoming active participants who are involved in and responsible for their own health care; and (3) increasing care coordination and patient engagement as a result of a focus on wellness and chronic care and disease management (Care Continuum Alliance, 2012). To accomplish this, proactive care needs to be given between encounters, relying heavily on technology and care managers or navigators that support individuals in their efforts to manage their own health. High-risk patients will be supported by care managers who hope to prevent the individual from becoming unhealthier and experiencing complications.

Primary care is the core of public health, but the shortage of primary care physicians offers a space where a team of providers—including advanced practice nurses, nurses, medical assistants, dieticians, health coaches, care managers, physical and occupational therapists, and pharmacists—will be charged to coordinate services to meet patient needs (Grumbach & Grundy, 2010). No single provider or setting of care will be sufficient to accomplish this work (Margolius & Bodenheimer, 2010).

The work flow in the future will be very different from what we have today. Out-of-office contacts will become the norm, supported by interactions via email, group visits, centering practices, and technology-enhanced intervention (Margolius & Bodenheimer, 2010). Aside from the oversight of hospital operations, nurse leaders will need to be expert in managing programs and projects across the continuum. Big data and analytics will be coupled with predictive modeling to prioritize and guide patient-centered, timely interventions. In light of this, nursing will be positioned to reclaim its focus on health promotion and educating patients and families. It will be critical for nurses to practice to the full scope of their licenses educational preparation, and certification standards. Care manager, health coach, and care coordinator are only a few of the roles that nurses assume in assisting patients with decision making and self-care management. Advanced practice nurses will continue to serve as preferred healthcare providers, particularly in rural and primary care settings.

POSITIONING NURSES FOR SUCCESS

Nurse leaders at all levels of organizations, in communities, and in policy settings at state and national levels will be called upon to shape new work cultures. In addition to shaping, managing, and leading change in the care delivery processes, they will be called upon to ensure the clinical competency of those providing care. New, revised, and refined skills in leading and managing teams will become central to success. Clarity in language, a commitment to continuous learning, and practicing resilience, which are essential during change, will be paramount in the delivery of care and services across care settings. Nurse leaders will set and articulate the vision to inspire nurses in fulfilling expectations that are inherent in the healthcare reform paradigm.

The recommendations from the Institute of Medicine (IOM) in *The Future of Nursing: Leading Change, Advancing Health* (2010) provide the foundation and a springboard for nurses to practice to the full scope of their education and licensure, achieve higher levels of education and training, become full partners with physicians and other healthcare professionals in redesigning the U.S. healthcare system, and contribute to workforce planning and policy making. Population health, technology-enhanced practices, and a willingness to enact elements of the profession that are held in high regard by both nurses and patients harken back to historical events in public health and community activism. Nurses will have the opportunity to demonstrate leading teams, enact flexible evidence-based practices in the community, expand health literacy, and execute plans that engage others in health promotion.

Transformational leadership has been shown to be the most influencing factor in leading and sustaining change in organizations and systems. In *Good to Great,*

Collins and a team of graduate students studied successful organizations over a 15-year time span (Collins, 2001). Without fail, the organizations that sustained growth and success had transformational leaders at the helm. Collins (2001) also defined five levels of leadership. The highest-level leader (level five) is one who transforms the organization by developing transformational leaders.

In health care, transformational leadership is needed now more than ever. Transformational nurse administrators are positioned to play a key role in the future of health care. In this exciting yet challenging time, nurse leaders have the opportunity to positively influence the face of health care as we know it. Nurses, by nature, are creative, caring communicators and collaborators. These attributes will serve them well as they establish transformative leadership styles. The American Organization of Nurse Executives (AONE) offers a dynamic evidence-based model for leading and transforming health care in an era of reform.

AONE NURSE LEADER COMPETENCIES

AONE outlined key competencies for current and aspiring nurse leaders as a template to drive toward its vision of shaping the future of health care through innovative nursing leadership. The competencies are categorized into overarching domains, with specific competencies established within them. The domains are communication and relationship building; knowledge of the healthcare environment; leadership; professionalism; and business skills. Specific skills and attributes are further explicated for each domain (American Organization of Nurse Executives [AONE], 2005).

Leadership

AONE's core competencies in nursing leadership are foundational thinking skills, personal journey disciplines, the ability to use systems thinking, succession planning, and change management. Foundational thinking skills address ideas, beliefs, or viewpoints that should be given serious consideration. These skills recognize methods of decision making and the role of beliefs, values, and inferences. Being able to critically analyze organizational issues after a review of the evidence is essential to problem solving. Maintaining curiosity and an eagerness to explore new knowledge and ideas further promotes nursing leadership as both a science and an art. The model of strengths-based leadership begins within and provides a framework for visionary thinking on issues that impact healthcare organizations.

Personal Journey Disciplines

Personal journey disciplines are the essential skills and self-reflections that are critical to nurse leaders if they are to bring value to the healthcare team, the patient experience, and the healthcare delivery system at large. AONE (2005) describes these essential components as follows:

- Value and act on feedback that is provided about one's own strengths and weaknesses.
- Demonstrate the value of lifelong learning through one's own example.
- Learn from setbacks and failures as well as successes.

- Assess one's personal, professional, and career goals and undertake career planning.
- Seek mentorship from respected colleagues.

Knowing one's strengths is essential to professional development. This does not mean individuals should ignore their weaknesses but they should leverage their strengths to build capacity for improvement. A visual tool, such as in the following example, can be useful in identifying personal strengths and opportunities for improvement. This tool can also be utilized when identifying team members who will bring diverse skills and contribute to a well-rounded team. The following steps, which are accompanied by examples that illustrate how to apply the model, provide a framework for identifying strengths, areas for improvement, and opportunities for growth and development:

1. Identify the individual's strengths (gifts) and weaknesses (opportunities for growth). In the example, the nurse leader's strengths are identified, including emotional intelligence, communication, and creativity, which denote an excitement for taking on projects. The nurse leader is easily distracted, loses track of time, and may lose focus. This knowledge can help teams prepare to maximize capacity.
2. Identify traits that are required for success of the individual or team. Note the attributes and the relative strengths or weaknesses of each member, as well as the overall team, to see a visual representation of what may be needed to balance the traits of individuals and teams. Using a scale (1–5) for each attribute could be helpful in determining how to best leverage skills. The higher the level, the greater the skill.
3. Plot the strengths and weaknesses in emotional intelligence, communication, problem resolution, organizational skills, creativity, and time management. **Figure 5-1** illustrates the attributes and strengths of Nurse A, which indicates the individual's strengths and areas for further growth, development, and coaching.

FIGURE 5-1   Attributes and strengths of Nurse A

Emotional Intelligence	Communication	Problem Resolution	Organizational Skills	Creativity	Time Management

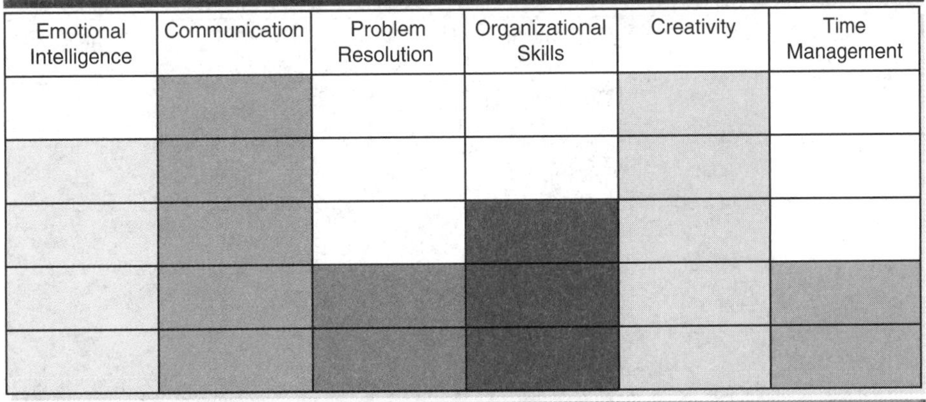

Each team member can be color coded and compared to other team members to discover skills that may be missing from the team. The attributes and strengths of Nurse B are shown in **Figure 5-2**.

Nurse B ranks high (level 5) for resolving problems through organizational skills and time management. Creativity, communication, and emotional intelligence are low level, thereby necessitating a balance of team members who demonstrate the capacity to solve problems creatively and communicate options for improvement. Emotional intelligence could be enhanced through modeling and coaching, particularly by team members who demonstrate high levels of emotional intelligence. Although it is desirable for all nurse leaders to be well rounded, it is a rare occurrence. In the figure, gaps are readily visible and can serve as a strategy for leadership development. Nurse A will need to share his or her creativity, communication, and emotional intelligence skills with the organization while striving to develop organizational skills and time management. When working on projects or interviewing potential teammates, Nurse A should seek an individual who will complement the existing skill set.

Leaders often tend to hire themselves; that is, they seek individuals who are similar to themselves. However, hiring those who complement the traits of the leader or the team will enable more diversity and success.

Nurse leaders model and encourage lifelong learning. Nurse leaders stay abreast of current best practices and standards of care and gain much from experiences played out in the healthcare world. Interactions with patients, their families and loved ones, physicians, and administrators can provide an education that is invaluable. Knowledge becomes wisdom when it is applied, integrated, and embedded in daily operations. Classrooms cannot prepare nurses to master the political environments they may encounter. Some lessons are hard learned, but the greatest growth can be realized from mistakes, setbacks, disappointments, or choices one regrets. The challenge is to take these life lessons and transform them into not only a personal growth experience but one that others can learn from as well. During these trying times, strength and valuable advice can be sought from respected and

FIGURE 5-2 Attributes and strengths of Nurse B

Emotional Intelligence	Communication	Problem Resolution	Organizational Skills	Creativity	Time Management

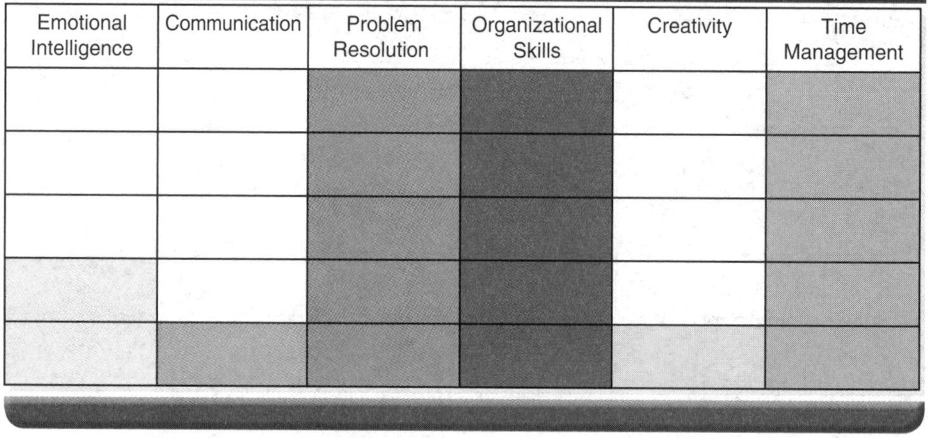

trusted mentors. The development of these valuable relationships is a hallmark of successful nurse leaders.

The Joint Commission set a standard that must be adhered to by participating hospitals. Nurse administrators are responsible not only for leading the department or division of nursing but also for setting the pace for healthcare collaboration, moving systems forward, and enabling the success of all healthcare team members for the benefit of healthcare recipients. To achieve this level of collaboration, nurse administrators must be emotionally mature individuals who are self-aware, reflective, and devoted to continuous growth and development.

Communication and Relationship Building

In the IOM (2010) report *The Future of Nursing: Leading Change, Advancing Health*, complex issues that face U.S. health care and recommendations for nursing's role and contributions moving forward are detailed. One of the core recommendations is that "nursing should be full partners, with physicians and other health professionals, in redesigning health care in the United States" (p. 2). The development and mentoring of present and future leaders within nursing and other disciplines is essential to successful organizations and their members. Building trusting and collaborative relationships is an essential competency for nurse executives.

Communication and relationship building provide competencies that guide nurse leaders in their quest to develop teams, to better collaborate, and to work cohesively. For example, a new physician department chair may have extensive surgical expertise but may not have previously served in a leadership position. The success of the new chair as a leader is essential to the success of the residency and the Department of Surgery. Recognizing this, the nurse administrator partners with the new chair, meeting weekly to set goals, determine areas of desired improvement, research best practices, and strategize areas of future growth. **Table 5-1** provides example action plans and anticipated outcomes for the Bariatric Center of Excellence and performance ratings for core measures.

Relationship building among all healthcare disciplines is essential to the success of the organization. Frontline nursing staff, all healthcare disciplines, students, physicians, and community leaders can build relationships to enrich the health of community members. Nurse executives are often charged with mobilizing diverse resources to benefit improved systems. While organizations often cite benefits from these relationships, community members also describe how the interactions brought them greater focus and awareness about where synergies exist.

Another example of communication and relationship building includes work with heart failure patients that are readmitted within 30 days of discharge. Readmission rates affect reimbursement and may result in financial penalties. It is the responsibility of healthcare providers to consider the continuum of care and correctly prepare patients for discharge to prevent avoidable readmissions. In the following example, the nurse executive brings a team together to address heart failure readmissions. The team consists of the members shown in **Table 5-2**.

The team utilized the Plan-Do-Study-Act (PDSA) model for process improvement. Goals were set for 30, 60, 90, and 120 days. **Table 5-3** identifies goals, including identifying the gap, educating, implementing, and evaluating, and ensuring sustainability.

TABLE 5-1 **Bariatric Center of Excellence**

Develop Bariatric Center of Excellence (BCOE)	Perform 100% on SCIP core measures	100% passing rate for surgical residents	Increase knowledge of new chair related to hospital administration

1. Develop business plan
  a. Offer competitive pricing
  b. Offer cash payment for bariatric procedures
  c. Determine breakeven, profitability of service
	1. Develop training sessions
	  a. OR staff, anesthesia staff, surgical residents, PACU and ICU staff
		1. Develop plan for simulation lab training, essential skills
		  a. Suture lab: Develop competencies
		  b. Laparoscopic simulation: Develop competencies
			1. Enroll chair in IHI open school core curriculum for leadership, safety, and PI

2. Develop clinical pathways based on best practices
  a. Partner with PACU nurses, postsurgical unit nurses, dieticians, pharmacists, and interdisciplinary team
	2. Develop concurrent monitoring tool
	  a. Tool should hold individuals accountable
	  b. Develop methods to provide timely feedback to all staff
		2. Identify and hire highly qualified surgical faculty to train residents
		  a. Ensure that faculty hold residents accountable
		  b. Must have a passion for mentoring others, teaching
			2. Appoint chair to Patient Safety Committee
			  a. Mentor chair to lead PI Council in the upcoming year
			  b. Chair will progress to lead Med Exec Committee in year two
			  c. Chair will mentor one physician as replacement committee lead

3. Identify a bariatric team coordinator
  a. Research requirements, identify barriers to becoming a BCOE
	3. Develop quality council to review fallouts, identify system failures, and redesign, retrain, and develop improvements to system	3. Include surgical residents on key committees (interdisciplinary collaboration)
		  a. Infection Prevention Committee
		  b. Rapid Response/Code Committee
		  c. EBP Committee
		  d. Readmissions Committee
			3. Chair to accompany administrative team to national summit, such as IHI or UHC, to network with other physician leaders and observe best practices

4. Develop bariatric OR team
  a. Training from surgeon
  b. Training from vendors
  c. Research best practices
  d. Assess equipment, instruments, and supplies, including pre- and postoperative units
	4. Develop order sets to incorporate SCIP measures
	  a. Ensure e-orders and paper downtime order sets match
	  b. Ensure old paper order sets are identified and eliminated
		4. Develop system to evaluate progress, provide rich feedback, remediate, and foster continual growth and development of residents	4. Consider TeamSTEPPS training or master training
			  a. Chair to share new skills with other department chairs and residents

TABLE 5-2	Nurse Executive Team				
Nurse executive	Clinical pharmacist	Nurse educator	Social worker	Biomedical librarian	Staff nurse
Cardiologist	Cardiology nurse practitioner	Nurse manager	Nurse informaticist	Administrator clinic	Assistant CFO

For example, an investigation of best practices revealed that in successful models, patients who were unable to afford prescriptions were provided with a 2-week supply of critical medications at discharge to prevent readmissions for heart failure. The cardiologist and nurse practitioner provided data demonstrating that when their patients were readmitted, it was often because they could not fill their prescriptions and take medications as prescribed. The team agreed to find a way to adopt the best practice, and formulated a plan. **Table 5-4** shows the actions, core justifications, and anticipated results.

Lessons learned from this experience include that engaging and leading a team toward improved outcomes results in the entire team gaining valuable leadership skills. The cardiologist learned the importance of financially justifying giving medications to patients to maintain wellness and prevent recurrent hospitalizations. The team learned to collaborate with other disciplines and respect the expertise of each team member. The team also learned to research evidence and implement a best practice. The collecting of baseline data and comparing them to postimplementation data clearly demonstrated the success of the project and the potential value of replicating the process with other chronic diseases (AONE, 2005).

Professionalism

AONE outlines core competencies of professionalism, including personal and professional accountability, career planning, and ethics. To be personally and professionally accountable, nurse leaders create an environment that facilitates the team to initiate actions that produce results; hold self and others accountable for actions and outcomes; create an environment where others are setting expectations and holding each other accountable; and answer for the results of one's own behaviors and actions (AONE, 2005). The nurse leader's responsibility in career planning is to develop his or her own career plan and measure progress according to that plan;

TABLE 5-3	Team Goals		
30-day goals	**60-day goals**	**90-day goals**	**120-day goals**
1. Research best practices 2. Outline current practices; collect baseline data 3. Perform gap analysis	1. Formulate plan 2. Education plan 3. Implementation plan	1. Roll out plan 2. Concurrent evaluation; review data 3. Revise and retrain as appropriate	1. Ensure sustainability 2. Report to administration 3. Share with other disciplines

TABLE 5-4   Reducing Heart Failure Readmissions: Actions and Results

Actions	Results
1. Cardiologist and nurse practitioner to determine crucial generic medications required to prevent readmissions.	■ Nine months postimplementation revealed only two heart failure readmissions, which were unrelated to heart failure.
2. Nurse executive and assistant CFO to determine cost avoidance of prevented readmissions and justification for providing free medications.	■ All heart failure patients who were provided with medications at discharge were taking medications appropriately at the first postdischarge clinic visit.
3. Nurse educator will train nursing on new practice.	■ All 9-month heart failure readmissions compared to previous year were reduced.
4. Nursing alerts nurse practitioner of all heart failure admissions.	
5. Nurse practitioner assesses heart failure patients' ability to purchase heart failure medications at discharge.	■ Project was determined to be successful and will be disseminated to other services. This model may also be useful in other patient populations, such as diabetic patients.
6. Nurse practitioner sends a request to pharmacy for heart failure home medications 48 hours before discharge when possible.	
7. A pharmacist delivers the medications to the bedside and educates the patient on each medication, using a teach-back technique.	■ Data will continue to be collected to ensure sustainability.
8. Nurse practitioner will call each heart failure patient within 72 hours of discharge and see each patient in clinic within 2 weeks of discharge.	
9. Nurse practitioner will coordinate care with community resources to provide medication assistance.	
10. Nurse practitioner and cardiologist will continue to collect readmission data to review with the team and administration and finance.	
11. Nurse executive and assistant CFO will review the financial benefits of the pilot program and provide results to the team and administration.	

Cost Justification:

- Cost to care for heart failure patient per day (non-ICU) ($500). Average length of stay of 6 days ($3,000) and average costs of Emergency Department visit preadmission ($500).   Total = $3,500
- Previous 12-month heart failure readmission costs (21 patients at $3,500).   Total = $73,500
- Heart failure readmission related to lack of medicine funds; potential avoidable readmission costs avoidance; total estimated annual costs to provide medications ($1,022 x 21 patients).   Total = $21,462
- By implementing an evidence-based best practice, patients with heart failure would be able to take critical medications required to prevent readmissions while potentially saving the healthcare system avoidable expenses.

Total estimated potential annual savings = $52,038

coach others in developing their own career plans; and create an environment in which professional and personal growth is expected (AONE, 2005).

The ethical component of professionalism includes articulating the application of ethical principles to operations and integrating high ethical standards and core values into everyday work activities (AONE, 2005). For nurse leaders, articulating the connection to the ANA Code of Ethics (2010) to emphasize the commitment and responsibility we have to the public is aligned with our decisions and actions.

Professionalism can be reflected in an example of a newly appointed chief nursing officer (CNO) at a university hospital who is asked to collaborate with the College of Nursing (CON) faculty as part of a national improvement science research study. The goal of the study was to identify interruptions in nursing care on medical–surgical units. The CNO gained consensus with the medical–surgical nurse managers and agreed to serve as a principal coinvestigator with a senior faculty member. The CNO created an environment that facilitated the team to initiate actions that produce results; held herself and others accountable for actions and outcomes; created an environment in which others are setting expectations; and answered for the results of their own behaviors and actions.

In an environment sensitive to team strengths and cultural diversity, the study provided an excellent opportunity for team building. The study incorporated tally cards that were carried by the staff nurses, who would record each interruption as it occurred for a 2-week time frame. The data from the cards were entered into a database, and the results were to be shared at some point in the future. After the cards were collected, the CNO approached the CON faculty about meeting with the frontline staff to begin resolving some of the issues they had identified during the study. A core faculty group partnered with the CNO, and the Frontline Innovations (FI) research group was formed. Delegates were asked to join the FI group, and the disgruntled or disillusioned squeaky wheels were invited too. Both shifts of nurses were represented. To build team cohesiveness, the group met at lunch once a month. Nurse managers and nurse educators agreed to relieve the staff so they could attend the meeting, and lunch was provided by the administration. Many frontline improvements were made with the support of the CNO and the faculty.

One project the staff adopted was missed medications. According to the FI nurses, medications were often missing at the time they were due to be administered. Much time was spent contacting and communicating with the pharmacy, making calls, and sending repeated fax notifications. Additionally, medications were not given on time. Coming together to better understand the processes and outcomes provided a venue in which interprofessional teams could be developed and empowered to lead and coach other staff members along the way.

Working through the study with newly created teams, baseline data were collected for 1 week by utilizing a tool created by the nurses. After the results were reviewed, the nurses invited representatives from the pharmacy to their next meeting. Nursing voiced mistrust of the pharmacy, but after one meeting with the pharmacist and technician, a partnership of collaboration was born. Over the course of the year, processes for daptomycin, heparin infusions, patient-controlled analgesia (PCA), and an interdisciplinary vancomycin protocol were developed by this team. Nurses learned to research best practices, collect data, collaborate with other disciplines, and improve processes. They began to believe in an empowered nurse workforce and saw the ability to determine their destiny.

Building on the success of the team's initial work and interprofessional team involvement, a core CON faculty member suggested the team apply for a small grant and consider moving toward a shared governance model. In collaboration with the CON, including the biomedical librarian, articles about shared governance were distributed to staff nurses, and all agreed to a site visit at an institution with a well-developed shared governance structure. Upon returning from the site visit, the FI staff requested they lead the frontline meetings from that point forward. A governing council was formed, bylaws were written, and the first Nurse Congress was born. Recruitment during the Nurses' Week breakfast was a joint effort between the governing council and the CON faculty. All units were included rather than only the medical–surgical units.

To get a stronger picture of the ongoing success of this collaborative work, a survey for readiness was conducted by the governing council, and it was determined that nurses throughout the organization were ready and interested in shared governance. Within 1 year, the Nurse Congress held a pinning ceremony to celebrate the membership and success of the Nurse Congress. Many evidence-based improvement projects have resulted from the work of the Nurse Congress. Members are presenting their work at conferences and evidence-based practice summits, and nursing is seen throughout the organization as an innovator and driver of healthcare improvement and excellence. Professionalism was demonstrated through the various processes, actions, and follow-up planning.

Professional accountability underscores the importance of creating an environment that enables the team to initiate actions that produce results; hold itself and others accountable for actions and outcomes; create an environment in which others are setting expectations and hold one another accountable; and answer for the results of one's own behaviors and actions. Working with staff nurses provided career planning opportunities for the CNO and frontline staff, including coaching the development of others by creating an environment in which professional and personal growth is an expectation. Facilitating an ethical milieu underscores the ethics of the organization. By articulating the application of ethical principles to operations and integrating high ethical standards and core values into everyday work activities, the CNO was able to live the story.

COMPLEXITY SCIENCE AND HEALTH CARE: IMPLICATIONS FOR NURSE LEADERS

The science of complex adaptive systems provides important concepts and tools for responding to the challenges of health care in the 21st century. Clinical practice, organization information management, research, education, and professional development are interdependent and are built around multiple self-adjusting and interacting systems. In complex systems, unpredictability and paradox are ever present, and some things will remain unknowable. New conceptual frameworks that incorporate a dynamic, emergent, creative, and intuitive view of the world must replace traditional reduce-and-resolve approaches to clinical care and service organization (Plsek & Greenhalgh, 2001).

SUMMARY

Nurse leaders are being offered an opportunity of a lifetime during this time of healthcare reform. What remains to be seen is whether we will capitalize on this moment to elevate and showcase what many nurses believe is their claim to health promotion, care delivery, and service. Transformational leaders will embrace the complexity, uncertainty, and clean slate offered by healthcare reform to enact competencies outlined by AONE for nurse executives based on the IOM *Future of Nursing: Leading Change, Advancing Health* report to practice to the full scope of our education and use data to mobilize an interdisciplinary workforce to establish outcomes that are demonstrative of the health and well-being of patients and their families. With technology as an enabler and using ourselves as an instrument of change, the possibilities are endless!

REFLECTIVE QUESTIONS

1. Identify a nurse leader you believe embodies transformational leadership abilities and has been courageous in implementing innovative care delivery change. What attributes does this nurse leader have that has allowed him or her to accomplish this work? Use the AONE competencies as a guide to your evaluation.
2. Reflecting on your experiences, identify a situation in which you have demonstrated elements of the personal journey disciplines to achieve a goal. What were your strengths, and what would you like to develop more fully?
3. Examine The Joint Commission National Patient Safety Goals in light of TeamSTEPPS. What steps could you take to move toward the structures and processes to engage a team?

CASE STUDY 5-1   Aligning Strengths and Opportunity to Lead Effective Teams

Stephanie Burnett

Jackie is a new nurse manager. She had no prior experience in a management position, but she was eager to accept the challenge of managing her own unit. She had been frustrated in her past positions as a staff nurse, staff educator, and nurse coordinator, feeling powerless to make significant change. She had enjoyed great success in these roles leading hospital projects, and she had received rave reviews from her peers and supervisor. Therefore, though she had no expertise in the specialty of her new unit, when this new nurse manager position became available and the opportunity was offered to her, she jumped at the chance to move to the next level into a real leadership role. She had heard that the staff was a very cohesive team, and she was eager to finally have authority to bring about change and influence.

She entered into the nurse manager position very enthusiastic to make immediate changes, in hopes of improving staff accessibility and greater utilization of technology when possible. In the first few

(continues)

CASE STUDY 5-1   Aligning Strengths and Opportunity to Lead Effective Teams (Continued)

months, after a brief orientation to the department, Jackie made many changes, such as changing the staff work patterns and scheduling process, quickly filling all vacant positions, eliminating the staff break room/lounge, and eliminating routine monthly staff meetings.

With each change, Jackie felt great pride in the changes she'd made, believing the staff would accept and appreciate the value in the changes, and she awaited the subsequent improved outcome. However, in less than 6 months, half of the new staff she'd hired had resigned, along with four existing staff members, creating an even greater vacancy rate. Staff call-ins increased by 50%, and the staff felt disconnected, unappreciated, and distrustful of Jackie. Many reported feeling that she was frequently unavailable and did not support them or appreciate their opinions or input. Jackie found that she was very uneasy having direct communication with the staff. She perceived all voiced concerns or complaints as a challenge to her nurse manager skills and authority, and she resisted all suggestions from them. When members of the interdisciplinary team approached her with areas that needed improvement, she felt personally attacked. She realized she had not anticipated how much personal contact the staff seemed to require. She was even more unprepared for how much supervision was necessary to monitor care delivery, patient and family satisfaction, and adherence to policy. Yet Jackie was eager for the staff to like her and feel friendly toward her.

Case Study Questions

1. What leadership principles did Jackie fail to apply when managing an effective team?
2. How would individual and team evaluations be useful in determining strengths and opportunities for each member?
3. How might Jackie's director best coach and mentor her in addressing her own strengths and opportunities to better manage and lead her nursing staff?

REFERENCES

Agency for Healthcare Research and Quality. (2008). TeamSTEPPS: National implementation. Retrieved from http://teamstepps.ahrq.gov/

American Nurses Association. (2010). *Guide to the code of ethics for nurses.* Silver Spring, MD: Author.

American Nurses Association. (2014). *Healthcare transformation: The Affordable Care Act and more.* Retrieved from http://www.nursingworld.org/MainMenu Categories/Policy-Advocacy/HealthSystemReform/AffordableCareAct.pdf

American Organization of Nurse Executives. Nurse executive competencies. Retrieved from http://www.aone.org/resources/leadership%20tools /nursecomp.shtml

Care Continuum Alliance. (2012). Advancing the population health improvement model. Retrieved from http://www.fiercehealthit.com/story/hennepin-health -project-looks-build-countywide-ehr-program-national-implica/2012-01-10

Centers for Medicare and Medicaid Services. (2010). *Affordable Care Act update: Improving Medicare cost savings.* Retrieved from http://www.cms.gov/apps /docs/aca-update-implementing-medicare-costs-savings.pdf

Collins, J. C. (2001). *Good to great.* New York, NY: HarperCollins.

Commonwealth Fund. (2014). *Mirror, mirror, on the wall: How the performance of the U.S. health care system compares internationally.* Retrieved from http:// www.commonwealthfund.org/~/media/files/publications/fund-report/2014 /jun/1755_davis_mirror_mirror_2014.pdf

Dahl, D., Reisetter, J., & Zismann, N. (2014). People, technology, and process meet the Triple Aim. *Nursing Administration Quarterly, 38*(1), 13–21.

Executive Office of the President Council of Economic Advisers. (2009). *The economic case for health reform.* Retrieved from http://www.whitehouse.gov /assets/documents/CEA_Health_Care_Report.pdf

Felt-Lisk, S., & Higgins, T. (2011). Exploring the promise of population health management program to improve health. *Mathematica Policy Research Issue Brief.* Retrieved from http://www.mathematica-mpr.com/~/media/publications /PDFs/health/PHM_brief.pdf

Gorman, A., & Appleby, J. (2014). Obamacare round 2: States gear up for start of next enrollment period in November. Health & Science, *Washington Post.* October 5, 2014. Retrieved from http://www.washingtonpost .com/national/health-science/obamacare-round-2-states-gear-up-for-start-of -next-enrollment-period-in-november/2014/10/05/031f0522-4b44-11e4-a046 -120a8a855cca_story.html

Grumbach, K., & Grundy, P. (2010). Multistakeholder movement needed to renew and reform primary care. Retrieved from http://www.rollcall.com /news/45890-1.html

Health Management Academy. (2013). *The cost and use of healthcare for baby boomers and generation Y: The role of payment models.* Retrieved from http:// www.hmacademy.com/pdfs/The_cost_and_use_of_healthcare-The_Health _Management_Academy_Policy_Brief.pdf

Institute for Health Technology Transformation. (2012). *Population health management: A roadmap for provider-based automation in a new era of healthcare.* Retrieved from http://ihealthtran.com/pdf/PHMReport.pdf

Institute of Medicine. (2010). *The future of nursing: Leading change, advancing health.* Washington, DC: National Academies Press.

Johnson, N., & Johnson, L. (2010). *Care of the uninsured in America.* New York, NY: Springer.

Kessler, G. (2014, July 24). Do 10,000 baby boomers retire every day? *Washington Post.* Retrieved from http://www.washingtonpost.com/blogs/fact-checker /wp/2014/07/24/do-10000-baby-boomers-retire-every-day/

Kindig, D., & Stoddart, G. (2003). What is population health? *American Journal of Public Health, 93*(3), 380–383.

Margolius, D., & Bodenheimer, J. (2010). Transforming primary care: From past practice to the practice of the future. *Health Affairs, 29*(5), 779–784.

Mor, V., Caswell, C., Littlehale, S., Niemi, J., & Fogel, B. (2009). *Changes in the quality of nursing homes in the US: A review and data update.* Retrieved from http://www.ahcancal.org/research_data/quality/documents/changesinnursing-homequality.pdf

Murray, C., Phil, D., & Frenk, J. (2010). Ranking 37th—measuring the performance of the U.S. health care system. *New England Journal of Medicine, 362*(2), 98–99.

Nix, K. (2012). But wait, it gets worse: The Medicare actuary's realistic outlook for the program. Retrieved from http://www.heritage.org/research/reports/2012/06/the-medicare-actuarys-realistic-outlook-for-the-program

Plonien, C., & Baldwin, K. (2014). Medical tourism: A nurse executive's need to know. *AORN, 100*(4), 429–434.

Plsek, P. E., & Greenhalgh, T. (2001). The challenge of complexity in health care. *British Medical Journal, 323*, 625–628.

Schultz, E., Pineda, N., Lonhart, J., Davies, S., & McDonald, K. (2013). A systematic review of the care coordination measurement landscape. *BMC Health Services Research, 31*(119). Retrieved from http://www.biomedcentral.com/1472-6963/13/11

The Joint Commission. (2015). 2015 national patient safety goals. Retrieved from http://www.jointcommission.org/standards_information/npsgs.aspx

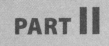

PART II

Leading the Business of Health Care: Processes and Principles

CHAPTER 6

Organizational Structure and Accountability

Anne Longo and Linda Roussel

LEARNING OBJECTIVES

1. Describe change in complex adaptive systems.
2. Synthesize the inputs and outputs in monitoring organizational effectiveness.
3. Examine the key components in developing organizational structures that maximize efficiency and profitability.
4. Evaluate the types and characteristics of organizational structures.
5. Synthesize the characteristics of a culture, particularly a culture of safety.

AONE KEY COMPETENCIES

I. Communication and relationship building
II. Knowledge of the healthcare environment
III. Leadership
IV. Professionalism
V. Business skills

AONE KEY COMPETENCIES DISCUSSED IN THIS CHAPTER

II. Knowledge of the healthcare environment
III. Leadership
IV. Professionalism

II. **Knowledge of the healthcare environment**
- Clinical practice knowledge
- Patient care delivery models and work design knowledge
- Healthcare economics knowledge
- Healthcare policy knowledge
- Understanding of governance
- Understanding of evidence-based practice
- Outcomes measurement
- Knowledge of, and dedication to, patient safety

- Understanding of utilization and case management
- Knowledge of quality improvement and metrics
- Knowledge of risk management

III. Leadership
- Foundational thinking skills
- Personal journey disciplines
- Ability to use systems thinking
- Succession planning
- Change management

IV. Professionalism
- Personal and professional accountability
- Career planning
- Ethics
- Evidence-based clinical and management practices
- Advocacy for the clinical enterprise and for nursing practice
- Active membership in professional organizations

FUTURE OF NURSING: FOUR KEY MESSAGES

1. Nurses should practice to the full extent of their education and training.
2. Nurses should achieve higher levels of education and training through an improved education system that promotes seamless academic progression.
3. Nurses should be full partners with physicians and other health professionals in redesigning health care in the United States.
4. Effective workforce planning and policy making require better data collection and information infrastructure.

Introduction

The International Council of Nurses (2014) defines nursing as encompassing "autonomous and collaborative care of individuals of all ages, families, groups and communities, sick or well and in all settings. Nursing includes the promotion of health, prevention of illness, and the care of ill, disabled and dying people. Advocacy, promotion of a safe environment, research, participation in shaping health policy and in patient and health systems management, and education are also key nursing roles" (para. 1). The very definition of nursing demonstrates the complex adaptive system in which nurse leaders work. Using influence with knowledge and skills allows nurse leaders to be accountable for creating and sustaining organizational structures that continue to change.

Nursing has been designated as the change agent to transform the U.S. healthcare system. This is a daunting task, yet no other profession has an understanding of the patient as a whole. Nurse leaders work within their own organizations to accomplish change. The challenge is to keep in mind the key messages of the Robert Wood Johnson Foundation and Institute of Medicine's initiative on the future of nursing as outlined in *The Future of Nursing: Leading Change, Advancing Health* (Institute of Medicine [IOM], 2011), which include the following:

- Nurses should practice to the full extent of their education and training.
- Nurses should achieve higher levels of education and training through an improved education system that promotes seamless academic progression.
- Nurses should be full partners, with physicians and other health professionals, in redesigning health care in the United States.
- Effective workforce planning and policy making require better data collection and improved information infrastructure.

The decisions and changes made by the nurse manager of a unit and the nurse leader of an organization will undoubtedly have upstream and downstream effects on patient populations as a whole.

OVERVIEW

Nurse leaders desire to keep abreast of the ever-changing framework of health care and determine how this work environment fits into the strategic management of larger organizations. As health care continues to move from the inpatient setting to ambulatory and home care settings, skilled nursing facilities, and palliative care settings, nurse leaders must determine how and what care clinical nurses will provide within their work settings that impact overall patient outcomes.

In the United States today, $2.5 trillion is spent on health care, twice the amount spent by any other industrialized nation per capita. Yet the United States ranks 49th in the world for life expectancy, with substantial gaps in how Americans use recommended healthcare services and the quality of care they receive. Nearly 40% of U.S. deaths are caused by preventable conditions each year, but clinical interventions to prevent these conditions reach only 20–50% of the people who need them.

Nurse leaders working in all areas of the care continuum need to understand the need for a shared model and shared accountability for the individual patient to receive the appropriate care, from preventive measures to end of life.

The Patient Protection and Affordable Care Act was enacted with the goal of increasing access to care and decreasing U.S. spending on health care. Healthcare reform emphasizes interprofessional collaborative care teams that provide patient-centered, service-line-based, mutually accountable care.

The overall goal of transforming the healthcare system is to develop a seamless, coordinated care approach for patients. The outcomes for the healthcare system, as defined by the Institute for Healthcare Improvement (IHI), are known as the Triple Aim (Stiefel & Nolan, 2012):

- Improve the health of populations
- Provide a better care experience for patients, including quality and satisfaction
- Lower costs through continuous improvement

The Triple Aim is a framework that describes an approach to optimizing healthcare system performance by designing the work around five concepts (Stiefel & Nolan, 2012):

- Focus on individuals and families
- Redesign of primary care services and structures

- Population health management
- Cost control platform
- System integration and execution

Nurse leaders must keep the concepts and goals of the Triple Aim at the center of each decision. Using change theory and strategic and business management skills as part of continuously improving the work environment will impact the satisfaction of both the patient and the caregiver as well as the outcome of care.

Nurse leaders have an opportunity to influence the redesign of the healthcare system by implementing the four key messages from the Institute of Medicine (IOM, 2001) Future of Nursing report. Additionally, nurse leaders who have the knowledge and skills to develop the following structure within their own work environments will succeed in meeting the portion of the Triple Aim that is specific to populations they care for:

- Creating a healthy work environment for the caregiver
- Fostering use of the principles of a high-reliability organization
- Using best evidence to inform best practice
- Following the cycle of continuous improvement
- Framing work within change management theory
- Incorporating quantitative and qualitative data about systems, the public, the point of care, and payers into all aspects of leadership
- Understanding the Triple Aim and its impact on the work environment

ORGANIZATIONAL STRUCTURES

Having an appreciation for standard organizational structures and how to evaluate them will guide nurse leaders as healthcare reform continues with the creation of new models in integrated care and methods of payment. There are several types of organizational structures:

- Functional structure is when each portion of the institution is organized around a specific purpose. Small businesses are often set up this way. Issues that may cause concern are coordination and communication among departments. As smaller physicians' offices are being purchased by larger corporations, the issues of functional structures may increase.
- Divisional structure can be found in larger organizations and within larger systems. In such a structure, needs can often be met quicker. As in functional structures, communication may be an issue because the staff works in different areas.
- Matrix structure is a combination of functional and divisional structures. There can be power struggles in this type of structure.

Since one of the goals of healthcare reform is the redesign of primary care services and structures, nurse leaders will need to consider the types of organizational structures and where interconnectedness and interrelatedness take place.

COMPLEX ADAPTIVE SYSTEMS

The use of various types of intelligence as part of managing change is critical to leaders working in a complex adaptive system. A complex adaptive system is often characterized by dynamic relationships among many agents, influences, and forces. The concept of complex adaptive systems comes from a body of literature known as complexity science, chaos theory, or network science. According to Olney (2005), the key traits of complex adaptive systems are as follows:

- An entangled web of relationships among many agents and forces, both internal and external; causes constant change, adaptation, and evolution of the system in an unpredictable, nonlinear manner
- Self-organizing
- Chaotic and do not move predictably toward an end goal
- Communication laden, which are heaviest at the boundaries of a system
- Observable system-wide patterns of behaviors
- Feedback loops as the mechanisms for change in a system
- Repeated patterns of behavior at different levels of a system and across systems

Plsek and Greenhalgh (2001) reported the following additional concepts:

- Tension and paradox are natural phenomena, not necessarily to be resolved
- Inherent pattern of the system (patterning)
- Attractor behaviors, which are patterns that provide a comparatively simple understanding of what first seems to be extremely complex behavior

Nurse leaders must become adept at environmental scanning. Because of the nature of their work, they function within complex adaptive systems. Possessing the knowledge of one's own areas of influence and how they integrate into the system as a whole increases the likelihood of sustainable change throughout the entire change process (Plsek & Greenhalgh, 2001).

Nurse leaders must adjust and adapt their behavior to align with staff needs to best engage them in addressing the institution's mission; they must be constantly aware of cues for the need to change. They must become more flexible and deal with employees in individualized ways, and they must be candid and confront conflict by allowing nurses to express their feelings, thoughts, and reactions. Management styles change, as do policies, procedures, relationships with subordinates, and employment and compensation practices. Individual needs and group motivations should be considered. The changes in nursing management aim to promote the ideas of all people, to encourage attentive listening, and to reward people for becoming personally involved and committed to their work. Nurse leaders see themselves as agents of change functioning within a profession that draws its basic support from society. Nurse managers will have to act as change agents in moving organizations forward and utilize human-intensive skills to mobilize resources that are available to them and their professional nursing peers. All this effort will serve to define, implement, and evaluate the strategies and processes that will meet the healthcare needs of the future. Decision making and delegation are fundamental to working in complex adaptive systems.

DECISION MAKING AND SYSTEMS THINKING

Hewertson (2015) suggests five keys to guide decision making: knowing the specific decision to be made; whose decision it is; how the decision will be made (methods used to decide); the timing of the decision; and how, when, and to whom the decision will be communicated.

In addition, Hewertson (2015) describes four main categories within a decision-making protocol: the type of decision; the level of risk (high, medium, low); the knowledge needed (high, medium, low); and the authority and job level involved in the decision-making process (high, medium, low). For example, the types of decision making may include autocratic, inclusive, participative, democratic, consensus, delegated, and no decision:

- Autocratic decision making means the leader makes the decision. It is important that the team or department know from the outset that the leader will decide.
- Inclusive refers to the leader gathering information, input, and feedback from others before making the decision. The leader may not be looking for a recommendation but may gather input to inform the decision. If input is not necessary, or if it will not be considered, it is important for the leader to be transparent about the motives. Trust and credibility are on the line. The leader makes the final decision.
- Participative decision making is essentially a group recommendation that the leader will almost always honor. The leader does have veto power if the results conflict with the overall mission, core values, and philosophy. It is important that communication between the team and the leader is handled well and that there is clarity about the intent of the decision. This type of decision making can facilitate alignment and commitment to the decision by all involved.
- Democratic decision making means that each person gets one vote; it can also refer to a two-thirds vote, or a quorum. The leader does not have veto power.
- Consensus decision making is when everyone has to be able to live with and support the decision. "The key here is that the right people are having the discussion; no one is being 'railroaded,' and everyone's voice is fully heard" (Hewertson, 2015, p. 156). The leader does not retain veto power in this method.
- Delegated decision making means the decision is made by those who will be affected the most by the outcome; the leader retains no veto power or even attachment to the outcome.
- No decision is a decision; that is, a decision not to decide is a decision. Hewertson (2015) cautions leaders to use this type of decision making intentionally, not to avoid making a decision when one is needed.

Decisions can be unanimous (100% agreement); they can be put up for a vote (the number of voters can be agreed upon); they can be decided in multivoting (majority carries); or they can be made by consensus (everyone who voted agrees to live with and support the decision). Hewertson describes a voting tool called rule of thumb:

> Thumbs up: 100% on board
> Thumbs sideways: There is a concern or thought
> Hand raised: A decision cannot be made until questions are answered
> Thumbs down: Decision cannot be supported (Hewertson, 2015, p. 157)

If thumbs are sideways or down, it is important to open the decision for discussion so feedback can be shared, questions can be asked to discover thoughts about the subject, and the team can be involved in decision making.

DELEGATION

Hewertson (2015) defines delegation as planned and well-managed new learning opportunities for another person that transfers duties or responsibilities to that person for a mutually beneficial purpose. Factors that can guide delegation include the actual job or task, who delegated the task, why the task was delegated, the delegate's initial perception of being assigned the task, and the benefits (or gains) for the person delegating the task. The principles of delegation may include the following (Hewertson, 2015):

- Select the right person: Consider the person's capabilities, and choose the right person at the right time. It is important to consult the person before delegating the task. Delegation is a two-way street. If possible, include those being delegated to in the decision to transfer duties and responsibilities.
- Show and tell: Consider learning styles. Generally, we learn by doing rather than by being told what to do. Role modeling and coaching are key strategies that use this principle.
- Delegate good and new work: To increase motivation, commitment, engagement, and development, it is important to delegate interesting, rewarding, and challenging projects. If you delegate only what you would rather not do, your associates will readily pick up on this and not trust you to help them develop professionally.
- Take your time: Training and developing expertise takes time. Be realistic about how much time is needed to learn the work and to complete the task.
- Delegate gradually and monitor progress carefully: Typically it is difficult to let go. It is important to not transfer too much responsibility too quickly. Consider the individual and his or her level of experience, knowledge of the work, and learning curve.
- Match authority with responsibility: It is frustrating to have responsibility without the requisite authority to carry out the work. Make sure responsibility and authority are aligned. "By empowering employees who perform delegated jobs with both the responsibilities and authority to manage those jobs, leaders free themselves to manage more effectively and at a higher level of effectiveness" (Hewertson, 2015, p. 164).
- Delegate the whole: It is important, when possible, to delegate the complete project or task to one person rather than giving away only one part of the task. Share the larger conceptual view so that the goal can be pictured by the person who is now responsible for the work. Allow room to innovate and for mistakes to be made because new and better solutions might be generated through creative thinking.
- Delegate for specific results: Share anticipated outcomes and desired results.
- Avoid gaps and overlaps: Consider process flow. Creating a process map to help understand the process flow can do much to identify gaps and overlaps in the project.
- Trust the successful delegate: By preparing, being clear, and sharing the larger view, leaders should be able to trust delegates by allowing them the freedom to make day-to-day decisions and have free rein to use their own resourcefulness within the established boundaries.

It is important to put the plan in writing. A delegation worksheet can include such elements as the name of the delegate; the name of the delegator; the delegated job or task (describe in detail); authority granted to the delegate (with details); the agreed upon time frame (consider training and practice); milestones; communication plan; performance standards; risk factors; resources needed; signatures; and date (Hewertson, 2015).

UNDERSTANDING HEALTHCARE FINANCING

Nurse leaders must understand various factors that impact healthcare financing. The level of understanding should be in relation to the nurse leader's role. For example, what is the organizational structure within which the nurse leader is currently practicing? In an ambulatory setting, the focus might be on which larger organization is in a position to purchase physician contracts. Another example would be nurse leaders working in a skilled nursing facility who need to align themselves with inpatient settings to provide seamless care. What components of the legal structure do nurse leaders need to be aware of? If an organization is in the process of acquiring additional sites, will the role of nurse leaders change or go away?

Some large organizations are choosing to become accountable care organizations. They are willing to risk acting as an insurance company for a specific patient population, meaning they need to provide seamless care throughout the continuum, even if they began as a sole acute care hospital. Nurse leaders must be part of the discussion about which subsets of the population should be targeted and the prioritization of disease groups based on groups with the fewest members and highest cost. This fact alone is critical for nurse leaders to understand. Working for an accountable care organization requires an understanding of the number of patients who will be served, how many physicians will be employed or affiliated, and the role of care coordination.

Depending on the role of nurse leaders, they must understand the impact of the following topics:

- Medicare valued-based purchasing
- Medicare inpatient payment
- Potential penalty for readmissions
- Hospital-acquired conditions
- Performance data benchmarking

Even if a nurse leader works in a specialty area such as pediatrics, all the previously listed topics are important to gain an understanding of where the organization lies on the continuum of care. Regardless of the position, for example, director of an inpatient unit or an ambulatory setting, or the chief nurse, the nurse leader needs to recognize the risks and benefits of becoming a payer versus fee-for-service. The nurse leader needs to understand how clinical care and insurance coverage will be integrated through staffing and infrastructure. Thus, keeping abreast of patient care delivery models and work design will assist nurse leaders in meeting the Triple Aim of improving the health of populations; providing better care experiences for patients, including quality and satisfaction; and lowering cost through continuous improvement. This is the overarching framework that nurse leaders keep in mind to guide staff in the provision of care. For example, nurse leaders consider how to effectively engage patients in prevention measures to reduce hospital admissions. Knowledge of the use of information management and technology permits nurse leaders to consider using the most cutting-edge telemedicine strategies for improving access and reducing costs for patients with chronic illness.

In addition, nurse leaders must maintain vigilant awareness of changes introduced by various regulatory agencies, such as The Joint Commission or the Centers for Medicare and Medicaid Services (CMS). For example, in 2014 CMS rewrote the hospital interpretive guidelines on discharge planning. Nurse leaders must understand how these new planning guidelines will affect the goal of reducing readmissions in a specific patient population along the continuum of care. A related competency is knowing how regulatory requirements of the Stark Law, Anti-Kickback Act, and False Claims Act impact relationships between physicians and the nurse leader's organization.

Nurse leaders can have the latest evidence delivered to them via email. For example, nurse leaders must be knowledgeable about The Joint Commission leadership standards topics such as the following:

- Conflicts of interest
- Contract management
- Disruptive behavior
- Patient safety standards
- Failure mode effects analysis (FMEA) standard
- Patient flow
- Conflict management

Nurse leaders can plug these search terms in to a browser, along with the Boolean terms "and" and "or" and the patient population or clinical setting to make sure they are not left behind.

Communication with hospital administration is key for nurse leaders who want to excel in understanding healthcare financing. In a recent issue of *HealthLeaders* magazine, Betbeze (2014) noted a skill set that chief executive officers say is important for nurse leaders. Nurse leaders need to be knowledgeable about the following to effectively communicate about their own work with other leaders:

- Mergers, acquisitions, partnerships
- Cost containment
- Skills that come from a clinical background
- Ability to align physicians and the hospital
- Performance metrics
- Leading a multisite operation
- Risk management
- Optimizing results along a continuum of care

At a bare minimum, nurse leaders need to know how their administration defines each listed item and, within each item, what the nurse leader controls.

HUMAN RESOURCE MANAGEMENT AND DEVELOPMENT

Nurse leaders are required to have some knowledge of business skills regardless of their role. The relationship among staffing, productivity, excellence, and performance is well documented in the literature. A Google Scholar search of those four terms yields articles about how nurse leaders influence the work environment; an example of using a nursing productivity committee to achieve cost savings and improve staffing at all levels; the impact of performance-based payment incentives on hospital nurses; and hundreds more. Nurse leaders strive to understand the implications of these factors within their own work environments. Answers to questions—such as, What is the skill mix necessary to achieve sustainable National Database of Nursing Quality Indicators? and How does my area's data impact the overall strategic goals of the hospital?—guide nurse leaders in mapping out a strategy for providing a sustainable, healthy work environment that is cost effective and provides the best patient outcomes.

Nurse leaders' skills in human resource management and development will directly impact nursing's work in designing the care management infrastructure. Very little is taught in academic settings about the use of medical homes, group visits, patient portals, and so forth. Understanding nurses' workload is more than the skill mix of a unit, such as the number of medical assistants, RNs, LPNs, monitor techs, health unit coordinators, paramedics, and so forth. Nurse leaders must know each discipline's scope of practice, which disciplines can be cross-trained to meet patient needs, and what the impact on patient care will be. What will the role of an advanced practice nurse be in the patient population for which the nurse leader is responsible? How will staff be educated to understand the importance of the tasks they perform for each patient in a caring manner? Failure to document the care and its impact on patients in the population will be critical to tracking and trending patterns.

Knowledge and skill in human resource management and development are directly related to the IOM key message that nurses should be full partners, with physicians and other healthcare professionals, in redesigning health care in the United States. For example, if the institution decides to use group visits to educate patients as part of their delivery model, what is the role of both patients and the staff to ensure the best outcomes? How will the outcomes be measured? What will happen if the patient is noncompliant? How do the rest of the care providers along the continuum participate in reinforcing the teaching? What will the role of technology be in assisting patients with self-management?

The greatest role nurse leaders have in the adventure of healthcare reform is that of champion for both the staff and patients. When nurse leaders step out of their comfort zone by learning more business skills and knowledge of the healthcare environment, both the staff and patients will be more satisfied. Nurse leaders need to draw a diagram of their world and post it at their desk as a frame of reference when making decisions that affect the patient population and the staff and when prioritizing which topic or issue should be addressed through continuous improvement.

What framework should nurse leaders use to create an environment in which the staff is willing to work toward significant changes that are required in the new healthcare environment? One strategy is to incorporate the standards of the American Association of Critical-Care Nurses *Healthy Work Environment* to answer the call for change. The six standards and their corresponding elements were developed in response to the 2001 IOM report titled *Crossing the Quality Chasm*:

- Standard 1: Skilled communication. Nurses must be as proficient in communication skills as they are in clinical skills.
- Standard 2: True collaboration. Nurses must be relentless in pursuing and fostering true collaboration.
- Standard 3: Effective decision making. Nurses must be valued and committed partners in making policy, directing and evaluating clinical care, and leading organizational operations.

- Standard 4: Appropriate staff. The staffing mix must ensure an effective match between patient needs and nurse competencies.
- Standard 5: Meaningful recognition. Nurses must be recognized and must recognize others for the value each person brings to the work of the organization.
- Standard 6: Authentic leadership. Nurse leaders must fully embrace the imperative of a healthy work environment, authentically live it, and engage others in its achievement.

Adaptation to change has always been a job requirement for nurses. Change is the key to progress and to the future; often that change begins with a focus on technology, without consideration for human relationships and political sensitivities. It is the task of nurse leaders to develop complimentary nursing systems that encompass new technology, improve patient care, and ultimately give greater satisfaction to nursing workers.

Thus, nurse leaders must seek a skill mix of staff members that are capable of providing care based on the *Nurse's Essential Role in Care Coordination* (American Nurses Association, 2012). The care coordination competencies include the following:

- Organization of care plan components
- Management of care to maximize independence and quality of life
- Assistance in identifying care options
- Communication with healthcare consumers, their families, and members of the healthcare system, especially during care transitions
- Advocacy for delivery of dignified care by the interprofessional team
- Documentation of coordination of care

Nurses' scope of practice within states and regions may dictate care delivery within the new healthcare system. For example, nurse leaders need to know the difference between accountable care organizations and medical homes. At their core, both are primary care models that strive to improve outcomes through care coordination. Both have defined populations, and both look at cost and quality. Nurse leaders need to work with risk management to learn risk mitigation skills and develop innovative programs to meet the needs of the population; care coordination can be part of that mix.

Patient engagement in accountable care organizations means the following:

- Involve patients in policy decision making
- Provide consistency throughout the care continuum
- Assess patient readiness to be active in the healthcare plan
- Foster better provider–patient communication
- Target patient transitions; that is, look at hand-offs of care

Nurse leaders need to know their role in patient engagement from a data collection, staffing resource, and strategic plan perspective.

SCOPE AND STANDARDS FOR NURSE ADMINISTRATORS: FRAMEWORK FOR PRACTICE

In a joint position statement on nursing administration education, the American Association of Colleges of Nursing and the American Nurses Association (ANA) outlined core abilities that are necessary for nurses in administrative roles. They include the abilities to use management skills that enhance collaborative relationships and team-based learning to advocate for patients and community partners, to embrace change and innovation, to manage resources effectively, to negotiate and resolve conflict, and to communicate effectively using information technology. Content for specialty education in nursing administration includes such concepts and constructs as strategic management, policy development, financial management and cost analysis, leadership, organizational development and business planning, and interdisciplinary relationships. Mentoring by expert executive nurses, engaging in research, and enacting evidence-based management (such as tracking the effectiveness of care, the cost of care, and patient outcomes) are also critical to the education of nurse administrators.

The ANA's *Nursing Administration: Scope and Standards of Practice* (2009) provides a conceptual model for educating and developing nurses in the professional practice of administrative nursing and health care. This document serves as a framework for this text, which focuses on the levels of nursing administration practice, standards of practice, and standards of professional performance for nurse administrators. Consideration of the scope and standards, the role of certification, Magnet recognition, and best practices are also included from this frame of reference. Management and leadership theory further reinforces the concepts required for nursing administrative practice. Such concepts are essential to managing a clinical practice discipline.

THE NURSE ADMINISTRATOR

The nurse administrator has been identified as a registered nurse whose primary responsibility is the management of healthcare delivery services and who represents nursing service. Nurse administrators can be found in a wide variety of settings, with entrepreneurial opportunities available throughout the healthcare arena. In addition to hospitals, home care, and skilled care, nurse administrators can also serve in such settings as assisted living, community health services, residential care, and adult day care. In these settings, the nurse administrator must be adequately prepared to face challenges in diverse fields such as information management, evidence-based care and management, legal and regulatory oversight, and ethical practices.

Spheres of Influence in Nursing Administrative Practice

The ANA conceptually divides nursing administration practice into spheres of influence: organization-wide authority; unit-based or service-line-based authority; program-focused authority; and project- or specific-task-based authority. Each has a particular focus that makes a unique contribution to the management of healthcare systems. The nurse executive's scope includes overall management of nursing practice, nursing education and professional development, nursing research, nursing administration, and nursing services. Nurse executives have the responsibility to manage within the context of the organization as a whole and to transform organizational values into daily operations, yielding an efficient, effective, and caring organization. Particular functions of nurse executives include leadership, development, implementation, and evaluation of protocols, programs, and services that are evidence based and congruent with professional standards.

Nurse managers are responsible to nurse executives and have more defined areas of nursing service. Advocating for and allocating available resources to facilitate effective, efficient, safe, and compassionate care based on standards of practice are the cornerstone roles of nurse managers. Nurse managers perform these management functions to deliver health care to patients. Nurse managers or administrators work at all levels to put into practice the concepts, principles, and theories of nursing management. They manage the organizational environment to provide a climate that is optimal to the provision of nursing care by clinical nurses and ancillary staff.

Management knowledge is universal; so is nursing management knowledge. It uses a systematic body of knowledge that includes concepts, principles, and theories that are applicable to all nursing management situations. A nurse manager who has applied this knowledge successfully in one situation can be expected to do so in new situations. Nursing management occurs at organization-wide, unit, or service-line levels; it is program focused and is based on projects or specific tasks. At the organization-wide level, it is frequently termed administration; however, the theories, principles, and concepts remain the same.

With decentralization and participatory management, the supervisor or middle management level has been largely eliminated. Nurse managers of clinical units are being educated in management theory and skills at the master's level. Clinical nurses are being educated in management skills that empower them to take action in managing groups of employees, as well as clients and families. Clinical nurse managers perform more of the coordinating duties among units, departments, and services. Nurse managers are responsible for the environment in which clinical nursing is practiced. Standards of practice and standards of professional performance serve as priorities for nurse administrative practice.

The standards of practice (as a framework for this text) include the following:

- Standard 1: Assessment. Collects comprehensive data pertinent to the issue, situation, or trends. Considers data collection systems and processes. Analyzes workflow in relation to effectiveness and efficiency of assessment processes. Evaluates assessment practices.
- Standard 2: Identifies issues, problems, or trends. Analyzes the assessment data to determine the issues, problems, or trends. Considers the identification and procurement of adequate resources for decision analysis. Promotes interdisciplinary collaboration. Promotes an organizational climate that supports the validation of problems and formulation of a diagnosis of the organization's environment, culture, and values that direct and support care delivery.
- Standard 3: Outcomes identification. Identifies expected outcomes for a plan that is individualized to the situation. Considers the interdisciplinary identification of outcomes and the development and utilization of databases that include nursing measures. Promotes continuous improvement of outcome-related clinical guidelines that foster continuity of care.
- Standard 4: Planning. Develops a plan that prescribes strategies and alternatives to attain expected outcomes. Considers development, maintenance, and evaluation of organizational systems that facilitate planning for care delivery. Fosters creativity and innovation that promote organizational processes for desired patient-defined and cost-effective outcomes. Collaborates

and advocates for staff involvement in all levels of organizational planning and decision making.

- Standard 5: Implementation. Considers the appropriate personnel to implement the design and improvement of systems and processes that ensure that interventions are carried out safely and effectively. Considers the efficient documentation of interventions and patient responses.
- Standard 5A: Coordination. Coordinates implementation and other associated processes. Provides leadership in the coordination of multidisciplinary healthcare resources for integrated delivery of care and services.
- Standard 5B: Health promotion, health teaching, and education. Employs strategies to foster health promotion, health teaching, and the provision of other educational services and resources.
- Standard 5C: Consultation. Provides consultation to influence the identified plan, enhance the abilities of others, and effect change.
- Standard 6: Evaluation. Evaluates progress toward attainment of outcomes. Considers support of participative decision making. Develops policies, procedures, and guidelines based on research findings and institutional measurement of quality outcomes. Conducts evaluations, including the integration of clinical, human resource, and financial data to adequately plan nursing and patient care.

Standards of professional performance such as quality of practice, education, professional practice evaluation, collegiality, collaboration, ethics, research, resource utilization, leadership, and advocacy are also integrated in the framework. These standards provide continuity of processes and systems of nursing administration.

Magnet Recognition Program and Scope and Standards for Nurse Administrators

The American Nurses Credentialing Center provides guidelines for the Magnet recognition program. This program's purpose is to recognize healthcare organizations that have demonstrated the very best in nursing care and professional nursing practice. Such programs have been recognized for having the best practices in nursing, and they also serve to attract and retain high-quality employees. A key objective of the program is to promote positive patient outcomes. This program also offers a vehicle for communicating best practices and strategies among nursing systems. Magnet designation allows consumers to locate healthcare organizations that have an evidence-based level of nursing care. Quality indicators and standards of nursing practice as identified by the ANA's *Nursing Administration: Scope and Standards of Practice* (2009) are the cornerstone of the Magnet recognition program. Qualitative and quantitative factors in nursing are also included in the appraisal process. In addition, the certification of nurse administrators is endorsed through the Magnet recognition program.

Qualifications of Nurse Administrators

Attaining the license, education, and experience required for various levels of nursing administrative practice is paramount to success in the role of nursing administrator. Nurse managers and nurse executives must have active registered nurse licenses and meet the requirements in the state in which they practice. Nurse executives should hold a bachelor's degree and master's degree (or higher), with a major in nursing.

Nurse managers should have a minimum of a bachelor's degree with a major in nursing. A master's degree with a focus in nursing is recommended, along with nationally recognized certification in nursing administration with an appropriate specialty. The backgrounds of professional nurses who are nurse administrators include clinical and administrative practice, which allow these registered nurses to consistently fulfill responsibilities that are inherent in their respective administrative roles.

Certification in Nursing Administration

The American Nurses Credentialing Center offers two levels for nursing administration, including an advanced level. Both certification examinations include the following domains: organization and structure, economics, human resources, ethics, and legal and regulatory issues. The domain of organization and structure accounts for the highest percentage of questions for the advanced-level certification examination. For the nurse manager level, the domain of human resources ranks highest. Both certification examinations include 175 questions, with 150 questions scored. Review and resource materials for certification are available and can provide continuing education units for the certification examination.

The management theory depicted in the ANA *Nursing Administration: Scope and Standards of Practice* (2009) is the underlying framework that supports the work of nurse administrators.

Strategic Management

An institution's management determines what care will be offered for population health management and the contracts that will be put in place to deliver that care. These decisions set priorities for the investment plan and shape the care management infrastructure. Nurse leaders must participate in networking opportunities to stay abreast of how their work is impacted by other departments, contracted outside agencies, and state and federal government rulings.

From a broad strategic perspective, hospital administrators shape the organization through decisions made; for example, the purchase of physicians' offices, sale of the organization to larger systems, and entering into risk-based contracts. In addition, administrators rely heavily on nurse leaders to ensure the institution does not receive a financial penalty for not meeting performance benchmarks as part of the CMS Hospital-Acquired Condition (HAC) Reduction Program.

The HAC Reduction Program is an example of why nurse leaders must have business skills in human resource management to ensure they have hired staff members who understand their role in providing direct patient care.

Strategic management focuses on core planning, including developing the strategic plan, business planning, and forecasting and performance management. In other words, a strategy is defined to meet the desired outcomes. Surveying the macro environment is key: What are the industry trends? Who should we benchmark with? What is considered best practice? In essence, a gap analysis—or a strengths, weaknesses, opportunities, and threats (SWOT) analysis—of the institution's characteristics, objective data, and subjective elements is completed. A SWOT analysis also includes physicians' readiness for change (if they are educated and ready to focus on performance improvement, to use ambulatory electronic medical records, and to manage risk contracts), leadership readiness (if the system is ready for a shift to population risk), and infrastructure readiness (if IT tools are in place to monitor quality and facilitate data exchange, and if management staff is in place to address the complex needs of the patient).

Nurse leaders must understand that the healthcare market is changing faster than organizations can respond to meet needs of patients. For example, inpatient volumes will continue to decrease, and the importance of medical homes will increase.

Value-Based Purchasing

Value-based purchasing (VBP) describes a broad set of performance-based payment strategies that align financial incentives to providers' performance on a set of prescribed indicators. VBP strategies are used by both public and private payers as a means of spearheading quality improvement and reduced healthcare spending. This may not be enough in considering the larger systems view from a complexity perspective as holding providers accountable for care delivery may only serve as a small attempt at radical change. Providing financial means to incentivize provider performance using measures of health outcomes may also contribute to better outcomes; however, this may only provide a short-term win. It is important to find a balance of structure, process, and outcome measures from a global perspective. Value-based purchasing, which has been defined as a demand-side strategy, is a necessary step for clinical quality improvement (The National Business Coalition on Health, 2015).

One aspect of healthcare reform is a payment model in which fee-for-service becomes pay for physician performance and value-based purchasing, followed by bundled payments to be shared, and ultimately leading to global payments. Contracting for population health management will be in large part based on institutions obtaining a large portion of their business from risk-based contracts. Nurse leaders must understand that regardless of where they work, their piece of care management is critical to the financial success of both their own area and to the strategic success of their institutions. For example, care management relies heavily on documentation, and nurse leaders must work with the IT infrastructure across the continuum of care to ensure seamless transitions for patients.

Patient Care Delivery Models

Strategic management includes patient care delivery models, such as integrated care, coordinated seamless health care, and eventually a community-integrated healthcare system. The institution must analyze and strategize to become a risk-capable organization. The structure for managing organizations will be dependent on populations, costs, budgets, monitoring, and other factors that contribute to a transformational and seamless, integrated community healthcare system.

The role of nurse leaders is often to direct teams that are responsible for improving the patient experience. Understanding the origins of data that influences nurse leaders' work and how to use that data will impact nurse leaders' decisions about the responsibilities of the care team. When nurse leaders are conscious of costs, from staffing to removing waste from the system, they make decisions that impact the strategic direction of the institution.

Accountable Care Organizations

Nurse leaders must understand that the institution's strategic management will include how much risk the administration is willing to accept. If a nurse leader is working for an accountable care organization, which is a model of care delivery, he or she will focus on quality, cost, and managing performance against risk. In this model, payers and employers expect providers to assume more risk for the care they are providing to the covered populations. Improving costs includes decreased spending on drugs, decreased lengths of stay, and fewer readmissions and emergency department visits. Reducing variations in care patterns through the use of clinical pathways and evidence-based care guidelines will achieve the best possible outcomes for patients with chronic illness. Nurse leaders are driving care integration through the use of care coordination across the continuum.

Marketing

The standard definition of marketing is the five Ps: price, product, promotion, place, and people:

- Price: How much does the product cost in relation to the value received?
- Product: What are the healthcare consumers receiving in relation to their needs or wants? Are we exceeding expectations?
- Promotion: What information is available about physicians, the nursing staff, the cleanliness of the hospital, and so forth? In other words, what is the patient experience?
- Place: Is care being offered close to where patients live?
- People: What is the perception of how caring the staff is? Are healthcare consumers' cultural differences taken into account?

To nurse leaders, marketing is a complete awareness of how their work impacts the overall strategy of the institution in relation to the work. For example, since customers now have an array of choices for insurance and healthcare services, there is more competition based on cost, convenience, and quality of care. What will the driving factor be for patients as they make choices in light of continually increasing deductibles? For example, if the goal is to keep patients in the care network, nurse leaders must champion their staff's critical thinking ability and competency so patients are not subject to hospital-acquired conditions or readmissions that would incur penalties.

Information Management and Technology

The Institute for Healthcare Improvement (IHI) Triple Aim (Population, Experience of care, Per capita costs) provides strong aims that nurse leaders can champion to improve overall health care for citizens and reduce fragmentation in the healthcare delivery system. The Triple Aim aligns closely with the nursing process and serves as a framework for translating evidence-based practice and technological changes into patient care delivery.

The Triple Aim provides knowledge for asking hard questions to champion care. Nurse leaders understand how information and technology can be used as part of the nursing process (assess, plan, implement, and evaluate). Nurse leaders start by realizing that the IOM key message of effective workforce planning and policy making depends on better data collection and an improved information infrastructure, which requires nursing to venture into the relative unknown. Nurse leaders need to ask questions about the following topics, which will inform the care delivery model for the unit or patient population:

- Use of registry data to improve patient outcomes
- Use of electronic medical record data to validate or change nursing practice
- Use of physician data to inform the continuum of care
- Use of public scorecards for benchmarking
- Use of specific metrics to measure and share with the public

Nurse leaders are required to establish data-driven processes for responding to problems and poor outcomes and for communicating to administration, staff, and patients. Nurse leaders must assist caregivers in understanding the value of their roles, which can occur in part through the use of data. Is there a caregiver outlier whose practice could lead to a hospital-acquired infection? How does a nurse leader help this caregiver, or the entire staff, change?

Collection and Development of Data

Nurse leaders need to gather both hard and soft data about the current work for discussion with stakeholders. Nurse leaders need to participate in determining what benchmarks—such as those from the National Database of Nursing Quality Indicators and Leapfrog—their organization will participate in for staff satisfaction, patient satisfaction, and payer satisfaction. Coupled with anecdotal evidence (an example of soft data), the data are analyzed and used to effect change when indicated. Personnel, particularly managers, can be educated to make and manage change. They will learn about labor power planning and use rather than leaving this function entirely to the human resources department. They will learn about financial management rather than depend on the accounting department to take care of it. These are areas in which effective strategies can be developed to foster external cooperative efforts among chief nurse executives in similar institutions and organizations within a community. Such concepts can be expanded to clinical services. If a division of nursing cannot afford to use such specialists, such as a full-time mental health nurse practitioner, several organizations can collectively contract for the services of one specialist. Thus, change becomes a cooperative venture.

Advocating for hard wiring of needed data components into an electronic medical record will provide nurse leaders with a much-needed source to plan and ultimately drive change as organizations become engaged in building accountable care organizations.

For example, in a 2012 article funded by the Commonwealth Fund, Van Otters and colleagues (2012) developed a table noting organizational capabilities that nurse leaders need to have knowledge of, as well as how their own organizations are choosing to implement these aspects of accountable care from a data perspective. Key organizational capabilities that facilitate delivery of accountable care include health information technology, care management strategies, and quality and performance improvement strategies. For example, organizational capabilities in health information technology might include disease registries, data warehousing, and predictive modeling to identify high-risk patients. Care management strategies might include disease management programs (diabetes, asthma), hospitalists, care navigators, patient navigators for cancer patients to support care transitions, home care, urgent care centers, inpatient care managers, and multidisciplinary care teams. Quality and performance improvement strategies include Six Sigma, physician champions, physician-level performance data that are reported internally, Lean, Plan-Do-Study-Act, and standardization.

Nurse leaders must know what measures are in use from a strategic perspective. What is the organization tracking and why? What measures is the discipline involved with, and what is expected of the particular work environment? Is there room for integration of measures? Where are the data posted? How often are results given to the staff?

Core Set of Health Care Quality Measures for Adults Enrolled in Medicaid is a 174-page document that nurse leaders must be aware of in terms of which measures impact their specific patient population, who is accountable, and where the information is documented. For example, nurse leaders must understand documentation of the percentage of Medicaid enrollees aged 18 to 64 years who received an influenza vaccination between July 1 of the measurement year and the date when the Consumer Assessment of Healthcare Providers and Systems (CAHPS) 5.0H survey was completed. For nurse leaders working within integrated care systems, something this simple can have an impact when it is not completed.

There are three types of measurements that are often used in improvement efforts. The IHI describes them in the following manner:

Outcome Measures
How does the system impact the values of patients, their health and wellbeing? What are impacts on other stakeholders such as payers, employees, or the community?

- For diabetes: Average hemoglobin A1c level for population of patients with diabetes
- For access: Number of days to 3rd next available appointment
- For critical care: Intensive Care Unit (ICU) percent unadjusted mortality
- For medication systems: Adverse drug events per 1,000 doses

Process Measures
Are the parts/steps in the system performing as planned? Are we on track in our efforts to improve the system?

- For diabetes: Percentage of patients whose hemoglobin A1c level was measured twice in the past year
- For access: Average daily clinician hours available for appointments
- For critical care: Percent of patients with intentional rounding completed on schedule

Balancing Measures (looking at a system from different directions/dimensions)
Are changes designed to improve one part of the system causing new problems in other parts of the system?

- For reducing time patients spend on a ventilator after surgery: Make sure re-intubation rates are not increasing
- For reducing patients' length of stay in the hospital: Make sure readmission rates are not increasing (Institute for Healthcare Improvement, 2014, Three Types of Measures section)

The use of data in measuring and managing healthcare quality measures requires creative thinking, innovation, and change management.

Change Management

Changing organizations for excellence requires a change in the ways people think and interact to create workplaces and systems that are purposeful and are aligned with evidence-based results. Whether nurse leaders are involved in research, education, or administration, the use of change theories as a means of creating a healthy work environment is considered.

The American Organization of Nurse Executives (2005) competencies include change management as part of the leadership skill set. The responsibilities of nurse leaders in using change management are as follows:

1. Use change theory to plan for the implementation of organizational changes.
2. Serve as a change agent, assisting others in understanding the importance, necessity, impact, and process of change.
3. Support staff during times of difficult transitions.
4. Recognize one's own reaction to change and strive to remain open to new ideas and approaches.
5. Adapt a leadership style to fit situational needs.

Using the change management theories addressed in this chapter provides nurse leaders with guidance in how to creatively think while solving problems on a daily basis. Hewertson (2015) describes five responses to change, stated as characteristics: victim, critic, bystander, charger, and navigator. Descriptions of these characteristics are as follows:

- The victim exhibits behaviors that consistently resist change and feels angry, depressed, or miserable. The victim often reverts to his or her old ways of doing work and will often whine, making statements such as, "Why is this happening to me?" and "Why can't things stay the same?" The victim can move forward by taking charge of and being responsible for what is happening in his or her life.
- The critic looks for reasons why the change will not be a success and fails to see any positive outcomes from the change. Critics believe they know better than anyone else. Statements that critics would make might include, "This has never worked before, and it won't work now," and "They don't know what is going on or what they are doing." If you are a critic, you can move out of this response by thinking about positive possibilities and opportunities that could occur because of the change. It is important to consider how and what could be done to influence change. Hewertson describes the difference between a critic and a resistor. Critics tend to be naysayers without positive intent or solutions, whereas "resistors come with ideas for alternative solutions and share their concerns based on positive intent" (2015, p. 212). Hewertson notes that it is important to listen to resistors because they have important information or important reasons, whether they turn out to be right or wrong.

- The bystander is reluctant to get involved, waits for others to take the lead, and does not offer input, solutions, or ideas. The bystander plays it safe. A bystander might say, "If I ignore this long enough, maybe it will go away," and "I'll wait until others have made the decision." A bystander may move forward by asking for more details and information and finding out what role he or she might play in the change efforts, not withholding, and finding ways to share ideas.
- The charger often leaps before looking and may push others too hard, force the issue, not listen to others, and ignore new and important information. The charger may say, "I know best, and I'll just force this to happen and be done with it!" The charger can improve his or her ability to work with change by considering how the change may affect others and trying to be empathic. The charger can ask questions to get input and engage others by listening carefully before making changes.
- The navigator looks for ways to reduce negative reactions, explores reasons for the change and how it might impact those involved, and is alert to culture shifts. The navigator finds ways to be useful, looks for opportunities to improve, and forms positive and supportive relationships with those affected by the change. The navigator may say, "This change presents opportunities to do things differently" and "I'm bound to make mistakes, but I'll learn from them." Being a navigator means helping yourself and others successfully move through change. The navigator can have a positive impact and influence the process.

Hewertson notes that "it is not uncommon for a person to react to change by experiencing and expressing all five responses in a relatively short time" (2015, p. 214).

Hewertson shares eight characteristics that change efforts have in common:

- Create a shared vision beginning with the end in mind and enroll stakeholders in the vision.
- Engage key stakeholders and build consensus for the need for change.
- Bring to awareness and share explicitly the change model and process you will be using.
- Create the plan: what, how, who, when?
- Begin the plan and processes and bring to awareness some quick wins.
- Provide ongoing surveillance and streamline the process along the way.
- Embed the new realities organizationally.
- Celebrate! Garner support for new and desired behaviors. (Hewertson, 2015)

Hewertson identifies three strategies that can lead to successful change:

1. Engage all the people affected by the change in the vision, design, planning, implementation, and evaluation of the changes.
2. Empower all the people affected by the change to take risks, innovate, and take action.
3. Embed what works within your systems, processes, and policies, and eliminate what does not work. (Hewertson, 2015, p. 218)

Strategies for Overcoming Obstacles to Change

Drucker notes that change cannot be managed; however, by understanding patterns and change, a manager can stay ahead of expected trends. Drucker suggests that managers lead change and view it as an opportunity. Nurse managers can lead change and act as change agents. One strategy nurse leaders can use is to hire a consultant to make a diagnosis and recommend programs, with the goal of improving the productivity of nurse personnel while giving them job satisfaction. The decision to hire a consultant must be tempered with the economic climate and the number of initiatives the nurse leader or manager has chosen to implement.

Effectively led change results in improvement of patient care services, better morale, increased productivity, and meeting patient and staff needs. Change is an art, the mastery of which can be exhilarating, refreshing, challenging, and exciting, because it represents opportunity. Change is facilitated when nurse employees are assigned to adapt to changing job requirements.

Leading Change

There are many change theories for nurse leaders to choose from when working in a complex adaptive system. Choosing a theory as a framework also requires nurse leaders to understand why change fails and the steps that can be taken to mitigate the potential for failure. Kotter (1995) outlines eight steps to transform an organization. Almost 2 decades later, those steps continue to be championed by many who are working to ensure their healthcare organizations continue to thrive. The steps are as follows:

1. Establish a sense of urgency by examining market and competitive realities. To nurse leaders, after a SWOT analysis is completed, there is a greater understanding of their role, which can include directing teams, integrating care across systems, and more.
2. Form a powerful guiding coalition by creating an interprofessional team capable of leading the change. Having champions who understand the rationale for why the change is being driven and being able to reinforce the change on a daily basis are important to making change sustainable.
3. Create a vision for the nurse leader's work that is supportive of the strategic plan. Developing care strategies to ensure the work performed by each staff member results in a positive patient experience is an example of how nurse leaders support the larger vision.
4. Communicate the vision as a means of embedding the change into the culture of work, which requires nurse leaders to market to their own staff. Providing a rationale of how their work impacts the patient experience and the budget and having a shared mental model to communicate the changes are important to the transformation.
5. Empower others to act on the vision by removing obstacles and changing systems that are not supportive of the vision, which requires nurse leaders to work with all levels of staff.
6. Plan for and create short-term wins, which involves meaningful recognition for staff who are implementing the change. Implement the principles of continuous improvement while working toward creating change that results in a high-reliability culture.

7. Consolidate improvements and produce still more change.
8. Institutionalize new approaches.

Nurse leaders who are change agents must understand how each decision will ultimately affect the satisfaction of both nurses and patients.

Evidence-Based Practice

Kalisch and Curley (2008) describe a case study in which an organization identified its strengths, weaknesses, opportunities, and threats through an analysis process. A transformation process was illustrated that included five phases: (1) setting the stage for change, (2) management training, (3) strategic planning, (4) developing and implementing changes at the organizational level, and (5) developing and implementing changes at the unit level. Lessons learned included the following: support from the top, adequate resources, willingness to face the brutal facts, early attention to sustainability, infusion into the grass roots, unrelenting communication, emphasis on building and maintaining trust, ensuring early wins, not declaring success too soon, and recognizing that you cannot fully know how. Encouraging nursing personnel to become involved in new nursing endeavors at work, in the community, and in professional organizations, as well as undertaking other activities will increase knowledge and skills in change management. Additionally, encouraging risk taking and acceptance of personal responsibility will increase accountability for quality, safety, and process improvement. The need for change and appreciating the ongoing challenge and continuing efforts to transform were underscored in this case study.

Successful companies hire and keep creative employees. They keep people by knowing how to manage, motivate, and reward them. Nurse leaders seek to create teams of managers who offer different creative skills. One nurse manager may assist a nurse leader in the people portion of the planned change; another may be creative on the technical or data side. Nurse leaders have nurse managers who are practical problem solvers and team players. All must be decisive.

In essence, change is all about critical thinking because nurse leaders must think through all aspects of planning the change by answering the following questions:

- What is the desired outcome? Is there evidence to support the change and how will it be measured—via research, performance improvement processes, or evidence-based practice projects?
- Who are the stakeholders, and how will they be involved?
- What change theory will be used?
- Has a baseline needs assessment been performed?
- How and where does this planned change fit in to strategic initiatives, such as implementation of the American Association of Critical-Care Nurses' *Healthy Work Environments*?
- Will there be variations among the implementation plans depending on location?
- What is the level of understanding (dual processing) and commitment (social and emotional intelligence) of staff?
- Who needs to be involved in the design of the change process?
- Have the complex adaptive system issues been taken into consideration during implementation?

Change involves nursing leaders' continued awareness of all aspects of their nursing environment. It requires planning by using any of the various change theories. Nurse leaders use communication, leadership, and motivation theory to overcome resistance and gain support to make the change work. The implemented change is continually evaluated to make it sustainable and effective. Prior to each new change, nurse leaders must have predetermined how the new change will be integrated into the current work environment.

Nurse leaders who use evidence as part of change management can facilitate innovation. Evidence-based decision making is not just for use by direct-care clinicians. Communication, shared decision making, and quality improvement are all pieces of transformational leadership, which promotes change in diverse healthcare systems. There are many evidence-based frameworks from which the nurse leader can choose to determine which evidence to use (Melynk & Fineout-Overholt, 2014).

High-Reliability Organizations

Many organizations are on the journey to becoming high-reliability organizations (HROs). An HRO is an organization that operates under very trying conditions all the time and yet manages to have fewer than its fair share of bad concerns. Reliability is the probability that a system will work correctly, as it should. Safety is defined as the absence of harm. Patient safety keeps reliability as a priority so that when possible, standardized care practices are consistently delivered without harm each and every time. In conjunction with both staff and hospital administration, nurse leaders determine what behaviors staff need to demonstrate in order to have a culture of safety.

The characteristics of an HRO are as follows:

- Preoccupation with failure
- Reluctance to simplify
- Sensitivity to operations (HROs distinguish themselves in this characteristic)
- Commitment to resilience
- Deference to expertise

An example from an HRO is a nurse leader who chooses to learn from the staff how a change is being accepted. Deferring to expertise is an example of effective decision making, which is a standard of a healthy working environment. If the environment has a shared governance model, nurse leaders have a ready way (sharing experiences) to explore the specific issue that needs to be addressed.

The IHI offers tools on their website that allow nurse leaders to create a framework for staff to use to ensure that care is standardized and consistent to prevent poor patient outcomes.

Culture of Safety

A culture of safety must surround the nurse leader's change efforts. The characteristics of a culture include the following:

- Shared and transmitted: A culture of safety holds both staff and patients free from harm as the core value. Nurse leaders work with staff in a shared governance model to determine expected safety behaviors that are shared as newly hired RNs are socialized into the culture.

- Social and symbols: In today's environment nurse leaders use tools such as whiteboards, rounding, safety huddles for each shift, and a daily organizational brief to embed a safety culture into the social fabric of the unit or area.
- Learned and acquired: Policies and procedures are written with both patient and staff safety at the heart in the context of standardizing best practice.
- Ideational: Nurse leaders use the forum of shared governance as the creative process of generating, developing, and communicating new ideas at the point of care. This leads to staff members owning their practice and valuing their contribution to a healthy work environment.
- Gratifies human needs: Caregivers, by the very nature of their work, desire to help others. Nurse leaders must keep the requirement of business skills, such as healthcare financing and the need for data, within the context of relationship-based care in a healthy work environment. Often this can be a source of concern because individual patient needs might not be perceived as most important.
- Adaptive: Nurse leaders must be cautious when considering adaptation within a safety culture. Standardization of care through the levels of high reliability, such as the creation of checklists or hard wiring requirements into the electronic medical record, will ensure that nurse leaders follow the overall safety culture requirements. Just as a unit policy can be more stringent than an institutional policy, so should a culture of safety.
- Tends toward integrating a society: As nurse leaders work as team members transforming health care, keeping the patient front and center in the continuum of care will provide a focus for effective decision making across the continuum. For example, how will the role of the care manager interact with the role of the clinical inpatient RN, the RN navigator in the community, and the ambulatory RN working in an outpatient clinic?
- Cumulative: Having a cumulative safety culture requires nurse leaders to work toward sustainability of expected safety behaviors, knowledge of current policies and procedures, and the importance of communicating using a shared mental model. For example, The Joint Commission notes that the predominance of serious safety events is rooted in communication issues. Working toward having the entire interprofessional staff use the same communication techniques will potentially reduce these communication errors.

Tools and strategies that have been noted to be effective in facilitating a culture of safety include:

1. SBAR: Communication begins with noting the Situation, the Background of the issue, the Assessment of the issue or patient, followed by the suggested Recommendation.
2. STAR: Stop, Think, Act, Review is a form of mindfulness that is very appropriately used by caregivers who may need to review a procedure they have not recently performed.
3. ARCC: Ask a question, Request a change, voice a Concern, and use the Chain of command.

For nurse leaders, a culture of safety provides a blueprint for decision making as it provides solidarity. An organization's culture is noted to be a predominating force in impacting change and sustained improvement. A longtime organizational guru, Drucker has been noted to communicate that culture trumps knowledge. For nurse leaders, being aware of the need for an embedded culture of safety to use as a framework for change is critical to the success of sustainable change.

Organizational Environment

Nurse leaders can be more successful by paying attention to the organizational environment in which change is introduced and the manner in which it is done. Leaders need to be committed to a change and to support it by actions that express their attitudes. When nurse leaders attempt to impose change in an authoritarian manner, people often resist it. Concern for employees is as important as concern for patients. Leaders can establish an environment for change by doing the following:

- Emphasizing relationships with and among groups
- Bringing out mutual trust and confidence
- Emphasizing interdependence and shared responsibility
- Containing group membership and responsibility by preventing individuals from belonging to too many groups and ensuring that the same responsibilities are not given to several groups
- Sharing control and responsibility widely
- Resolving conflict through bargaining or problem-solving discussions (Longo, 2013)
- Permitting job movement to facilitate careers
- Anticipating and rewarding change, thus institutionalizing it (Longo, 2013)
- Modifying the nursing organizational structure to accommodate changes that provide growth and development
- Promoting a can-do attitude
- Providing predictability and stability by maintaining job security, sharing bad news early, and shifting concern to teamwork and process improvement (Longo, 2013)

When the organizational climate changes, employees change their behaviors. A desired organizational climate fosters high-quality patient care (Longo, 2013).

SUMMARY

Nurse leaders strive to use knowledge and skill to drive staff accountability for implementing and sustaining organizational change. Providing staff with the rationale for why changes being made at the strategic level are filtering to the point-of-care level assists caregivers with understanding their own value in meeting the IHI's Triple Aim of improving the health of populations, providing a better care experience for patients (including quality and satisfaction), and lowering costs through continuous improvement. Implementing new models of patient care delivery requires nurse leaders to be knowledgeable of healthcare financing, human resource management, strategic management, marketing, and information management and technology. By having these business skills, nurse managers can do the following:

- Create a healthy work environment for the interprofessional care team to implement evidence-based best practice
- Foster the use of principles of an HRO by following the cycle of continuous quality improvement
- Frame the work of a complex adaptive system within change management theory
- Incorporate quantitative and qualitative data from the organizational system, public sector, and payers into all aspects of leadership

By being accountable for the required changes, nurse leaders implement two of the key messages of the IOM (2011) report on the future of nursing: nurses should be full partners with physicians and other healthcare professionals in redesigning health care in the United States, and effective workforce planning and policy making require better data collection and improved information infrastructure. Nurse leaders have the opportunity to champion safe, effective, and efficient care delivery.

REFLECTIVE QUESTIONS

Nurse leaders consider the following questions as they work to be full partners in the creation of an organizational structure that is accountable to the strategic plan:

1. How does a complex adaptive system affect day-to-day decision making? What factors need to be taken into account when creating a climate for change?
2. What data inputs and outputs are used to monitor the work to ensure effectiveness for implementation of the Triple Aim?
3. What is the type of organizational structure within which nurse leaders work? Are you aware of the status of each characteristic?
4. How does awareness of a culture of safety impact the care provided by individual caregivers? How does it impact the strategic plan?
5. What are the key components of developing an organizational structure that maximizes efficiency and profitability?
6. What is the importance for nurse leaders of having business skills related to marketing, information management, and human resources?
7. What impact does having knowledge of evidence-based practice have on the overall healthcare climate of the organization?
8. How does the use of quality improvement tools impact care?
9. Why is it important for nurse leaders to work with interprofessional care teams to redesign health care in the United States?
10. What is the importance of governance in a work design that results in a new patient care delivery model?
11. Why should nurse leaders be involved in data collection and improving the infrastructure as a means of workforce planning and policy making?

CASE STUDY 6-1   Future of Nursing

Susan Allen

In response to the IOM's (2011) *Future of Nursing* recommendations for nurses to achieve higher levels of education and training, one midwestern pediatric and academic medical center set annual targets for increasing the number of clinical nurses with bachelor of science (BSN) in nursing degrees and increasing the number of clinical nurses who have specialty certifications.

During the most recent fiscal year, the percentage of BSN-prepared clinical nurses (72.2%) outperformed the goal of 70%. A generous tuition reimbursement policy, RN-to-BSN cohorts, including an on-site program, and other collaborations with local colleges of nursing supported nurses returning to school to earn a BSN degree. The BSN degree is a requirement in the Nursing Clinical Advancement program for attainment of the second-level position, Registered Nurse II.

In contrast, the percentage of specialty-certified clinical nurses dropped, and the fiscal year goal of 35% was not met. At the beginning of the fiscal year, 31.2% of clinical nurses were certified, and currently that number has dropped to 27.9%. The hospital provides free on-site certification review courses for many specialty certifications and provides reimbursement for certification examination fees (with proof of passing the exam) and reimbursement for recertification fees. For the pediatric nurses' specialty certification exam (the most common certification that clinical nurses hold at this hospital), nurses do not have to pay any upfront costs. Recognition of all certified nurses occurs annually on March 19, Certified Nurses Day, and via multiple weekly, monthly, and quarterly internal hospital publications, in addition to unit-based recognitions. Currently, specialty certification is not a requirement in the Nursing Clinical Advancement program. The hospital provides many no-cost, on-site continuing education opportunities for nurses to meet their recertification educational needs, in addition to generous endowed education funds to support education conference travel for clinical nurses.

During annual performance management time, managers work with clinical nurses to establish performance goals for the coming fiscal year and provide coaching opportunities for nurses' professional growth. Anecdotal reports have been received from managers about clinical nurses' dissatisfaction with having to provide upfront costs for recertification and a perceived lack of importance of specialty certification, resulting in certification lapses. There is a painful awareness about low numbers of certified clinical nurses this fiscal year, which has focused attention on this issue.

Case Study Questions

1. What is the role of the nurse leader in addressing declining specialty certification numbers?
2. How do internal and external motivators play a role in specialty certification and recertification?
3. What unit-based actions or activities to increase specialty certification and recertification can the nurse leader recommend?
4. What hospital-wide actions or activities to increase specialty certification and recertification can the nurse leader recommend?
5. How does the nurse leader determine whether increasing RN certifications will impact patient outcomes?
6. What factors does the nurse leader take into consideration to justify the expenditure necessary to increase the percentage of certified RNs?

CASE STUDY 6-2   Shared Governance

Anne Longo

The implementation of a shared governance structure and strengthening this structure as it matures and adapts within an organizational culture are a never-ending process. The cultural changes that occur in an organization with shared governance are significant (Porter-O'Grady, 2009). Currently, such cultural shifts are compounded by the additional changes happening due to the internal and external political and economic forces evident in today's healthcare environment (IOM, 2011). Nursing leadership is critical to creating improvements in health care (IOM, 2011). Changes in the culture of the healthcare environment are needed to strengthen nursing practice and better position nurses to be the leaders they need to be to improve patient care delivery and manage the environment of care. Clinical nurses' participation in a shared governance structure, and shared decision making with nursing managers within that structure, may be one way for this to occur.

Cincinnati Children's Hospital Medical Center has had a nursing shared governance structure since 1989. An allied health shared governance structure was added in 1999. These parallel structures remained functional but separate until 2008, when an enhanced interprofessional shared governance was launched (Hoying & Allen, 2011). A qualitative study was recently conducted to explore the experiences of clinical nurses as they moved into formal nursing shared governance chair and chair-elect positions in the nursing governance structure (Allen, 2013). Two findings in this study confirmed the importance of the nurse executive and manager roles in these young leaders' professional development.

1. Moving from "Just a Staff Nurse" Self-Perceptions

To discover the leader within them, the clinical nurse council leaders often needed to overcome the belief of being "just a nurse," a common and deeply held conviction by clinical nurses in an organizational culture. As one study participant noted, "I was probably sometimes intimidated to open up, when you were saying like, how, you know, I think in some of the forums you feel like, 'hmm, I'm just a nurse.'" Another said she had confidence in herself as a nurse, but this confidence did not extend to her role as a leader: "I'm a very good nurse, I don't, I have a hard time giving myself that credit, I can't, I have a hard time doing that, so to step up to a leader role, it was hard and I think it's taking time to have that confidence." Many of the council leaders stated it was a nursing manager who assisted them to realize their own importance in their participation in the governance of the organization. These managers encouraged them to speak up and share their knowledge and experiences to influence decision making.

2. Seeing the Big Picture

Many clinical nurses have had little exposure to what goes on in the healthcare environment beyond the area in which they work. Nursing leaders have a critically important role in providing the organizational context and connecting the work of the councils with that of the larger organization. Nurse managers have knowledge of the strategic directions, human and financial resources and limitations, emerging healthcare trends locally and beyond, and the political and economic climate of their organization. Communicating this knowledge is essential for effective and pertinent decision making to occur in the shared governance councils.

The council chairs and chair-elects in the study (Allen, 2013) noted that partnerships with managers helped clinical nurses understand the big picture and advance their accountability for professional practice. A council chair shared an example of a discussion in Cincinnati Children's nursing divisional coordinating council about productivity, time keeping, and budgeting, concepts that were unfamiliar to the clinical nurses on the council, but essential factors in the operational and economic health of the organization. After deepening their understanding of these economic factors, the council

(continues)

CASE STUDY 6-2   Shared Governance (Continued)

members established a goal to partner with managers to ensure clinical nurse engagement and understanding of the economic factors of the big picture; that is, "why we are doing it, rather than just your manager saying you can't clock in before six minutes to. Or you can't do overtime . . . or our staffing is such that you've got to float here or do whatever." The council chair believed this kind of partnership between nurse managers and clinical nurses would lead to shared understanding of one another's roles and increase clinical nurses' caring about the economic health of the organization.

Lessons Learned

The role of the nursing manager is pivotal to the successful implementation and strengthening of shared governance, and indeed, the presence of managers who are visibly committed to its success may be an essential factor. As can be seen in the examples presented here, a second essential factor is the ability of those managers to develop clinical nurses to be the leaders they need to be for a shared governance culture to thrive.

Case Study Questions

1. Describe how your organization could replicate this qualitative study to enhance your existing professional practice model.
2. Identify effective strategies that you could use in your organizational system to change the "just a nurse" perception and to see the big picture in your professional nursing practice environment.

CASE STUDY 6-3   Culture of Safety

Lisa Keegan

Developing a successful culture of safety at the point of care is accomplished through staff working within the elements of an effective safety culture. Two units decided to create a safety culture. One unit cares for patients with complex GI issues and patients requiring colorectal, gynecological, and urological surgery; the other unit cares for patients who are listed for or have had kidney, liver, or small bowel transplants and patients who have had bariatric or other complex surgical procedures. The nurse leader supports the culture by creating a healthy work environment where there is a commitment of leadership to safety, all employees are empowered and engaged in ongoing vigilance, and there is organizational learning from errors and near misses (precursor events). On one unit, the nurse leader had implemented the following high-reliability processes:

- Organizational safety brief
- Rounding to influence
- Unit huddles
- Charge nurse huddles (flow, staffing, safety issues)
- Senior leader walks rounds
- Medical response team
- Safety team

The nurse leader also created a healthy work environment that includes the following:

- Interdisciplinary shared governance
- Clinical systems improvement
- Improvement science training

CASE STUDY 6-3   Culture of Safety (Continued)

- Rapid cycle improvement collaborative
- Crucial conversations training
- Safety coach training

How did the nurse leader put it all together? One example is a standardized shift huddle at 0700 and 1900 for about 5 minutes that includes reviewing the state of the unit, which addresses a review of safety data, current status (census, watchers, staffing), a look ahead (admits, discharges, potential problems, regulatory visitors), a look back (any concerns from the prior shift), and tracking safety issues.

Another example is standardization of the shift report, including in-room safety checks, introduction, checking the patient's ID bracelet, review of fluids and medications, emergency equipment, and review and edit of the patient plan of care.

Another component of the safety culture is night talks, where the resident and charge nurse discuss information obtained from nurses by the charge nurse, including RN concerns, family concerns, and unclear orders. In addition, the resident meets with family members or assesses patients as needed.

The patient and family remain at the center of all decision making, leading to better patient outcomes.

Case Study Questions

1. How would knowledge of marketing influence the creation of this safety culture?
2. What additional outcome measures could the point-of-care nurse leader use to ensure sustainability of the culture?
3. How does the nurse leader know when evidence updates need to be incorporated into the next change?

REFERENCES

Allen, S. R. (2013). *An ethnonursing study of the cultural meanings and practices of clinical nurse council leaders in shared governance* (Unpublished dissertation). University of Cincinnati, Ohio.

American Association of Critical-Care Nurses. (2015). *AACN Healthy Work Environment Initiative.* Retrieved from http://www.aacn.org/wd/hwe/content /hwehome.pcms?menu=hwe

American Nurses Association. (2009). *Nursing administration: Scope and standards of practice.* Silver Spring, MD: Author.

American Nurses Association. (2012). *Nurse's essential role in care coordination.* Silver Spring, MD: Author.

Aricca, D., Van Citters, B. K., Larson, K. L., Carluzzo, J. N., Gbemudu, S. A., Kreindler, F. M., … Fisher, E. S. (2012). *Four health care organizations' efforts to improve patient care and reduce costs.* Retrieved from http://www.commonwealthfund .org/publications/case-studies/2012/jan/four-health-care-organizations

Betbeze, P. (2014, May 13). Presidents, CEOs, and the new leadership model. Retrieved from http://www.healthleadersmedia.com/content/MAG-304260 /Presidents-CEOs-and-the-New-Leadership-Model

Drucker, Peter F. (1999). *Management challenges for the 21st century.* New York, NY: HarperBusiness.

Hewertson, R. (2015). *Lead like it matters, because it does matter.* New York, NY: McGraw-Hill Education.

Hoying, C., & Allen, S. (2011). Enhancing shared governance for interdisciplinary practice. *Nursing Administration Quarterly, 35*(3), 252–259.

Institute for Healthcare Improvement. (2014). Science of improvement: Establishing measures. Retrieved from http://www.ihi.org/resources/Pages/Howto Improve/ScienceofImprovementEstablishingMeasures.aspx

Institute for Healthcare Improvement. (2015). Tools. Retrieved from http://www .ihi.org/resources/Pages/Tools/default.aspx

Institute of Medicine. (2001). *Crossing the quality chasm: A new health system for the 21st century.* Washington, DC: National Academies Press.

Institute of Medicine. (2011). *The future of nursing: Leading change, advancing health.* Washington, DC: National Academies Press.

International Council of Nurses. (2014). Definition of nursing. Retrieved from http://www.icn.ch/about-icn/icn-definition-of-nursing/

Kalisch, B., & Curley, M. (2008). Transforming a nursing organization: A case study. *Journal of Nursing Administration, 38*, 76–83.

Kotter, J. (1995, March/April). Leading change: Why transformation efforts fail. *Harvard Business Review* (Reprint 95204).

Longo, A. (2013). Change, complexity, and creativity. In *L. Roussel (Ed.), Management and leadership for nurse administrators* (6th ed., pp. 121–159). Burlington, MA: Jones & Bartlett Learning.

Medicaid. (2014). *Core set of health care quality measures for adults enrolled in Medicaid (Medicaid Adult Core Set).* Retrieved from http://www.medicaid.gov /Medicaid-CHIP-Program-Information/By-Topics/Quality-of-Care/Downloads /Medicaid-Adult-Core-Set-Manual.pdf

Melnyk, B., & Fineout-Overholt, E. (2014). *Evidence-based practice in nursing and healthcare: A guide to best practice,* (3rd ed.). Philadelphia, PA: Lippincott Williams & Wilkins.

National Business Coalition on Health's Value Purchasing Council. (2015). *Value-based purchasing: A definition.* Retrieved from http://www.nbch.org /Value-based-Purchasing-A-Definition

Olny, C. (2005). Using evaluation to adapt health information to the complex environment of community-based organization. *Journal of the Medical Library Association, 93*(Suppl. 1), S57–S67.

Plsek, P. E., & Greenhalgh, T. (2001). Complexity science: The challenge of complexity in health care. *British Medical Journal, 323*, 625–628.

Porter-O'Grady, T. (2009). *Interdisciplinary shared governance: Integrating practice, transforming health care* (2nd ed.). Sudbury, MA: Jones and Bartlett.

Stiefel, M., & Nolan, K. (2012). *A guide to measuring the Triple Aim: Population health, experience of care, and per capita cost.* Cambridge, MA: Institute for Healthcare Improvement. Retrieved from http://www.ihi.org/resources/Pages /IHIWhitePapers/AGuidetoMeasuringTripleAim.aspx

Van Otters, A. D., Larson, B. K., Carluzzo, K. L., Gbemudu, J. N., Kreindler, S. A., Wu, F. M., . . . Fisher, E. S. (2012). Four healthcare organizations' efforts to improve patient care and reduce costs. The Commonwealth Fund. Retrieved from http://www.commonwealthfund.org/publications /case-studies/2012/jan/four-health-care-organizations

Strategic Planning and Change Leadership: Foundations for Organizational Effectiveness

Patricia L. Thomas and Roland Loup

LEARNING OBJECTIVES

1. Consider applications and demonstrations of strategic planning in contemporary organizations.
2. Define the mission and purpose statement as it pertains to nursing services and managing teams.
3. Differentiate between strategic planning and tactical planning.
4. Explore change leadership and organizational learning as key drivers for implementing strategic plans.

AONE KEY COMPETENCIES

I. Communication and relationship building
II. Knowledge of the healthcare environment
III. Leadership
IV. Professionalism
V. Business skills

AONE KEY COMPETENCIES DISCUSSED IN THIS CHAPTER

II. Knowledge of the healthcare environment
III. Leadership
IV. Professionalism
V. Business skills

II. **Knowledge of the healthcare environment**
- Clinical practice knowledge
- Patient care delivery models and work design knowledge
- Healthcare economics knowledge
- Healthcare policy knowledge
- Understanding of governance
- Understanding of evidence-based practice
- Outcomes measurement

- Knowledge of, and dedication to, patient safety
- Understanding of utilization and case management
- Knowledge of quality improvement and metrics
- Knowledge of risk management

III. Leadership
- Foundational thinking skills
- Personal journey disciplines
- Ability to use systems thinking
- Succession planning
- Change management

IV. Professionalism
- Personal and professional accountability
- Career planning
- Ethics
- Evidence-based clinical and management practices
- Advocacy for the clinical enterprise and for nursing practice
- Active membership in professional organizations

V. Business skills
- Understanding of healthcare financing
- Human resource management and development
- Strategic management
- Marketing
- Information management and technology

FUTURE OF NURSING: FOUR KEY MESSAGES

1. Nurses should practice to the full extent of their education and training.
2. Nurses should achieve higher levels of education and training through an improved education system that promotes seamless academic progression.
3. Nurses should be full partners with physicians and other health professionals in redesigning health care in the United States.
4. Effective workforce planning and policy making require better data collection and information infrastructure.

Introduction

Strategic planning is essential for organizations because it is the process by which the future of the organization is charted. By establishing a strategic plan, goals and action plans to focus the work in an organization can be undertaken. Healthcare organizations engage in strategic planning relevant to the overall future success of the organization. Nurse leaders commonly use the organization strategic plan to derive a nursing department strategic plan that aligns nursing activities and outcomes to the organizational plan.

In 2010, the Institute of Medicine (IOM), in collaboration with the Robert Wood Johnson Foundation, published *The Future of Nursing: Leading Change, Advancing Health*. This report highlights the opportunities nurses have to transform health care through strategic initiatives emphasizing seamless, affordable care that is accessible, patient centered, evidence based, and demonstrated through quantifiable outcomes. As the largest segment of the healthcare workforce, nurses have an opportunity and obligation to shape healthcare reform, and the report serves as a blueprint for strategic planning and action for nurses. Four overarching recommendations were offered to guide and shape planning and action by nurse leaders: (1) ensure that nurses can practice to the full extent of their education and training, (2) improve nursing education, (3) provide opportunities for nurses to assume leadership positions and to serve as full partners in healthcare redesign and improvement efforts, and (4) improve data collection for workforce planning and policy making. Each of these recommendations offers opportunity for strategic, operational, and business planning within organizations and in collaboration with external stakeholders and organizations. Likewise, they present opportunities for nursing leaders to collaborate with other disciplines and stakeholders to actualize members of the nursing profession as an equal partner in future healthcare delivery systems.

When considering strategic planning approaches, nurse leaders are challenged by scarce resources and past practice. Historically, strategic planning was undertaken by senior leaders in a top-down approach. Today, organizational practices emphasize inclusive planning with all employees engaging in a deliberate, systematic, interdisciplinary approach to these activities (Flanagan, Smith, Farren, Reis, & Wright, 2010; Kash, Spaulding, Johnson, & Gamm, 2014). Examples are found in quality and safety initiatives where members of interdisciplinary teams are brought together to address current and future issues that prevent accomplishment of shared goals and desired outcomes within a health system. This necessitates unlearning silo or department-specific planning approaches to enable interdependency among disciplines and departments in achieving organizational goals.

Although past practice and experience with strategic planning distinguished between conceptual exercises and actual practice, the current healthcare environment demands an integrated approach. Appreciative inquiry provides a framework for strategic planning, highlighting current trends in the organization and the industry within a spirit of inquiry and with acknowledgment of past accomplishments. This approach allows leaders to tap the creative energy of participants as a springboard to organizational change.

Nurse leaders benefit from shared language that is found in National Patient Safety Goals and the IOM's six safety aims to highlight contributions made by nurses as partners in achieving defined, measurable collaborative goals (Institute of Medicine [IOM], 2001; The Joint Commission, 2015). Strategic threads centered on safety, quality, cost reductions, and interdependent departments and disciplines emphasizing efficiency and effectiveness offer opportunities for nurse leaders to demonstrate the influence of professional nursing practice on organizational outcomes through measurement and defined metrics. Specific strategic initiatives, clear objectives, and defined tactics found in quality improvement philosophies create a framework for action. Specific interventions and rapid cycle improvements like those found in Transforming Care at the Bedside (TCAB); Small Troubles, Adaptive Responses (STAR-2); and Donabedian's Structure-Process-Outcomes (SPO) model (1980) are excellent examples of best practices using sound evidence. Additionally, Lean, Six Sigma, and Plan-Do-Study-Act offer disciplined approaches for nurses at all levels of an organization to participate in planning for and evaluating care (Donabedian, 1980; Miles & Vallish, 2010; Nelson, Batalden, & Godfrey, 2007; Rutherford, Lee, & Greiner, 2004).

The Patient Protection and Affordable Care Act and the Health Care and Education Reconciliation Act of 2010 represent federal statutes broadly described as healthcare reform laws. Within these acts, the concept of accountable care organizations is introduced, outlining how networks of physicians and hospitals will commit to sharing responsibility in providing care to patients. These laws center on health insurance reform, in areas such as access to care and coverage for all U.S. citizens, coverage for preexisting conditions, improving prescription drug coverage in the Medicare population, and a shift from illness and disease care in emergency departments and hospitals to wellness and the management of chronic conditions in the most appropriate setting. Inherent in the law is an expectation to reduce costs and improve the coordination of care through efficient and effective applications of evidence-based practices supported by technology, electronic health records, streamlined communication, and effective use of the human resources that comprise the healthcare team. Significant attention is being paid to accountable care organizations, which are believed to be the structure to bring together the component parts of patient care, including primary care, specialists, hospitals, home care, and community services in a coordinated and streamlined fashion (Zuckerman, 2012). Nurses need to position themselves and engage in policy development and strategic planning to ensure a place at the table with other members of the healthcare team who will determine national health policies for the future (American Nurses Association [ANA], 2014).

Proprietary changes have brought innovation and competition to the healthcare industry. Moving from a hospital-based industry to a market-driven industry will require attention to community-based services and the coordination of care across settings. With this come business techniques, new corporate structures, service lines, for-profit and not-for-profit organizations, and diversification (Zuckerman, 2012). In light of this profound shift in how we envision our role in health services, nurse leadership within organizations will need to engage in dynamic and future-oriented strategies rather than focus on maintenance of existing missions, entities, and history.

Nurse leaders continue to emphasize the continuum of care and the unique contributions nurses make in care coordination and managing transitions of care among settings, specialties, and the component settings of integrated systems. New roles are emerging for those with a background in nursing as payers and healthcare systems respond to pay for performance and at-risk contracting for payment (Naylor, 2012). The knowledge and skills of nurses have gained prominence by industry leaders who recognize the need for clinical assessment, triage, and access to service at the most appropriate location for care using the least costly option. Nurses play a key role in supervision and oversight of delegated tasks to unlicensed personnel, commonly identified as coaches or navigators, for services provided in settings beyond acute care and telephonically. Attention to systems thinking and the redesign of care delivery highlight the important role nurse leaders will play in creating successful models in the reformed healthcare industry.

With the Affordable Care Act, renewed attention to health promotion, health education, care transitions, and nurse autonomy to practice to the full extent of their education has occurred. Shifting focus from acute care to elements of the care continuum and community has emerged. Patient-centered medical homes, care provision in the home and retail settings, and technology-supported applications for information and access to care offer opportunities for nurse leaders to demonstrate the influence of professional nursing practice on outcomes through measurement and defined metrics. Inherent in this process is recognition that human resource planning ensures effective use of a scarce commodity, the professional nurse.

Many nursing organizations have embraced the Magnet model and domains as a framework for strategic planning. Magnet designation, offered by the American Nurses Credentialing Center as an independent arm of the American Nurses Association (ANA), is achieved by less than 10% of hospitals in the United States (American Nurses Credentialing Center [ANCC], 2014a). The Magnet model domains are Transformational Leadership, Structural Empowerment, Exemplary Professional Practice, Innovation and New Knowledge, and Empiric Outcomes. As a strategic road map, the Magnet model emphasizes the need for transformative leaders at all levels of an organization, empiric demonstration of outcomes of nursing care, innovation, quality improvement, and an empowered workforce across practice settings (ANCC, 2014c).

The framework offered by the Magnet model has evolved from research conducted in the 1980s that examined the practices of hospitals that are able to attract and retain nurses in a time of nursing shortage (ANCC, 2014b). Predicated on strategic plans, structures, processes, and outcomes of exceptional clinical practice, Magnet designation has been described as a journey that engages nurses at all levels of an organization to enact professional nursing values in concert with interdisciplinary team members that translates into accomplishment of national imperatives in the provision of healthcare services.

WHAT IS STRATEGIC PLANNING?

A strategic plan is the blueprint an organization uses to build future success. The process is inclusive and considers current trends, forecasts, and innovations to set in action activities that need to continue, expand, or be developed to remain competitive in the healthcare industry. The future orientation of a strategic plan is intended to inspire, excite, and connect employees to the contributions they will make in the achievement of the organization's vision for the future (McNamara, 2009; Zuckerman, 2014). Having a strategic plan does not leave success to chance and attempts to prevent the status quo or overwhelming demands from third-party payers, regulators, and other departments in the organization from paralyzing nursing progress.

Although traditionally done by senior leaders, strategic planning is now an essential skill for all nurse leaders. Nurse leaders need to be actively involved in the strategy development and execution for the organization because nursing is an integral part of any patient care activity. Nursing's participation in the organization strategic planning process is essential to the success of the plan and its execution. Participation in the organization strategic planning process also prepares nurse leaders to articulate and align resources to lead and execute initiatives that demonstrate the necessity for nursing services (Drenkard, 2012).

Developed to support the organizational strategic plan, nursing strategic plans identify objectives for the contributions nursing will make (stated in the future tense), typically spanning a 1- to 5-year time frame. In light of the profound proposed changes to healthcare delivery systems centered on the need to cut costs, increase access, and demonstrate outcomes for reimbursement for core measures, and the Patient Protection and Affordable Care Act, planning beyond 5 years will likely not be fruitful (Zuckerman, 2012).

Focused on being coldly objective, strategic plans focus attention on necessary outcomes and elements of the work of the nursing discipline that are required for future success, and they serve as a means to establish and evaluate contributions nurses make. Components of a strategic plan include statements of mission, vision, values, objectives, and operational or tactical plans (McNamera, 2009). Nurse leaders at all levels of an organization, irrespective of setting, use varied combinations of these documents as guideposts to accomplish the work of nursing.

The development of these plans and their acceptance and achievement are best accomplished by engaging a broad set of constituents and stakeholders to build commitment to the plan's goals and objectives so people will do the change work to implement the plan and then work in the new systems, structures, and processes that result from the change. A lack of staff engagement in the planning processes is one of the major reasons that strategic planning fails. Failure is often not a fault of the plan itself but rather of poor execution. Though strategic plans are dispassionate, the work needed to execute the plans is emotionally charged and laden with fear, frustration, loss, disappointment, pride of achievement, excitement, and elation (Drenkard, 2012; McNamera, 2009; Zuckerman, 2014).

The strategic planning process yields the direction for an organization's future; that is, goals and objectives and how the plan will be executed through initiatives and other actions, including the resources that will be needed to execute the plan. The initiatives and additional actions outline how managers, staff, and other healthcare team members will be involved. Inherent in the initiatives is what must be done to manage the changes needed in processes, structures, systems, and technologies as well as capital and human resources (Drenkard, 2012; McNamera, 2009; Zuckerman, 2012).

Another way to think of this is consideration of what must be done to execute the strategic plan, which is work that is essentially different from daily operations. Strategic plans address what must be different for future success inclusive of resources for daily operations and those necessary to conduct the change initiatives to accomplish the goals and objectives in the strategic plan.

A clearly articulated strategic plan with the commitment of leaders and staff throughout the organization helps an organization define its future success and provides direction for operational plans. A strong strategic plan is necessary, but not sufficient, for organizational success. Because execution requires actions that effect major shifts in the way the organization functions, it can be argued that the cornerstone for organizational achievement rests in leadership's ability to make, manage, and thrive in implementing change.

Strategy is a plan for getting from a point in the present to a point in the future knowing there will be uncertainty and resistance. In health care, the economic, political, technological, societal, and regulatory landscapes often shift before a strategic plan is fully implemented. The knowledge gained in the planning process gives leaders a strong base to respond to these ever-shifting environments (Zuckerman, 2012).

Planning the strategy of an organization is essential to all businesses, including those providing health care. Nursing is beginning to embrace this business strategy as a vehicle for defining the contributions nurses make to the healthcare industry, recognizing it affords the opportunity to determine how capital and human resources are allocated when aligned to the mission and purpose of the organization. Through business and project plans, organizations establish communication strategies, budgets, an engagement strategy, metrics and measures of success, training requirements for staff, technology needs, and a road map for executing elements of the strategic plan (Drenkard, 2012; Studor, 2004).

In this unprecedented time of change, appreciative inquiry (AI) can help leaders create a space for members of an organization to participate in the future-oriented thinking necessary to develop a strategic plan. Cooperrider and Whitney describe AI as follows:

> Appreciative Inquiry is about the coevolutionary search for the best in people, their organizations, and the relevant world around them. In its broadest focus, it involves systematic discovery of what gives "life" to a living system when it is most alive, most effective, and most constructively capable in economic, ecological, and human terms. AI involves, in a central way, the art and practice of asking questions that strengthen a system's capacity to apprehend, anticipate, and heighten positive potential. It centrally involves the mobilization of inquiry through the crafting of the "unconditional positive question." . . . In AI the arduous task of intervention gives way to the speed of imagination and innovation; instead of negation, criticism, and spiraling diagnosis, there is discovery, dream, and design. AI seeks, fundamentally, to build a constructive union between a whole people and the massive entirety of what people talk about as past and present capacities: achievements, assets, unexplored potentials, innovations, strengths, elevated thoughts, opportunities, benchmarks, high point moments, lived values, traditions, strategic competencies, stories, expressions of wisdom, insights into the deeper corporate spirit or soul—and visions of valued and possible futures. Taking all of these together as a gestalt, AI deliberately, in everything it does, seeks to work from accounts of this "positive change core"—and it assumes that every living system has many untapped and rich and inspiring accounts of the positive. Link the energy of this core directly to any change agenda and changes never thought possible are suddenly and democratically mobilized. (Cooperrider & Whitney, 2005, p. 3)

From this overview, Cooperrider and Whitney (2005) developed a four-dimension model in discover, dream, design, and destiny to guide AI work. Using AI in strategic planning allows participants to start with a clean slate and a spirit of inquiry and possibility thinking based on past accomplishments and aspirations as foundations for strategic planning. Within the AI framework, participants are encouraged and expected to explore and develop the work of their future with a spirit of curiosity and opportunity rather than a critical review of past goals and what was not accomplished.

ELEMENTS OF A STRATEGIC PLAN

Although the form and format of strategic plans may vary, the elements are generally consistent. The mission, vision, values, and objectives are the building blocks to bring a preferred future state into tangible activities and outcomes. Written statements of mission, vision, values, and objectives are transferred into tactical plans as blueprints for effective management in an organization. The components of tactical planning exist at all levels of management and guide operational decisions and performance evaluation across an enterprise. The forecasting of events and the laying out of a stream of activities for accomplishing the work of nursing in an organization are requisite for success. In an environment of changing technology, rising costs, and multiple priorities, clear executive nursing leadership to articulate the vision and support subordinates in the accomplishment of the plan is essential (McNamera, 2009; Zuckerman, 2012).

Mission

Every organization exists for specific purposes and to fulfill specific social functions. The mission of an organization describes the purpose for which that organization exists. Mission statements provide information, direction, and inspiration that clearly and explicitly outline the way ahead for the organization (McNamera, 2009; Zuckerman, 2012). The mission or purpose statement may incorporate the culture of the organization, including strong leadership, rules and regulations, achievement of goals, and the notion that people are more important than work.

Articulation of a mission statement is the first step in the strategic planning process. Industry leaders have learned that customers are the most critical stakeholders and frequently note this fact in their mission statements. Of late, strategic plans have called out the engagement of the community, emphasizing patient centeredness as a foundational premise to guide decision making. With reimbursement tied to care coordination, patient satisfaction, and the experience of care, learning how our organizations are experienced by the patient, customer, or consumer offers a different perspective from that of clinician providers and administrators. Organizations have embraced this in strategic planning by having patients who have received care in the organization participate in the process or serve on committees so the voice of the patient can be blended with that of the provider and administrators (Zuckerman, 2012).

Mission statements in successful business and industrial organizations incorporate socially meaningful and measurable criteria to provide a clearly defined reason for being. These simple yet crucial statements move the organization forward and are formulated for performance, products, and services. They contain statements of ethics, principles, and standards that are understood by workers. Workers who clearly perceive that they are pursuing meaningful and worthwhile goals through their individual efforts are more committed and dedicated than those who do not. The mission of an organization moves, guides, and delivers the organization to its perceived goal.

A nursing mission needs to align with the organizational mission and articulate the nature of nursing, its value, and the stakeholders to be satisfied. Defining a mission is foundational for the performance of nursing within the organization to be evaluated. The mission is the framework to guide nurse leaders' actions grounded in a commitment to professional nursing standards. It explains how professional practice is defined and conceptualized and the unique contributions nurses make to achieve organizational outcomes. Central to the nursing mission is the ability to articulate the metaparadigm of nursing (person, health, environment, and nursing) and the functions of nurses' enactment of social policy statements, professional standards of care, and evidence-based practices (ANA, 2010).

A further mission of nursing is to provide a public good. This purpose should be indicated in the mission statement of the nursing entity. Because it gives the reason for their employment, the mission statement is written so that all people working within the organizational entity can understand and abide by it. An ultimate strategy is to have nursing personnel participate in developing mission statements and in keeping them updated so that nurses are empowered to fully support the mission.

The mission should be known and understood by other healthcare practitioners, by clients and their families, and by the community. A statement of purpose must be dynamic, giving action and strength to evolving statements of philosophy, objectives, and management plans. Statements of purpose can be made dynamic by indicating the relationships among the nursing departments or divisions, units, patients, personnel, and community.

Statements of mission and objectives for nursing services support each other at different organizational levels—from the unit to the service or department, the division, the organization, and finally the system and community levels—and provide the rationale for the unique contributions nurses make. Often, as part of the nursing strategic plan, the philosophy of nursing is developed from the ANA Code of Ethics, the ANA standards of practice, and nursing theories that guide nursing actions and interventions. The nursing mission statement pertains to the clinical best practice of nursing supported by research, education, and management across clinical specialties, service lines, and levels of care. It is translated into patient-centered action by nursing personnel.

Vision

The vision of an organization should be an image of a successful future the organization seeks to create. It is not an abstract goal but a set of practical ideals that offer a platform for goals to be accomplished in terms that can ultimately be assessed and evaluated. It is a mental prediction of the fulfillment of the organization's success. The vision statement is created with the customers' needs in mind. External customers include those who purchase the products or services of the organization. In nursing, external customers are prospective patients and their families, accreditation and licensing officials, faculty and students, donors, regulators, and even taxpayers and shareholders. Internal customers include employees, physicians, members of the interdisciplinary team, and staff who work in support departments.

While external market pressures and regulation shape the vision of care providers, a vision statement offers an opportunity to marry expectations imposed by external forces with specific internal practices. Perhaps most important is the connection of the aspirations of the leaders and staff in the organization to the vision. The vision paints a picture of the preferred future that captures the hearts and minds of the members of an organization and inspires them to make changes to improve the patient experience, quality, safety, and outcomes, thereby transforming the organization.

Employees who participate in developing the vision statement believe in their own abilities and are more committed to the organization than employees who do not participate. The vision statement is shared throughout the organization so employees can live the vision. It is regularly updated to keep pace with technology and trends.

Values

Values are concepts of perceived worth or importance that drive the institution and inform its mission, vision, and goals. Examples of values are commitment, creativity, honesty, quality, respect, integrity, and caring. Values are the moral rationale for business; therefore, value statements make employees feel proud and managers feel committed. Values give meaning to the right way to do things and contribute to employee motivation, enthusiasm, and energy. Values bond people and set behavioral standards. Values represent actionable terms that align to guiding principles that support the work of the organization.

Objectives

Objectives are statements about measurable results that are specific to an organizational goal. To be effective, objectives need to be specific, measurable, attainable, realistic, and time bound. Typical categories for nursing objectives include the use of resources (human, physical, and financial), staffing, requisition of supplies and equipment, planning of educational programs, innovation, evaluation of provided care, and evaluation of personnel.

Objectives need to be dynamic, meaningful, relevant, and functional. Moore (1971) states, "If objectives are presented in terms of what can be observed, they can serve as useful tools for evaluation of nursing care and personnel performance, and as a basis for planning educational programs, staffing, requisition of supplies and equipment, and other functions associated with the nursing department" (p. 13). As such, objectives should provide for the abandonment of unneeded or outdated nursing services and provide leverage for new services, products, service lines, or patient populations aligned with the organizational goals. Inherent in objectives are opportunities for research, generation of new knowledge, best practice, and professional development. Objectives provide for attractive job and career opportunities and for activities to manage employee assignments and productivity. They are the means by which productivity in nursing can be measured and demonstrate a discharge of responsibility to the public. Leaders use objectives to define short-term and long-term activities they aspire to accomplish.

In light of reform and the future landscape of health care, nursing strategic and operational plans could shape significant contributions to future care delivery systems. Highlighting the contributions of professional nurses at all levels of an organization by emphasizing the ways in which nurses address the needs of patients and populations—supported by the ANA Code of Ethics, Scope and Standards of Practice, and technology-enhanced, consumer-driven wellness strategies—is being done by many organizations across the country.

TACTICAL, FUNCTIONAL, AND OPERATIONAL PLANNING

Operational planning is the process that puts thought into action. Nurse leaders initiate communication, engage staff to develop a shared understanding of the future state, and identify needed change so human and fiscal resources can be attained to enact elements of the plan. The major purpose of planning is to make the best possible use of personnel, supplies, and equipment to support the fulfillment of organizational goals. Tactical or functional planning is intended to convert objectives or project plans into action through discrete activities, timelines, deadlines, and assignments of responsibility and accountability. Typically, these plans are enacted daily, weekly, or monthly and provide data about results and points of accomplishment for celebration with staff as they implement the change. Planning within the nursing organization is intended to assist in fulfilling the mission of the healthcare facility and meshes with the plans of all other departments contributing to the provision of all healthcare needs, ultimately demonstrating support of the nursing agency.

Planning is a continuous process that starts with setting goals and objectives, followed by laying out a plan, reviewing processes and outcomes, and concluding with feedback to staff. A decision is then made about whether modifications are needed, and the process is initiated again. As plans are put into action, the management functions of leading, organizing, implementing, and evaluating are undertaken. Planning promotes analytic thinking within a framework for decision making and orients people to action rather than reaction. It provides a basis for managing organizational and individual performance aligned to senior leader objectives. It promotes improved flexibility and decision making in a cost-effective manner and provides clarity in uncertain times.

Engaging employees in the development of plans increases the likelihood of success. Tactical, functional, and operational plans are based on goals and on their achievement. A nurse leader's style influences whether goal setting and planning will be top-down or bottom-up. Bottom-up goal setting is participatory and empowers staff to identify human, fiscal, and capital needs necessary for the provision of care. Participatory goal setting and planning is believed to increase workers' commitment and achievement of organizational goals. Increased participation leads to greater group cohesiveness, which in turn fosters increased morale, increased motivation, and productivity.

BUSINESS PLANS

As an extension of strategic and functional planning, business plans are detailed descriptions of the process to implement a new product or product line, project, unit, or service (Williams & Simmons, 2012). Several of the key elements are the same, although a business plan is more detailed than a strategic plan. Their purpose is to provide information to decision makers about the proposed service and to motivate those involved in the implementation toward the measurement of performance. Business plans are the road map for new ventures and support the allocation of fiscal and human resources within an organization. Developing a business plan is not unlike outlining strategies for a project plan. A business plan uses a project management methodology and has a beginning and an end, is designed to specify the market or community need to be addressed (after completion of a formal needs assessment), and is an evidence-based proposal to support a change, with metrics and measurement to establish expected outcomes and demonstrate effectiveness to an organization. Elements of a business plan include the introduction, background, description or proposal for the new service, market or community assessment, research and development plans and outcomes, operational plan, and detailed evaluation plan.

BALANCED SCORECARDS

Balanced scorecards have been used by many businesses for several decades. As an extension of this work, healthcare organizations have adopted balanced scorecards to monitor financial, clinical, and operational outcomes at a unit, department, service-line, and organizational level (Ball, Garets, & Handler, 2003; Nash et al., 2010). Third-party payers and regulators have started using this concept to establish payment for services rendered based on the quality of the outcomes achieved. The Centers for Medicare and Medicaid Services initiated public reporting of critical elements of care and defined metrics for home care and long-term care facilities (Centers for Medicare and Medicaid Services [CMS], 2013). Accessed through the Internet, applications allow consumers to review measurements and metrics of care quality and safety in hospitals, nursing homes, and home care agencies across the United States.

The balanced scorecard approach has been linked to functional and tactical plans to support pay-for-performance measures that are reported publically. Examples of indicators include provider-preventable conditions like wrong site surgery, retained foreign objects after surgery, pressure ulcers, falls, trauma, catheter-associated urinary tract infections, vascular catheter-associated infection, poor glycemic control, and development of deep vein thrombosis or pulmonary embolism following hip or knee replacement surgery (CMS, 2011, 2014).

ORGANIZATIONAL CULTURE

The organization's values and vision form two major elements of an organization's culture. The third component is the assumptions and beliefs that leaders and staff operate under as each works in the organization. Schein, one of the leading thinkers and writers about organizational culture, said, "The term culture should be reserved for the deeper level of basic assumptions and beliefs that are shared by members of an organization, that operate unconsciously, and that define in a basic 'taken-for-granted' fashion an organization's view of itself and its environment" (Schein, 1985, p. 6).

An organization's strategy is like a fish that lives in the water of organizational culture. The water determines the fish's ability to live and thrive, and when toxic, it can even kill the fish. The fish is unaware of the water and how that water determines its success or failure to achieve its intention, but the fish's naivety does not exempt it from being affected.

Organizational culture is an intangible force that influences how a strategy is formed and executed and can determine whether a stated strategy can be achieved. For a strategy to have any chance of successful implementation, the organizational culture must allow and support what needs to be done to create and, more importantly, to execute that strategy.

Organizational culture is a mixture of many subcultures, such as professions, ethnic origins of leaders and staff, cultures created by founders, ongoing governance cultures, and religious sponsors. This combination of values, assumptions, and beliefs makes organizational culture a complex, unique, vibrant, ever-shifting entity within an organization. Because assumptions and beliefs that are the cultural foundation operate unconsciously among leaders and staff in the organization, culture is difficult to be aware of, to discuss, and to change.

Every strategy requires certain assumptions and beliefs. As an example, medical record documentation for many years was on paper, and the handwritten chart was the source of truth containing essentially all information about a patient. With the advent and implementation of computer-based electronic health records, patient care documentation required a different set of assumptions and beliefs by nurses, physicians, and members of the healthcare team. Shifting the old assumptions and beliefs required significant culture change.

Leaders must be aware of the culture needed to achieve the strategic results and must build and sustain that culture. Essential elements of a culture that are needed to execute strategy successfully are accountability for decisions and actions, continual organizational learning, accepting ongoing change as a part of everyday organizational life, using diversity of thought and opinion among leaders and staff to make and implement decisions, engaging people throughout the organization in decisions and actions to make change, and ensuring that decisions are made at the right level of the organization thereby driving decisions down into the organization. Establishing and maintaining the right culture provide the biggest challenge for leaders in the successful execution of a strategic plan.

STRATEGIC THINKING

Organizational strategic thinking is a leadership process for developing possibilities and options that will help ensure the viability of the future of the enterprise. Strategic thinking informs the decisions made by leadership in creating the strategic plan, that is, in making the final decisions on the mission, vision, values, and objectives. Strategic thinking also gives leaders a common knowledge base that prepares them to make major decisions quickly and intelligently in rapidly shifting environments, in essence making the organization more agile.

Organization executives lead long-term and short-term strategic thinking. Long-term strategic thinking encompasses 5 to 20 years and generally informs the mission, vision, and strategic goals. Short-term strategic thinking encompasses 1 to 5 years and informs the objectives and major initiatives that are undertaken to accomplish the organization's strategy.

Long-Term Strategic Thinking

The purpose of long-term strategic thinking is to inform leaders and staff about events, developments, and trends over 5 to 20 years that may offer threats or opportunities to the organization's future. Understanding major events, developments, and trends that may affect the organization in the long run helps leaders gain a broader context for thinking about the future, both in the short term and in the long term.

Short-Term Strategic Thinking

Short-term strategic thinking informs the strategic plan through gathering data about the events, developments, and social, political, and economic trends in the organization's environments that can affect the future of the organization. Short-term strategic thinking involves gathering and analyzing data, adding context and assumptions to the analysis to form information, and then creating future options or scenarios for the organization based on that information. This data-driven, analytical process is complemented by adding the aspirations for the organization of the leaders and staff. The resulting future options are then based on current data and include the results that those in the organization believe will help it accomplish its mission. The organization's vision, as a statement of a picture of organizational success in the future, is a major source of information about the aspirations of leaders and staff.

The values in the strategic plan guide how strategic planning is carried out and the decisions about future options that result from it. The values and vision provide major components of the framework for the organizational culture, the most important factor in the execution of the strategic plan.

To be most effective, short-term strategic thinking must be an intentional process that is championed by leadership and has essentially the same import to the organization as the budgeting process. That is, it must be systematic, well defined, driven by leadership, accepted by all management and staff, and well executed (Loup, 2014).

Foundational to this thinking process is a commitment to individual and organizational learning. Recognizing that some of the skills and attributes that made us successful in the past will need to be revised, refined, or abandoned is key to leading in a learning organization. Leaders at all levels will need to be skilled in learning and unlearning old behaviors to role model new behaviors for their staff (Kerman, Freundlich, Lee, & Brenner, 2012).

CHANGE LEADERSHIP AND STRATEGIC PLANNING

With the adoption of the Patient Protection and Affordable Care Act and the Health Care and Education Reconciliation Act of 2010, the pace of change in the healthcare industry and within healthcare organizations will quicken. Healthcare organizations will need to continually adapt to major shifts in their environments in shorter time intervals. Leaders in healthcare organizations will need to have the skills and competencies to lead and manage those changes.

There are two major components to change leadership. The first is developing a strategic plan that will help ensure future success in these rapidly shifting environments; the second is executing the strategic plan.

The importance of and the components of a strategic plan have been described. A well-articulated mission accepted by all in the organization forms the backbone of the strategy. A clear vision that everyone in the organization can understand and see their part in gives a picture of success. The 1- to 5-year goals provide focus areas for resource commitment throughout the period of the plan, and objectives provide measureable, achievable results that show achievement of the mission and vision.

The strategic plan needs to describe a culture that allows for rapid organizational change to meet constantly shifting stakeholder needs and to respond to changing environments. Bossidy and Charan (2002) highlight execution as a core element of organizational culture and emphasize that without execution, the strategic plan is like a car in the driveway: full of potential energy but not going anywhere. Building and sustaining the discipline of execution is one of the major skills required of all executives today.

Nurse leaders need to participate actively in organizational strategic planning and execution, lead strategic planning for their organizations, and ensure the execution of the nursing strategic plan. As previously discussed, leading initiatives for change and establishing and implementing business plans for new products and services are major activities in executing a strategic plan.

Organizational change occurs first at the individual level. Stakeholders need to commit to the proposed change before they will take actions to effect the change. One model of building commitment to change is the road to commitment, which consists of three stages (Loup & Koller, 2005):

1. Awareness and understanding of the change, how it may happen, and its intended results based on knowledge of different aspects of the change. This stage can be thought of as engaging a person's head in the change.

2. Belief that this change will have a positive benefit to me, my organization, and my customers, and that the organization will actually make the change. These beliefs require thought, discussion, and challenges to current assumptions and beliefs about the organization and how we do our work. Coming to these beliefs requires a person to engage his or her heart in the change.

3. Commitment to the change, exhibited by taking necessary actions to do the work needed to bring about the change and then to do the new work after the change efforts are complete. Commitment means that the person will engage body, mind, and spirit to do the work necessary to effect the change.

Figure 7-1 shows that engaging employees in the right change work at the right time is the major success factor in overcoming resistance and gaining commitment to any organizational change.

Without coming to the beliefs in the accompanying list, a stakeholder will not commit but will instead live in some level of compliance and not do the required work to make the change. Leaders must build commitment to change by creating awareness and understanding of the change and guide people through examining their beliefs about the change. Not all people will come to the required beliefs, but not all are needed to make the change. The leader needs to build beliefs among a critical mass of people who will then do the work of change.

ORGANIZATIONAL LEARNING

Organizational learning is now a well-accepted success component of organizational culture. In this technology era, we are inundated with information. There is too much information for any one person to even see, much less understand.

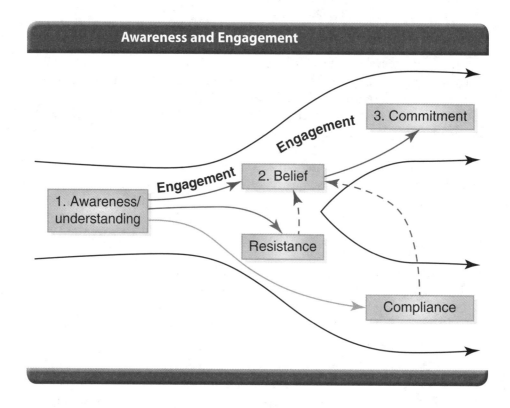

Awareness and Engagement

We are in an age of information overload. It has been likened to standing under Niagara Falls with your mouth open and hoping to get a drink of water.

Organizational learning can be loosely defined as the result of interactions among people in the organization and with their stakeholders to gain knowledge and understanding that can be applied to planning, management, and operations. Deming and Juran, in their work on quality in the 1970s and 1980s, included organizational learning as essential to improving processes and quality. Still, organizational learning is not a usual act in many organizational cultures that emphasize planning and action more than learning (Provost, 2011).

Organizational learning must be part of the way the organization operates, insisting that people take the time to examine and learn from failures and successes to be more effective in the future. The learning processes can occur anywhere at any time in the organization, for example, after an interaction with a customer, after an action is taken, as a major initiative unfolds, or after a process such as strategic planning has been completed.

Strategic thinking and strategic planning are important components of organizational learning because each process engages many people in the organization in the study of the organization's strengths, weaknesses, opportunities, and threats (SWOT) and its many environments. Sharing the knowledge gained in these processes, especially through direct interactions, can build a strong base of information for everyone in the organization as they plan and execute to make the organization successful.

SUMMARY

The major concepts discussed in this chapter are strategic planning, strategic thinking, organizational culture, execution of the strategic plan through initiatives and product and service development, change leadership, and organizational learning, which are important components of organization leadership. Leaders sponsor and ensure the implementation of strategic thinking and planning, build and sustain a culture that includes execution as a primary component, oversee the initiatives to execute the plan, and ensure that the leadership team executes all phases of the plan. In doing so, they create the space for ongoing organizational learning. Not all of these concepts are new to nurse leaders, but in the coming years, taken separately and together, they will play a significant role in successful nurse leadership.

REFLECTIVE QUESTIONS

1. Does your organization have a strategic plan? A nursing strategic plan?
2. If asked to create a nursing strategic plan, where would you start? What documents would you need to gather, and who would you ask to participate in the process?
3. List the common pitfalls of a strategic plan. Identify what strategies you would take to overcome them.

CASE STUDY 7-1   Creating a Common Nursing Vision and Strategic Priorities across a System

Joyce Young

XYZ Health System (HS) is one of the largest health systems in the United States, and it is continuing to grow. The health system comprises more than 56,000 full-time equivalent employees, which includes more than 11,000 active physicians (3,400 employed physicians and residents) and more than 16,000 registered nurses (RNs) practicing in 47 hospitals across 10 states. A shared mission and common values connect these 47 diverse hospitals. Additionally, XYZ HS understands the importance of a shared vision to bring leaders together in strategy and the pursuit of transformational change.

Creating a common nursing vision to determine and drive strategy across a large, diverse health system is clearly a challenge but is worthy of undertaking. The XYZ HS nursing leaders recognized the power of leveraging the talent bank of 47 diverse hospitals and nursing leaders toward a common vision and strategies; in fact, they saw this as critical to leading change and preparing for a reformed future of healthcare delivery. The leaders recognized that success in this endeavor required essential keys steps, beginning with awareness or understanding of the pivotal role of nursing. Only with awareness and understanding can an effective strategy be determined.

Awareness

Events of the past decade, and certainly since the Patient Protection and Affordable Care Act was signed into law on March 23, 2010, have fueled interest within the healthcare industry and in the nursing profession in understanding what a reformed healthcare delivery system looks like and how to position the industry and profession for success.

(continues)

CASE STUDY 7-1 Creating a Common Nursing Vision and Strategic Priorities across a System (Continued)

In the IOM and Robert Wood Johnson Foundation report *The Future of Nursing: Leading Change, Advancing Heath* (IOM, 2010), it was noted that the U.S. healthcare industry is fraught with fragmentation as well as barriers to care and the ability to provide cost-effective, high-quality care. The report said the solutions may reside in a transformed nursing profession. The report outlined recommendations directing not only nursing leaders but also policy makers, payers, licensing bodies, and other healthcare leaders to align the industry and care delivery system with the current era of reform. Similarly, the Advisory Board Company's report *Perfecting the Patient Care Services Strategic Plan* (2012) wove nursing innovation strategy throughout the five core components of service, quality, finance, people, and growth.

The universal theme in these reports clearly points to the pivotal role that nursing must play in designing the future of health care. In a seminal speech given at the Institute for Healthcare Improvement national forum, Berwick articulated what he called "the moral test" (Berwick, 2011). Berwick spoke to the impending changes that the healthcare industry is facing and stated, "This is the threshold we have now come to, but not yet crossed; the threshold from the care we have to the care we need. . . . Our vision is for healthcare that is just, safe, infinitely humane, and that takes only its fair share of our wealth" (2011, p. 11).

The vision Berwick spoke of was embraced by the XYZ HS nursing leaders. This vision became the impetus for unifying the XYZ HS nursing leaders' commitment to a system-wide strategic focus and transformational change. In an industry bombarded with high-velocity change, focus was quickly identified as the next key to success in this important strategic work.

Focus

Given the size and complexity of XYZ HS, along with the pace of change in the industry, the need for focus could not be understated. For XYZ HS, the ability to focus was fostered through the commitment of dedicated time (over several months) and to a clear understanding of the current state. Focus enables the ability to identify what is most important.

An appreciative inquiry approach was used to integrate feedback and information that had been gathered over a dedicated time period (Tagnesi, Dumont, Rawlinson, & Byrd, 2009). The numerous nurse leaders from the 47 diverse hospitals were then divided into three small work groups. In the spirit of shared leadership, each work group was tasked with identifying and proposing three to five strategic goals. The resulting 9 to 15 proposed strategic goals were then taken back to the full group for voting. The voting results served as the basis for determining three system-wide strategic nursing priorities.

Guided by a vision of health care that is just, safe, and infinitely humane, the three strategic priorities promoted the pivotal role of nursing. The size and scope of nursing leaders from 47 diverse hospitals across 10 states leveraged the profession in leading change and readiness for a reformed future of healthcare delivery. Focus ensured the appropriate strategic goal selection and prioritization; this set the direction for the work required to execute the strategy.

Commitment and accountability round out the keys to success in creating a common nursing vision and strategic priorities across a system. The XYZ HS leaders understood that it was through commitment and accountability that they would get where they desired to go. Accountable, empowered work teams were created to execute each strategic priority. Milestones were identified along with due dates, metrics, and reporting requirements. The process described in this case exemplar was grounded in the shared leadership principles of partnership, equity, commitment, and accountability.

One year later, progress is encouraging and the journey continues. Thanks to a common vision, thoughtfully determined strategic priorities, and empowered, accountable, highly committed leaders, the XYZ HS is successfully positioned to meet the challenges of the future.

> ## CASE STUDY 7-1   Creating a Common Nursing Vision and Strategic Priorities across a System (Continued)
>
> ### Case Study Questions
>
> 1. What lessons are learned from reviewing the strategic plan and progress made in XYZ HS?
> 2. What factors were most significant in driving 47 diverse hospital nursing leaders toward a common vision and strategic priorities?
> 3. Of the key steps articulated, which do you think was most important?
> 4. Are there other steps that you would advise employing in this process?
> 5. How does size and scope help or hinder strategic success?

REFERENCES

Advisory Board Company. (2012). Perfecting the patient care services strategic plan. Retrieved from http://www.advisory.com/Research/Nursing-Executive-Center/Resources/Posters/Perfecting-the-patient-care-services-strategic-plan

American Nurses Association. (2010). *Nursing's social policy statement: The essence of the profession.* Washington, DC: Author.

American Nurses Association. (2014). *Health care transformation: The Affordable Care Act and more.* Retrieved from http://www.nursingworld.org/MainMenuCategories/Policy-Advocacy/HealthSystemReform/AffordableCareAct.pdf

American Nurses Credentialing Center. (2014a). Growth of the program. Retrieved from http://nursecredentialing.org/MagnetGrowth.aspx

American Nurses Credentialing Center. (2014b). History of the Magnet program. Retrieved from http://nursecredentialing.org/Magnet/ProgramOverview/HistoryoftheMagnetProgram

American Nurses Credentialing Center. (2014c). Magnet model. Retrieved from http://nursecredentialing.org/Magnet/ProgramOverview/New-Magnet-Model

Ball, M., Garets, D., & Handler, T. (2003). Leveraging information technology towards enhancing patient care and a culture of safety in the U.S. *Methods of Information in Medicine, 6,* 503–508.

Berwick, D. M. (2011, December). *The moral test.* Presented at Institute for Healthcare Improvement National Forum, Orlando, Florida. Retrieved from http://www.ihi.org/resources/Pages/Presentations/TheMoralTestBerwickForum2011Keynote.aspx

Bossidy, L., & Charan, R. (2002). *Execution: The discipline of getting things done.* New York, NY: Crown Business.

Centers for Medicare and Medicaid Services. (2011). Affordable Care Act gives states tools to improve quality of care in Medicaid, save taxpayer dollars. Retrieved from http://www.cms.gov/Newsroom/MediaReleaseDatabase/Press-releases/2011-Press-releases-items/2011-06-01.html

Centers for Medicare and Medicaid Services. (2013). Hospital compare. Retrieved from http://www.cms.gov/Medicare/Quality-Initiatives-Patient-Assessment-Instruments/HospitalQualityInits/HospitalCompare.html

Centers for Medicare and Medicaid Services. (2014). Hospital value-based purchasing. Retrieved from http://www.cms.gov/Medicare/Quality-Initiatives -Patient-Assessment-Instruments/hospital-value-based-purchasing/index .html?redirect=/hospital-value-based-purchasing

Cooperrider, D., & Whitney, D. (2005). *A positive revolution in change: Appreciative inquiry.* Retrieved from http://appreciativeinquiry.case.edu/uploads /whatisai.pdf

Donabedian, A. (1980). *Explorations in quality assessment and monitoring: The definition of quality and approaches to its assessment.* Ann Arbor, MI: Health Administration Press.

Drenkard, K. (2012). Strategy as solution: Developing a nursing strategic plan. *Journal of Nursing Administration, 42*(5), 242–243.

Flanagan, J., Smith, M., Farren, A., Reis, P., & Wright, B. (2010). Using appreciative inquiry for strategic planning in a professional nursing organization. *Visions, 17*(1), 19–38.

Institute of Medicine. (2001). *Crossing the quality chasm: A new health system for the 21st century.* Retrieved from https://www.iom.edu/~/media/Files /Report%20Files/2001/Crossing-the-Quality-Chasm/Quality%20Chasm%20 2001%20%20report%20brief.pdf

Institute of Medicine. (2010). *The future of nursing: Leading change, advancing health.* Washington, DC: National Academies Press. Retrieved from http://www .iom.edu/Reports/2010/The-Future-of-Nursing-Leading-Change-Advancing- Health.aspx

Kash, B., Spaulding, A., Johnson, C., & Gamm, L. (2014). Success factors for strategic change initiatives: A qualitative study. *Journal of Healthcare Management, 59*(1), 65–82.

Kerman, B., Freundlich, M., Lee, J. M., & Brenner, E. (2012). Learning while doing in the human services: Becoming a learning organization through organizational change. *Administration in Social Work, 36*(3), 234–257.

Loup, R. (2014). Unpublished manuscript.

Loup, R., & Koller, R. (2005). The road to commitment: Capturing the head, hearts and hands of people to effect change. *The OD Journal, 23*(3), 73–81.

McNamara, C. (2009). All about strategic planning. Retrieved from http:// managementhelp.org/strategicplanning/index.htm

Miles, K., & Vallish, R. (2010). Creating a personalized professional practice framework for nursing. *Nursing Economics, 28*(3), 171–189.

Moore, M. (1971). Philosophhy, purpose, and objectives: Why do we have them? *Journal of Nursing Administration, 1*(3), 9–14.

Nash, M., Pestrue, J., Geier, P., Sharp, K., Helder, A., & McAlearney, A. (2010). Leveraging information technology to drive improvement in patient satisfaction. *Journal for Healthcare Quality: Promoting Excellence in Healthcare, 32*(5), 30–40.

Naylor, M. (2012). Advancing high value transitional care: The central role of nursing and its leadership. *Nursing Administration Quarterly, 36*(2), 115–126.

Nelson, E., Batalden, P., & Godfrey, M. (2007). *Quality by design: A clinical microsystems approach.* San Francisco, CA: Jossey-Bass.

Patient Protection and Affordable Care Act, 111th Congress Public Law 148, (2010). Retrieved from http://www.gpo.gov/fdsys/pkg/PLAW-111publ148 /html/PLAW-111publ148.htm

Provost, L. (2011). Analytical studies: A framework for quality improvement design and analysis. *BMJ Quality & Safety, 20,* i92–i96.

Rutherford, P., Lee, B., & Greiner, A. (2004). *Transforming care at the bedside* (IHI Innovation Series white paper). Boston, MA: Institute for Healthcare Improvement. Retrieved from http://www.ihi.org

Schein, E. (1985). *Organizational culture and leadership.* San Francisco, CA: Jossey-Bass.

Stevens, K. (2009). A research network for improvement science: The Improvement Science Research Network. NIH 1RC NR011946-01. Retrieved from https://isrn.net/https%3A/%252Fimprovementscienceresearch.net/about

Studor, Q. (2004). *Hardwiring excellence: Purpose, worthwhile work, making a difference.* Gulf Breeze, FL: Firestarter.

Tagnesi, K., Dumont, C., Rawlinson, C., & Byrd, H. (2009). The CNO: Challenges and opportunities on the journey to excellence. *Nursing Administration Quarterly, 33*(2), 159–167.

The Joint Commission. (2015). 2015 national patient safety goals. Retrieved from http://www.jointcommission.org/standards_information/npsgs.aspx

Williams, C., & Simmons, K. (2012). Boost nursing projects by creating a successful business plan. *OR Nurse, 6*(3), 9–13.

Zuckerman, A. (2012). *Healthcare strategic planning* (3rd ed.). Chicago, IL: Health Administration Press.

Zuckerman, A. (2014). Successful strategic planning for a reformed delivery system. *Journal of Healthcare Management, 59*(3), 168–192.

CHAPTER 8

Procuring and Sustaining Resources

Patricia L. Thomas, Linda Roussel, Val Gokenbach, Elizabeth Anderson, and Denise Danna

LEARNING OBJECTIVES

1. Examine concepts in the budgeting process, including direct and indirect costs; fixed, variable, and sunk costs; operating or cash budget; personnel; supplies; and equipment and capital budgets.
2. Identify steps in the budget planning process.
3. Explore the effects of reimbursement structures.
4. Explain value-based purchasing as it relates to quality and safety initiatives.

AONE KEY COMPETENCIES

I. Communication and relationship building
II. Knowledge of the healthcare environment
III. Leadership
IV. Professionalism
V. Business skills

AONE KEY COMPETENCIES DISCUSSED IN THIS CHAPTER

II. Knowledge of the healthcare environment
III. Leadership
V. Business skills

II. **Knowledge of the healthcare environment**
   - Clinical practice knowledge
   - Patient care delivery models and work design knowledge
   - Healthcare economics knowledge
   - Healthcare policy knowledge
   - Understanding of governance
   - Understanding of evidence-based practice
   - Outcomes measurement
   - Knowledge of, and dedication to, patient safety
   - Understanding of utilization and case management

- Knowledge of quality improvement and metrics
- Knowledge of risk management

III. Leadership
- Foundational thinking skills
- Personal journey disciplines
- Ability to use systems thinking
- Succession planning
- Change management

V. Business skills
- Understanding of healthcare financing
- Human resource management and development
- Strategic management
- Marketing
- Information management and technology

FUTURE OF NURSING: FOUR KEY MESSAGES

1. Nurses should practice to the full extent of their education and training.
2. Nurses should achieve higher levels of education and training through an improved education system that promotes seamless academic progression.
3. Nurses should be full partners with physicians and other health professionals in redesigning health care in the United States.
4. Effective workforce planning and policy making require better data collection and information infrastructure.

Introduction

Nurse leaders have a central role in determining the human and fiscal resources required to accomplish work. This is foundational to allocating available resources to approved projects or programs, which is rooted in the budgeting process. Budgeting is an ongoing activity in which revenues and expenses are managed to maintain fiscal responsibility and the fiscal health of an organization. Nurse leaders have financial responsibility, are accountable for managing the nursing budget, and make decisions about how to adjust the nursing budget based on organizational priorities. Inherent in this process is the ability to prioritize available resources, manage program costs, make recommendations for when to add or eliminate a program or service, initiate or expand contractual agreements, steward available resources, and advocate for resources within the nursing enterprise.

With limited resources and in a competitive market, healthcare organizations must use personnel and material resources wisely and efficiently. Enlightened nurses know that the person who controls the budget is the person who controls nursing services. Because the amount and quality of nursing services depend on budgetary plans, nurses and nurse leaders should become proficient in budgeting procedures. This proficiency provides the resources necessary for safe and effective nursing care. The costs of nursing services have been identified for many years, but the income earned from nursing services has been included in bed and board on the budget sheets (Davis et al., 2013).

With the enactment of the Affordable Care Act and ongoing healthcare reform in the United States, pressures to reduce costs, improve quality, and manage care across the continuum with greater coordination and fewer gaps and redundancies will be essential. Although it once centered on acute care hospitals and physician practice, the paradigm shift includes the community and populations, with care provision taking place within homes, long-term care facilities, long-term acute care hospitals, outpatient clinics, and retail storefronts. The principles of budgeting and procuring resources are key to the success of nurse leaders (Finkler & Jones, 2013). In this chapter, the principles of budgeting from an acute care perspective will serve as the starting point; however, unique attributes of budgeting for community-based care and care in settings outside the hospital will be offered.

BASIC PLANNING

In most organizations, planning yields forecasts for 1 year and for several years. The budget is an annual plan intended to guide effective use of human and material resources, products, or services and to manage the environment to improve productivity. Budgetary planning ensures that the best methods are used to achieve financial objectives. It should be based on valid objectives to provide a product or service that the community needs and for which it will pay. In nursing, budgetary planning helps ensure that clients or patients receive the nursing services they want and need from satisfied nursing workers. A good budget is based on objectives; is simple, flexible, and balanced; has standards; and uses available resources first to avoid increasing costs (Finkler & Jones, 2013).

There is no formula for the form, detail, or periods covered by budgets. Each budget system is designed for the situation at hand and must take into consideration the character of the company, the company's position, and the nature of the plans involved. Ordinarily, the budget system is most detailed in aspects of operations that are most important to the firm's success. Furthermore, the period covered by the budget varies with the nature of the plans and with the degree of accuracy possible in the preparation of estimates (Finkler & Jones, 2013).

A nursing budget is a systematic plan that is an informed best estimate by nurse administrators of revenues and nursing expenses. It projects how revenues will meet expenses, and it projects a return on equity, that is, profit or cost avoidance. The budget should be stated in terms of attainable objectives to maintain the motivation of nurses at the unit or cost center level. The nursing budget serves three purposes:

- Plan the objectives, programs, and activities of nursing services and the fiscal resources needed to accomplish them
- Motivate nursing workers through analysis of actual experiences
- Serve as a standard to evaluate the performance of nurse administrators and managers and increase awareness of costs

These purposes should include the organization's mission, strategic plans, new programs or projects, and goals. Managing the financial end of nursing through an operational budget can create a new sense of involvement for nurses. The budget can be a strong support for developing written objectives for the nursing division and for each of its units. It can provide motivation for effective planning and standards by which to evaluate the performance of nurse leaders and managers (Dunham-Taylor & Pinczuk, 2014). Effective planning provides for contingencies by indicating which programs or activities can be reduced or eliminated if budget goals are not met.

PROCEDURES

Decentralized budgeting involves unit managers and staff in the process. Nursing service is labor intensive, reflected in the fact that the first six of the following budget planning steps pertain to labor. Note that only steps 7 and 8 are concerned with nonlabor expenses. The steps are as follows (Penner, 2013):

1. Determine the productivity goal. The chief nursing officer (CNO) and the nurse manager determine the unit's productivity goal for the coming fiscal year. Changes to the organization's service line and patient outcome measure results all must be considered when planning the unit and overall nursing services budget.
2. Forecast the workload. The number of patient days expected on each nursing unit for the coming fiscal year is calculated.
3. Budget patient care hours. The expected number of hours devoted to patient care for the forecasted patient days is calculated.
4. Budget patient care hours and staffing schedules. The budgeted patient care hours are reflected in recommended staffing schedules by shift and by day of the week.
5. Plan nonproductive hours. Vacation, holiday, education leave, sick leave, and similar hours are budgeted for the coming year.
6. Chart productive and nonproductive time. To aid in the planning process, a graph is used to show nurses how the level of forecasted patient days, and therefore the staffing requirements, are expected to increase and decrease during the year. Productive time is the time spent on the job in patient care, administration of the unit, conferences, educational activities, and orientation.
7. Estimate costs of supplies and services. Consideration should be given to any new services or changes in patient mix. The supplies and services to be purchased for the year are budgeted.
8. Anticipate capital expenses. The expected capital investments for the coming year are included in the budget.

These eight steps result in a proposed budget that goes to the CNO for review. After preliminary acceptance, this budget is sent to the accounting department, where the forecasted patient days are translated into expected revenue. The budgeted productive and nonproductive times are converted into dollars, as are the costs for supplies, services, and other operating expenses that will be allocated to a given nursing unit for the coming year. A pro forma operating statement is then returned to the director of nursing for review with the nurse manager. After the CNO and the nurse manager accept the budget, it is returned to the accounting department and forwarded with the rest of the agency manager's budgets to administration and the board of directors (Finkler & Jones, 2013).

People who pay high prices for health care want accountability of both costs and quality of service. A recent trend in the literature is to approach a nursing budget as a shared responsibility between the leaders and the clinical staff. Although nurse managers provide the oversight and monitoring of the budget, the information is shared openly with staff whose actions determine whether or not the budget is met. Through input and participation in developing the budget, shared experience becomes an object of ownership, and staff put forth effort to work within its framework. Additionally, as nurses learn about budgets and are able to articulate budgetary principles and applications, their professional stature is enhanced (Finkler & Jones, 2013).

MANAGING COST CENTERS

A cost center is a given area of assigned accountability for both direct and indirect expenditures. A department of nursing is a cost center, as are each of its units. Other cost centers are each clinic, in-service education, surgical suites, long-term care, home care, and any other section with a nursing mission in which nurses provide services to clients.

Each cost center is an internal department dealing with distribution of services and products. The cost center manager is responsible for determining the cost of such services or products and how they are distributed within the organization. Two types of cost centers are mission, or revenue producing, and service. Examples of mission centers are radiology and laboratory departments. These centers have monetary income related to the purpose of the organization. A service center is a support center that provides a service to other units and charges for that service; no exchange of revenue takes place. The unit served adds the costs of these support services to its costs of output (Penner, 2013). Examples of support centers are food service, purchasing, and laundry.

Relationship of Budget and Objectives

One of the chief planning activities is to identify the objectives of the nursing division and each of its units, including developing a management plan with a budget for each objective. One of the first sources of budgetary information is nursing objectives. By using these objectives, nurse managers see the benefit of developing pertinent, specific, and practical budgeting objectives. These objectives must align and be monitored for changes with the organization's financial plan and objectives, third-party payer requirements for reimbursement to the organization, and accreditation obligations (Finkler & Jones, 2013).

BUDGET STAGES

For practical purposes, the nursing budget follows three stages of development: formulation, review and enactment, and execution. The entire budgeting process is given a specific time frame, and a target date is assigned for each step. During the fiscal year of the execution stage of budgeting, the formulation and review and enactment stages for the next fiscal year are carried out (Finkler & Jones, 2013).

Formulation Stage

The formulation stage is usually a set number of months (6 or 7) before the start of the fiscal year for the budget. During this period, procedures are used to obtain an estimate of the funds needed, funds available, expenses, and revenues. Financial reports of expenses and revenues of the previous fiscal year and the year to date are analyzed by the CNO, department heads, cost center managers, and financial or business analysts.

One of the first steps in writing a budget is gathering data for accurate prediction of expenses (costs) and revenues (income). This task can be developed into a system. The primary sources of data are the objectives for the division of nursing and for each cost center. Each program and activity needs to have an estimated cost placed on it. If in-service educators want new audiovisual equipment, they should not walk into the nurse administrator's office and expect to have it next week or next month. Purchasing this equipment should be planned 6 to 7 months before the next fiscal year begins, and it may be budgeted for any quarter or month within that fiscal year. In surveying the objectives, nurse administrators and managers evaluate the previous year, review the philosophy, and rewrite the objectives for the future.

Other data include programs from other departments that require the use or expansion of nursing resources, expansion of nursing clinics and client teaching programs, travel costs for attendance at professional and educational meetings, incentive awards, library requirements, clinical and office supplies and equipment, investment equipment and facilities modification on a 5-year plan, and contracts for items such as intravenous pumps and oxygen equipment. Data can be obtained from historical financial records of the organization.

Several cost center reports may assist nurse managers:

- Daily staffing reports
- Monthly staffing reports
- Payroll summaries
- Daily lists of financial categories of patients
- Workload and occupancy reports
- Biometric reports of workload
- Monthly financial summaries of revenues and expenses

Review and Enactment Stage

Review and enactment are budget development processes that put all the pieces together for approval of a final budget. After the cost center managers present their budgets to the budget council, the CNO consolidates the nursing budget. The budget officer further consolidates the budget into an organizational budget. The chief executive officer of the organization and the governing board then give their approval. Throughout this process, conferences are held at which budget adjustments are made. Nurses can sell a budget by using a marketing strategy, anticipating challenges, being persuasive without being emotional, and working toward a win–win situation (Finkler & Jones, 2013).

Execution Stage

The formulation stage and the review and enactment stage of the budget are planning activities. The execution of the budget involves directing and evaluating activities. The nurse administrators and managers who planned the budget execute it. Revisions in execution of the budget are scheduled at stated intervals, usually once or twice during the fiscal year. Contingency plans may be required by an organization to establish priority changes if the budget targets are not met, particularly if a cost center is volume driven. Having a line of sight between the budget targets and the achieved budget allows nurse leaders to shift course during a budget year to prevent year-end shortfalls.

Certain procedures are followed for evaluating the budget at cost center levels. Budgets are prepared for either a fiscal year that coincides with government budgets or a calendar year, depending on the policy of the organization. A clear understanding of the budget year is critical for effective monitoring and evaluation.

Cost Factors

Cost is money expended for all resources used, including personnel, supplies, and equipment (**Box 8-1**). The acuity and volume of services provided are the greatest factors affecting costs. Other factors include length of stay, salaries, material costs, case mix, seasonal factors, and efficiencies (such as simplification of procedures and quality management to prevent errors that increase patient complications and increase costs). Other factors warranting attention based on cost impacts are regulations, competition for market share, third-party payer requirements and contracts, the age and size of the agency, types and amounts of services provided, the agency's mission, and relationships among nurses, physicians, and other personnel.

Expenses

Expenses are the costs of providing services to patients. They are frequently called *overhead* and include wages and salaries, fringe benefits, supplies, food service,

---

BOX 8-1   Cost Factors in the Budgeting Process

- Patient acuity
- Volume of service
- Length of patient stay
- Salaries
- Price of materials
- Case mix
- Seasonal factors
- Efficiencies (prevention of errors; decreased patient complications)
- Regulation
- Competition for market share
- Third-party payers
- Age and size of agency
- Type and amount of services
- Agency mission
- Relationship of personnel (collaborative)

utilities, and office and medical supplies. As part of the budget, expenses are a collection or summary of forecasts for each cost center's account.

Full costs include both direct and indirect expenses. Although direct costs such as nursing can be traced to the source, indirect costs such as utilities, telephones, or purchased services are allocated to the source department by a standard formula within the organization.

Expense Budgeting

The purpose of expense budgeting is to outline the monetary needs of an organization through forecasting, recording, and monitoring manpower, materials, and supplies so each of the components can be controlled (Dunham-Taylor & Pinczuk, 2014) (**Box 8-2**). As such, the components of expense budgeting are each of the cost centers. Historical trends are the single best and most inexpensive indicator available to organizations for the prediction of present and future trends.

TYPES OF EXPENSES AND COSTS

Fixed, Variable, and Sunk Costs

Fixed costs are not related to volume. They remain constant as volume increases and decreases over a period of time. Among fixed costs are depreciation of equipment and buildings, salaries, benefits, utilities, interest on loans or bonds, and taxes.

Variable costs do relate to volume and census (patient days). They include items such as meals and linen. Supplies are usually volume responsive, meaning that total costs increase or decrease according to use. The cost of supplies varies by patient census, physician orders, clinical specialty, and patient diagnosis. For example, the cost of surgical dressings increases when a patient's wound has drainage and dressings must be changed frequently. Likewise, the cost of supplies increases or decreases with the census. For this reason, every cost center should have an established unit of measure for productivity. This unit may be numbers of tests, procedures, patients of a specific acuity type, hours or minutes of service, or discharges. Most activities include elements of both fixed and variable costs. For example, personnel costs and utility costs can be both fixed and variable because a minimum is required for each.

Sunk costs are fixed expenses that cannot be recovered even if a program is canceled. An example of this is advertising.

BOX 8-2   Purposes of Expense Budgeting

- Predict labor hours, material, supplies, and cash flow needs
- Establish procedures for making comparative studies
- Provide mechanism for change management

Direct and Indirect Costs

Direct costs are the costs of providing the product or service and are often considered to be those directly related to patient care, such as personnel costs and the variable cost of supplies. The definition of direct costs varies by department. In areas not involved in direct patient care, each department incurs its own category of direct costs.

Indirect costs are those incurred in supporting the provision of the product or service, are not directly related to patient care, and include utilities, administration, housekeeping, and building maintenance. As previously mentioned, however, they are direct costs for the source department. Some indirect costs are fixed, such as depreciation and administration. Others, such as laundry and accounting, are variable. All indirect costs are allocated or transferred by a specific method within the organization to the departments that use the service (Finkler & Jones, 2013).

Every hospital has a method to establish costs, including the Hospital and Hospital Health Care Complex Cost Report Certification and Settlement Summary, commonly known as the Centers for Medicare and Medicaid Services (CMS) Cost Report (2014a). As pressures surrounding expenses and costs have increased, sophisticated methods have been developed within organizations. As such, nurse leaders need to be vigilant and informed about methods favored by their organizations.

Cost Accounting

A cost accounting system assigns all costs to cost centers. Periodically, usually monthly, reports of costs are provided to cost center managers, but they do not reflect all costs. Many indirect costs are allocated only once a year in the CMS Cost Report. Included are costs of items such as utilities, accounting, administration, data processing, and admitting. Informed and influential nurse managers use these cost allocations when preparing budgets. Such allocations are usually hidden in the operational budget under the room costs category.

Cost assignments to cost centers are made on the basis of direct costing if they are direct costs of patient care. Otherwise, they are made by transfer costing from a patient care support department or by cost allocation if they are not related to direct patient care or support. Job order sheets are a method used to account for all services to patients. Direct overhead costs that cannot be identified with specific services rendered are allocated based on some other measurement, such as square feet of floor space.

Service Units

Service units are measurable units of productivity or volume for identifying and counting costs. They must be measurable, known to managers, and affected by volume. The number of service units produced measures productivity. They vary by location, clinical specialty, and level of care across the continuum. For example, psychiatric care in the emergency department, outpatient services, partial day programs, residential or housing services, and hospitals have defined service units depending on where the patient receives care.

Unit of Service

A unit of service is a measurement of the output of agency services consumed by the patient. In the surgical suite and recovery room it is measured in minutes or hours, in the emergency room it is the number of visits or time and procedures, and on nursing units it is based on the acuity category of patients and hours per day expressed as a targeted number. Types of measurement include procedures, patient days, patient visits, and cases. With the increased sophistication of data collection and management from electronic records and claims processing procedures, nurse managers have become involved with identifying and costing service units that can be quantified by hours of nursing care per category of acuity of the illness.

Chart of Accounts

A chart of accounts that includes a number and table for each cost center is subdivided into major classifications and subcodes. Examples are salaries and wages, employee benefits, medical and surgical supplies, professional fees, purchased services, utilities, other direct expenses, depreciation, and rent. These classifications are divided into further subcategories (Penner, 2013).

To assign items to the correct cost center, one must record all movement of labor and materials between cost centers. All benefits must be charged to the appropriate cost center by some established method, as must all purchases, including shared ones. This is usually done using allocated shares of service units.

Amortized expenses are deferred charges allocated to units over a specified period of time. They include depreciation charges for aging plant and equipment in addition to prepaid items. Prepaid items usually are charged monthly as service units. Other deferred expenses include unamortized borrowing costs and costs incurred for capital expansion or renovation programs (Finkler & Jones, 2013).

Financial Accountability

In accepting financial accountability, nurses' first duty is to their patients, who have given them their trust (Dunham-Taylor & Pinczuk, 2014). Nurses should be accountable to themselves for their work, to their professional peers, to their employers, and, in publicly funded institutions, to taxpayers.

In one way or another, patients pay the costs of health care. They may do so through insurance premiums, taxes, employee benefit packages, or from their own pockets. Financial accountability means that nurses and others can account for the efficient spending of the money paid for health care and demonstrate they have been responsible stewards of the money entrusted to them.

Nurse managers need information on the costs of all services provided by their own and competing institutions. In the past decade, the provision of care that was once offered only in acute care hospitals is now provided in long-term care facilities, outpatient facilities, or patient homes. As such, it has challenged nurse leaders and clinicians to become even more astute about why care needs to be provided in one setting versus another. As we step further into healthcare reform with greater public expectation of cost reductions and demonstration of value through outcomes, financial cost and reimbursement information needs to be provided to clinical nurses who know best what it costs to do their work. By establishing the costs for care, all of us become more cost conscious, and it supports efforts to reduce waste and demonstrate effective cost management (Penner, 2013). Some managers mistakenly believe that controlling nursing labor power and expenditures can control overspending. Holding nurses accountable for their budgets, including both revenues and expenses, can rectify this misconception (Dunham-Taylor & Pinczuk, 2014).

Cost of Nursing Care

To determine the cost of nursing care, one must consider several factors. Nursing charges should be quantifiable. A patient acuity system serves this purpose. The patient acuity system usually separates patients into four or five levels of nursing care and enumerates nursing requirements for each level. Charges could be set by level and negotiated with third-party payers. These costs could be separated from the cost of nonnursing requirements. Nonnursing tasks could then be reassigned to ensure that the charges for nursing care reflect the actual cost of providing such care.

A second method of costing nursing services is determining what share of total agency cost is attributable to nursing. This varies by medical severity diagnosis-related group. An industry-wide effort for each region could produce standards for nursing costs and charges. Otherwise, most healthcare institutions in the United States would need to undertake research to determine nursing costs and charges on an agency-specific basis. Multinational corporations, of course, can apply research studies across member institutions.

Activity-based costing accounts for the total process of doing business from personnel, supplies, material, and parts to installation and service of products. Healthcare organizations know and manage the costs of the entire economic chain, tying the costs to all sources of payment. To do this requires foundation, productivity, competence, and resource allocation information. Personnel perform to meet specific expectations, and they are evaluated accordingly. If activity-based costing is used, managers would turn data into information through analysis and interpretation. In this regard, activity-based costing allows action as it informs the redesign of care delivery models. As outdated structures are replaced with new cost centers that support activity-based costing, meaningful structures would emerge.

DEFINITIONS

Budget

According to *Merriam-Webster's Online Dictionary*, a budget is "a statement of the financial position of an administration for a definite period of time based on estimates of expenditures during the period and proposals for financing them" (Budget, n.d.). A budget is an operational management plan, stated in terms of income and expenses, covering all phases of activity for a future division of time. It is a financial document that expresses an operation's plan of action. In the division of nursing, it sets the limits of financial support, thereby controlling the extent and quality of nursing programs. The budget determines the number and kinds of personnel, materials, and financial resources available for patient care and for achievement of the stated nursing objectives. It is a financial policy statement. Budgeting is the process whereby objectives and plans are translated into financial terms and evaluated using financial and statistical criteria.

Revenue

Revenue is the income from sales of products and services. Nursing revenue traditionally has been included with room charges. It can be unbundled from the room rate as a separate charge per patient acuity category and per visit, day, or procedure (Finkler & Jones, 2013).

Revenue can include assets, such as accounts receivable and income-producing endowments. The latter can be restricted to specific purposes. Buildings, land, and other items can be assets if they produce income or are capable of producing income. Total income is frequently termed gross income; the excess of revenues over expenses is known as net income or profit.

Revenues also come from research grants, gift shops, donations, gifts, rentals of cots and televisions, parking fees, telephone charges, and vending machines. Revenues may be elements of product lines such as orthopedic services that include orthopedic nursing, traction equipment, and prostheses. In hospitals, revenue may refer to sources such as Medicare, Medicaid, third-party payers (insurance companies), and patients (Finkler & Jones, 2013).

Revenue Budgeting

Revenue budgeting, or rate setting, is the process by which an agency determines revenues required to cover anticipated costs and to establish prices sufficient to generate these revenues. Not all patients (purchasers) pay an equal share of an agency's costs, which complicates the process. To remain viable, any business must generate sufficient revenues to cover operating costs and make a profit. These revenues include increases in working capital, capital replacements, and inflation adjustments (Finkler & Jones, 2013).

Nonprofits use profits to improve plants and services; profits do not go to stockholders or owners. Profit appears as a positive balance on account ledgers (Finkler & Jones, 2013). Fundamental to the rate-setting process are adequate statistical data, historical and projected, for implementing the rate-setting method to be used. On a departmental basis, these data include volume of services, current rate, allocated costs, and rate increase constraints. The goal is to obtain the greatest impact from a minimum cumulative rate increase in a cost-management environment. This can be accomplished by increasing rates in high-profit departments while instituting rate reductions in low-profit departments so they offset each other. Revenues are often budgeted before expenses. This is necessary to determine how much revenue is available.

Patient Days

Patient days are used to project revenues. They are commonly used as units of service to compute staffing. Patient day statistics are usually derived from census reports that are done daily at midnight and summarized monthly for the year to date and annually. A patient admitted on May 2 and discharged on May 10 is charged for nine patient days. **Table 8-1** illustrates the number of patient days per unit for 1 month.

TABLE 8-1	Sample of Patient Day Census					
	Current Year			**Year to Date**		
Nursing Station	**May**	**OCC (%)**	**April**	**Current Year**	**OCC (%)**	**Previous Year**
3rd Floor	1,014	79.8	833	9,792	78.6	8,650
4th Floor	811	76.9	718	7,834	75.8	7,255
5th Floor N.	526	65.3	524	5,300	67.1	4,838
5th Floor S.	622	77.2	592	5,587	70.7	5,603
6th Floor	792	71	866	8,730	79.8	8,176
7th Floor	850	68.5	895	9,086	74.7	8,885
8th Floor N.	376	60.6	383	4,624	76.1	2,393
8th Floor S.	303	69.8	274	3,253	6.4	1,729
9th Floor N.	526	84.8	501	5,332	87.7	2,690
9th Floor S.	481	77.6	506	5,118	84.2	2,617
Burn Unit	173	79.7	188	1,723	81	1,912
CCU	206	83.1	148	1,848	76	1,937
Clinical Research Unit	137	73.7	132	1,342	73.6	1,361
EAU	23	0	7	390	0	634
Labor and Delivery	138	37.1	99	1,228	33.7	1,258
MICU	213	85.9	191	2,099	86.3	2,291
MINU	104	83.9	89	1,041	85.6	432
NTICU	209	84.3	87	1,891	77.8	2,277
PICU	169	54.5	112	1,612	53	1,834
SICU	229	92.3	207	2,175	89.4	2,302
SINU	73	58.9	84	964	79.3	471
Total	7,975	73.2	7,436	80,969	75.3	79,086

(*Abbreviations:* CCU: Critical Care Unit; EAU: Emergency Admit Unit; MICU: Medical Intensive Care Unit; MINU: Medical Intensive Nursing Unit; NTICU: Neurotrauma Intensive Care Unit; PICU: Pediatric Intensive Care Unit; SICU: Surgical Intensive Care Unit; SINU: Surgical Intensive Nursing Unit.)

Midnight census does not fully reflect the nursing resources required to accommodate outpatients that occupy a bed for 23 to 48 hours or swings in census that require nursing workloads to increase with admissions and discharges. Despite improvements with electronic documentation for admission, discharge, transfer, and patient location, the CNO and nurse manager are still required to track these trends manually to adequately plan resources needed because the systems are not yet sophisticated enough to distinguish between patients by name.

Fiscal Year

A fiscal year is the budgetary or financial year. It may be the calendar year in some organizations, beginning on January 1 and ending on December 31. Many organizations use October 1 to September 30 as the fiscal year. Some use July 1 to June 30 to coincide with budget decisions of state legislatures and the U.S. Congress.

Year to Date

The term *year to date* describes the accumulated units of service at a particular point in the fiscal year. If the fiscal year begins October 1, the year-to-date patient days for December 31 would be the summary for 92 days.

Average Daily Census

The census is summarized for a specific number of days and divided by that number of days. For example, the average daily census for the month of May is the total patient days for May divided by 31. In Table 8-1, the number of patient days for May is 7,975. When this number is divided by 31, the average daily census is 257.

Hours of Care

Hours of care have traditionally been the number of hours of care allocated per patient per day (24 hours) on a unit. With the use of patient acuity rating systems, hours of care can be determined to the hour or even to the fraction of an hour. Patients usually fall into one of four or five patient acuity categories, each of which is assigned a specific number of hours of care per patient day.

Caregiver

Each nurse who works with patients is called a caregiver. In nursing, the three common types of caregivers are registered nurses (RNs), licensed practical nurses, and nurse aides or extenders. Inpatient personnel budgets have a ratio of RNs to other caregivers and patients. Considerable research supports a high proportion of RN caregiver staff to patient safety and improved clinical outcomes (Penner, 2013). Despite this, the current cost management environment often makes this difficult.

Case Mix

The patients' acuity of services is known as a case mix. Case mix refers to the types of patients cared for by the institution. Some of the variables included in the case mix are diagnosis, comorbidities, and treatment patterns.

RESPONSIBILITY FOR CREATION AND MANAGEMENT OF THE BUDGET

Healthcare organizations are receiving less reimbursement for services than at any other time in the history of health care, and further cuts are projected for the future. Federal budget cuts also affect reimbursement, and Medicare payments are planned to decrease another 2% over the next several years. The Advisory Board Company (2012) said the total loss of reimbursement will be $11 billion to the Medicare program, with $5.8 billion cut from hospitals. Value-based purchasing has shifted reimbursement from volume to quality. The nursing staff is the largest cost in any hospital, and therefore it is the easiest and largest target for budget cuts (Ellerbee, 2013).

Nursing leaders must understand and become familiar with the literature on quality of care and the correlation of nursing staff to safe care delivery. Multiple studies have demonstrated that nurse staffing levels and skill mix has an impact on quality of care, failure to rescue, and patient satisfaction at the bedside (Aiken et al., 2012; Needleman et al., 2011; Patrician et al., 2011). It is important for nursing leaders to craft an effective message for all administrators about the importance of appropriate nurse staffing and the associated evidence.

Apart from an understanding of the literature on staffing, nursing leaders at all levels in the organization need to have a good grasp of the organization's financial processes. Although the fundamentals of finance are the same across all health-care organizations, the reporting structure and style might vary from institution to institution and there may be different approaches to budget formation. It is important to develop a collegial and strong relationship with financial leaders and their staff. These individuals are vital to providing support to nursing leaders for any financial needs.

BUDGETING APPROACHES

Zero-Base Budgeting

Zero-base budgeting is a method of budgeting used to control costs. In a zero-base budget, the budgeting process starts from zero, and everything must be justified in each new budget cycle (Finkler & Jones, 2013). A previous activity can be included in the budget, but its relation to the current organizational objectives must justify funding for it. In theory, each function in a zero-base budget must stand on its own merits, and the merits of each function are reviewed annually. All labor power and costs are recalculated, and decisions are made about whether to continue the function and at what levels.

Program Budgeting

Program budgeting is a part of budget planning. Items such as continuing education programs, employee benefits fairs, and health promotion programs should be incorporated into the annual budget. The budget for each program should enumerate fixed expenses, such as rent, advertising, fixed speaker fees, and department overhead and variable expenses, such as food, handouts, and per-person honorarium speaker fees. Some costs, such as those for advertising, are unrecoverable even if the program is canceled. They are sunk costs and should be in the cost center budget as well as in the individual program's budget (Finkler & Jones, 2013).

Program budgets should include a break-even analysis. If the cost of a program is $2,000 and the reasonable charge is $50 per participant, the break-even point is 40 participants. A break-even chart can be made for each program (**Figure 8-1**). Income above the break-even point is profit; below it is loss.

The point at which the cost to carry out a program is equal to the cost to cancel it is called the least-loss point (Dunham-Taylor & Pinczuk, 2014). If enough people have registered to pay the sunk costs, the net loss is the same whether the program is canceled or held. It may be good public relations to carry out a program at the least-loss point.

Flexible Budgeting

Flexible budgeting takes into account variations or ranges from low to high points (Finkler & Jones, 2013). This approach requires a well-prepared and

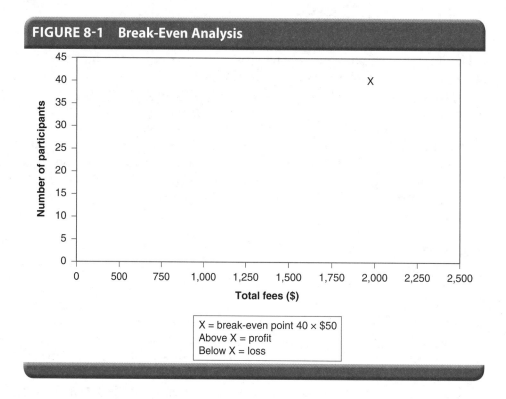

FIGURE 8-1   Break-Even Analysis

X = break-even point 40 × $50
Above X = profit
Below X = loss

educated nurse manager. It determines a range of volume instead of an actual volume, which is much more difficult to plan and manage.

Fixed Budgeting

A fixed budget is based on a fixed annual level of volume (Finkler & Jones, 2013). For example, the annual number of X-rays performed is divided by 12, giving a monthly average of X-rays. This approach to budgeting does not take seasonal or monthly variations into consideration.

TYPES OF BUDGETS

Operating Budget

The operating budget is the overall plan identifying expected revenues and expenses, both fixed and variable, for the forthcoming fiscal year. It is an annual budget that includes the cash budget and the capital budget. In addition, the operating budget identifies the source and nature of expected revenues and expenses. The operating budget determines the per diem and other charges to be made to the patient (Finkler & Jones, 2013).

Cost-to-Charge Ratios

Cost-to-charge ratios are convenient tools for computing the cost of providing a service. For example, if the charge to a patient for endoscopic laboratory services is $1,000, and the cost-to-charge ratio is 0.815626, then the cost to the hospital for these services is approximately $815.63. This cost includes the expense of running the endoscopic laboratory and a portion of the hospital's overhead cost. In some instances, the cost-to-charge ratio is greater than 1, which means the cost of operating these cost centers is greater than the charges.

Hospitals have two types of cost centers. The first is a revenue-producing cost center, such as the endoscopic laboratory, which bills patients for services provided. The second type is an overhead cost center, such as the accounting department, which exists to support the revenue-producing centers. The cost of overhead cost centers is allocated to revenue-producing centers by various statistical methods. For example, utility costs are allocated to revenue-producing departments based on the square footage of space they occupy. Accounting department costs, however, are allocated based on the size of the operating budget of each revenue-producing cost center. The cost-to-charge ratio is computed by dividing the total cost of the cost center, both direct and overhead, by the total charges for the same department.

Cost–Benefit Analysis

A cost–benefit analysis is a planning technique that answers the following questions: What are the costs of pursuing a goal, an objective, a program, or a specific nursing intervention? How do costs compare with benefits? Is the project worthwhile? A comparison of different nursing interventions for the same nursing diagnosis or problem results in using the least costly interaction to achieve similar or better results. The intervention used is then cost effective (Finkler & Jones, 2013).

Operating or Cash Budget

The cash budget is the actual operating budget in detail, usually excluding the capital budget (Finkler & Jones, 2013). A cash budget indicates whether the cash flow will be adequate to meet anticipated payments, such as debt obligations, including replacement and expansion of facilities, unanticipated requirements, payroll, payment for supplies and services, and a prudent investment program. Cash receipts come from third-party payers, tuition, endowment fund earnings, and sales of food, gifts, and services.

The cash budget is the day-to-day budget and represents money coming in and going out. It is advisable to have cash reserves so that cash flow and the money coming in pay the bills (Finkler & Jones, 2013). Otherwise, revenues must be sped up or the payment of bills must be slowed down.

Organizations often review their revenue cycle to ensure that cash and expenses are kept in the appropriate ratio. Cash reserves should not be excessive; they may represent money that should be working for the organization. Cash budgets show revenues and expenses, whereas operating budgets show plans. They are usually considered integrated entities (Finkler & Jones, 2013).

NEGATIVE CASH FLOW

Five major factors influence negative cash flow:

- There is a time lag between delivery of services and collection of payments.
- The timing of cycles between net income and flow of cash is different.

- Lag occurs because of the large up-and-down cycles of volume during different seasons (cash deficit during a busy census cycle or surplus during a low census cycle).
- Labor expense (60% to 70% of operating expense) paid out in salary and wages does not cycle concurrently with collections.
- Service-line costs have outpaced reimbursement, such as implants for certain cardiac and orthopedic procedures.

To maintain solvency, cash flow must be managed carefully, and cycles of cash shortage must be planned for appropriately. The cash budget should plan for the ability to borrow cash during shortfalls, the investment of excess cash, and the strict monitoring and reporting of lost charges and of the billing and collecting process. The cash budget is a part of the total budget and is apportioned to departments based on individual cost center activity (Dunham-Taylor & Pinczuk, 2014).

DEVELOPING THE OPERATING BUDGET

Operating budget information supplied to the chief nurse executive, department heads, and cost center managers includes a budget worksheet (**Table 8-2**). The budget worksheet depicts information by the account number and subcode of each cost center and lists prior year expense, original budget, and annualized expense. This form is usually provided during the new budget formulation stage, and the annualized expense is the projected total expense if current rates continue to the end of the fiscal year. The column headed "Budget Adjustments" is empty so the cost center manager can fill in the budget expenses for the projected fiscal year. The column "Approved Budget" is the budget that has been approved by the finance department and administration after they review the requested adjustments. Note in Table 8-2 that the cost center manager had projected an increased budget of $1,000 for subcode 6000, supplies. This amount was reduced to an annualized projection of $650 (subcodes 6100 and 6200) at the annual budget meeting.

Note that subcode 8200, maintenance and repairs, was increased by $100 (from $800 to $900). This increase was justified on the adjustment explanation (**Table 8-3**). Overall, increases were approved for subcodes 8200 (maintenance and repairs), 9200 (travel), and 9300 (airfare). A total budget for supplies and minor equipment for this cost center was approved for $2,925.

STAFFING PATTERNS AND PROCESSES

One of the biggest challenges for any leader is the management of effective staffing levels and defense of the need for those levels in situations of economic challenge. Because nursing has the largest budget in the organization, it is the largest target for staff reduction and budget cuts. The effects of nurse staffing on patient safety and satisfaction have been studied, with strong evidence supporting the need for adequate staffing to result in positive outcomes for patients. It is critical that nursing leaders understand the tenets of staffing as they relate to variables in their own organizations. The American Nurses Association (2014) defined an optimal nurse staffing model as one that assesses patient acuity, the levels of unlicensed assistive personnel, and the staff's level of skill and education.

TABLE 8-2   Budget Worksheet

Operating Expenses

Subcode	Description	Prior-Year Expense ($)	Original Budget ($)	Annualized Expense ($)	Budget Adjustments ($)	Approved Budget ($)
6000	Total—Supplies		0.00	1,000	915	650
6100	Forms	860	0.00	200		200
6200	Books	450	0.00	450		450
6434	Brochures	398	0.00	0.00		
6660	Film rental	100	0.00	0.00		
Total Supplies		**1,808**	**1,000**	**650**		
8000	Total—Repairs & Maintenance		0.00	1,360		
8200	Main & Repair	100	0.00	800	900	1,190
8310	Minor Equip.	675	0.00	100		100
8524	Telephone	185	0.00	190		190
Total Repairs & Main.			**960**	**1,360**	**1,090**	
9000	Total—OCE		0.00	1,370		
9200	Travel	1,345	0.00		685	1,085
9300	Airfare	800	0.00		200	400
9600	Entertainment	275	0.00		220	
Total Other Controllable		**2,420**	**1,370**	**420**		
Account Total		**5,188**	**3,730**	**2,160**		
Total $2,925						

The allocation of funds for effective staffing levels is one goal of nursing leaders; however, another important consideration is the level of turnover, vacancy rate, and time to fill positions. High levels of turnover contribute to the same safety and burnout problems as not having positions allocated in the first place. Nurse leaders must monitor their units for situations of high turnover rates; they must investigate the causes and follow through with strategies to decrease them. In situations

TABLE 8-3   Adjustment Explanation for Fiscal Year 2004

Emergency Department Budget Unit: Supplies and Minor Equipment, Fiscal Year 2004

Subcode	Description	Budget Adjustment ($)	Justification
8200	Maintenance and repairs	100	Ice machine is breaking more frequently
9200	Travel	685	Two extra conferences for TJC
9300	Airfare	200	As above

where cyclically large numbers of nurses leave areas for anesthesia or promotional opportunities, staffing strategies should account for the average number of vacancies, and hiring should begin far ahead of the vacancies.

Hours per patient day (HPPD) refers to the number of hours of care required over a 24-hour period. This measurement criteria was developed by the American Nurses Association for the National Database of Nursing Quality Indicators (NDNQI) to provide a way for organizations across the country to benchmark against one another to evaluate the effectiveness of their nursing model. Higher-acuity patients require an increased HPPD. The utilization of HPPD in the creation of the budget allows for a mathematical approach for analysis. The NDNQI values for the average HPPD are as follows:

Unit type: mean (SD), 25th percentile, median, 75th percentile
Adult Critical Care: 15.68(3.05), 13.83, 15.11, 17.08
Adult Step-Down: 8.01(2.16), 6.60, 7.63, 9.06
Adult Medical: 6.03(1.51), 5.07, 5.85, 6.82
Adult Surgical: 6.34(1.51), 5.37, 6.15, 7.02
Adult Medical-Surgical Combined: 6.12(1.60), 5.12, 5.91, 6.83
Adult Critical Access: 11.22(6.16), 7.12, 9.34, 12.21
Pediatric Critical Care: 19.05(3.82), 16.39, 18.73, 21.22
Pediatric Step-down: 10.97(2.04), 9.66, 10.86, 12.12
Pediatric Medical: 10.61(4.61), 7.92, 8.96, 12.05
Pediatric Surgical: 9.34(2.33), 7.94, 8.90, 10.76
Pediatric Medical-Surgical Combined: 10.87(4.78), 7.98, 9.45, 12.34
Well-baby Nursery: 6.20(2.67), 4.76, 5.97, 7.19
Level I Neonatal Continuing Care: 10.10(4.47), 8.16, 8.26, 10.78
Level II Intermediate Care: 12.64(4.72), 9.66, 11.64, 15.06
Level III/IV Critical Care: 11.64(2.51), 10.10, 10.17, 12.59
Psychiatric Adult: 4.26(1.58), 3.23, 4.04, 5.00
Psychiatric Child/Adolescent: 5.24(2.33), 3.87, 5.10, 5.98
Psychiatric Geripsych: 4.66(1.36), 3.83, 4.46, 5.45
Psychiatric other: 3.97(1.47), 3.01, 3.77, 4.81
Adult rehabilitation: 4.95(1.51), 3.99, 4.73, 5.68
Pediatric rehabilitation: 8.28(3.59), 4.00, 9.12, 10.60 (National Database of Nursing Quality Indicators, 2012, p. 4)

Acuity Models

In addition to the utilization of HPPD, another tool to help leaders allocate staffing appropriately is acuity assessment software. Such software is designed to apply a mathematical value to the care needs of a patient at the bedside, and it generates assignments made based on those needs. The idea of this strategy is to smooth out nursing staffing and to assign the appropriate numbers of patients to nurses based on what the assessment shows (Harper & McCully, 2007). Software tools are available for purchase, but they can be costly, so many organizations create their own. Regardless of the approach, there can be problems with overscoring and monitoring. An example of a web-based system is McKesson's Assignment and Workload Manager for ANSOS One-Staff. This software system uses objective clinical charting data to guide staff scheduling decisions. This hospital scheduling software module uses patient acuity and workload data to forecast staffing requirements for the current shift as well as for a 24-hour projection (Mckesson, 2015).

Mandated Ratios

The notion of nurse staffing legislation began with concerns about reducing levels of nursing at the bedside. The thinking was that if the government could mandate ratios, there would never be a concern for loss of nursing positions, and safe care at the bedside would be ensured. Lang, Hodge, Olson, Romano, and Kravitz (2004) studied the literature regarding outcomes of mandated ratios and published the evidence, which concluded that there was no support for minimum nurse–patient ratios with regard to quality and safety. However, the State of California implemented minimal staffing ratios in 2004, but since then no other states have adopted similar laws (Nelson, 2008). Twelve other states have implemented some form of regulation, but nothing close to the California approach.

Skill Mix

Another consideration for the development of an effective staffing plan is skill mix. Skill mix is defined as the combination of various categories or levels of staff, including professional and assistive. It is, however, important to realize that the substitution of a lower skill mix to achieve a more cost-effective approach to staffing can compromise, quality, safety, and patient satisfaction (Aiken et al., 2012).

PERSONNEL BUDGET

Most budgets for nursing personnel are based on quantitative workload measurements, such as a patient acuity system. A computer software program usually produces staffing requirements by shift and day. It produces an acuity index for each patient, and the formula indicates the needed staff by skill mix—RN, licensed practical nurse, nurse aide or extender—and by shift. It also compares actual staffing with required staffing, and a summary can be provided by month and year. Each day either the unit secretary or a nurse enters the acuity rating for each patient into a computer.

Table 8-4 is a nursing personnel budget based on a patient acuity rating system. The average daily census is obtained from records produced in the admissions office. It is the result of dividing the total patient days for a unit in 1 year by 365 days. Census reports are generated daily, monthly, and annually by a computer.

The application of a staffing formula for preparing the personnel budget for a specific unit is illustrated in **Box 8-3**. If the nursing department does not use an acuity system, HPPD can be used. Several organizations benchmark HPPD, comparing specific types of units and types of hospitals that can assist the CNO in determining if the HPPD need to be adjusted. Changes in the Medicare case mix index can also be used as a justification for HPPD adjustments.

In planning the personnel budget, the nurse has quantitative information related to staffing and can accurately predict the number of full-time equivalents (FTEs) needed for patient care. Other considerations must be weighed at the same time: Will there be a pay increase next year? If so, it must be calculated and

TABLE 8-4 Nursing Personnel Budget

Nursing Budget

1. The personnel budget is based on total number of hours of care needed, which is determined by the acuity levels (1–4).

   Patient Acuity Level HPPD (hours of care per patient day)

   1 4.0 hours

   2 6.4 hours

   3 10.5 hours

   4 16.0 hours

2. The staffing formula is

$$\frac{\text{Average census} \times \text{nursing hours} \times 1.4 \times 1.14}{7.5}$$

3. The total nursing personnel needed for an average daily census (ADC) and specific patient acuity is presented below. The total nursing personnel also includes unit secretaries.

Unit	ADC	Acuity	HPPD	RN	LPN	CNA	Other	Total
Medical								
Oncology	17.1	3.0	10.5	24	2	12	4	42
BMT	8.2	4.0	16.0	22	0	6	2	30
Telemetry	22.3	2.0	6.4	18	3	9	6	36
4S	19.4	1.0	4.0	9	2	6	3	20
MICU	8.0	4.0	16.0	27	0	0	3	30
Total				100	7	33	18	158
Surgical								
Orthopedics	30.0	2.0	6.4	26	5	10	6	47
SICU	8.0	4.0	16.0	27	0	0	4	31
4CW	20.3	2.0	6.4	22	0	6	3	31
5CW	26.7	2.0	6.4	28	1	7	3.5	39.5
Total				103	6	23	16.5	148.5
Women's & Infants								
NBN	18.4	2.0	6.4	21	0	4	4.0	29
NICU	19.3	4.0	16.0	65	0	0	4.5	69.5
L & D*	28	0				7	3.5	38.5
Women's	24.1	2.0	6.4	25	2	6	2	35
Total				139	2	17	14	172.0
Inpatient Rehabilitation								
3 East	11.7	2.0	6.4	9	1	6	4	20

* No acuity system.

Abbreviations: 4CW: 4 Center West; 5CW: 5 Center West; 4S: 4 South; BMT: Bone Marrow Transplant; L & D: Labor and Delivery; MICU: Medical Intensive Care Unit; NBN: New Born Nursery; NICU: Neonatal Intensive Care Unit; SICU: Surgical Intensive Care Unit.

The staffing formula is

$$\frac{\text{Average census} \times \text{nursing hours} \times 1.4 \times 1.14}{7.5}$$

Example: Oncology Unit

- Average daily census = 17.1
- HPPD = 10.5
- 1.4 is a constant representing 7 days in a week with a full-time employee working 5 days a week: $7 \div 5 = 1.4$

- 1.14 is a constant that allows for 0.14 FTE for vacation, sickness, etc. for each 1.0 FTE
- 7.5 is one workday

$$\frac{17.1 \times 10.5 \times 1.4 \times 1.14}{7.5} = 38\,\text{FTEs}$$

The budgeted staffing for the Oncology Unit consists of 24 RNs, 2 LPNs, and 12 CNAs. In addition, the unit has 4 unit secretaries.

budgeted. Will benefits increase or decrease? They must also be budgeted. If new programs are being implemented, do they require additional labor power? Will this labor power come from cutbacks in other programs or from added FTEs? **Box 8-4** provides a worksheet for adding new positions to the budget.

Personnel accounts for the largest portion of the nursing budget. When one is preparing budgets for clinics, emergency departments, recovery rooms, operating rooms, delivery rooms, and home care, quantitative data must be available, such as

1. Job Title:
2. Department:
3. FTE Status:
   - Exempt
   - Non-exempt
4. Expected Starting Date:
5. Hours/Shift:
   - Full time
   - Part time
   - Permanent
   - Temporary: If temporary, provide finishing date
6. Description of Essential Job Duties:
   _____
   _____

7. Justification for New Position (e.g., new program/increased volume):
8. Requirements Essential for Position (e.g., licensure, education):
9. Advertising:
10. Preferred Publication:
    - Yes
    - No
11. Approvals:
    Supervisor: Date:
    Human Resources: Date:

numbers of visits, procedures, and deliveries. Records of length of time required for each activity can be obtained by using management engineering techniques in which visits, procedures, or other activities are charted over a period of time.

Data should be collected over a representative period to show the actual hours worked by shift and by day. The data indicate fluctuations in the workload by shift and by day of the week. Use a second data sheet to determine the total number of patients in the emergency department at any one time, including patients in a holding status. Conversion of the data into graphs provides information to compare staffing with workload. The data provide the following information (Penner, 2013):

- Current nursing hours available per patient visit
- Fluctuations in available hours by shift and by day
- Fluctuations in workload by time of day
- Fluctuations in ratio of staffing levels to patient load

Basic staffing of an emergency room should be calculated to handle a critical mass, which is the staffing level required to handle an unexpected emergency. In addition to quantitative data, the CNO should collect qualitative data from the staff to assist in containing stress, determining staff mix, and improving support services. Data can be compared with data from other institutions. The result is then translated into personnel dollars (Finkler & Jones, 2013).

In the process of budgeting, the nurse manager knows how much each decision will cost and whether it involves numbers and kinds of personnel or amounts and kinds of supplies and equipment. Few nurse managers have the luxury of a budget that provides all the resources that can be used. Hard decisions must be made. These decisions are easier to substantiate when workloads are quantified. If the patient dependency or acuity system is reliable and valid and has quality checks on the raters, it will provide data that justify the personnel budget. When the number of adult patients of the highest-acuity level increases from 24 to 32 per shift and day, the budget must be adjusted. Comparisons must be made to determine whether other levels have decreased. Estimates must be made as to whether the increases and decreases are permanent or temporary. Then the budget decisions are made.

Nurse managers study fluctuation trends in patient census and use the data for minimum staffing requirements to determine the percentage of time to staff one nurse less and the percentage of time to staff one nurse more per shift. The salary expense for the one time that one nurse less per shift is needed should be subtracted from the budget. The salary expense for the one time that one nurse more per shift is needed should be added to the budget. The result is an improved salary expense budget result.

The following strategies can reduce budget overages (Finkler & Jones, 2013):

- Maintain good staff retention.
- Use nurse extenders to perform non-RN functions.
- Monitor and control unscheduled absenteeism.
- Implement an effective on-call system.
- Institute a flex team in related clinical areas to avoid overtime and agency nurse expenses.

- Create a large pool of part-time nurses.
- Budget according to trends.
- Negotiate for a reasonable budget that considers turnover and orientation.

NONPRODUCTIVE FULL-TIME EQUIVALENTS

Nonproductive FTEs are hours for which an employee is paid but does not work, such as vacation days, holidays, sick days, education and training time, jury duty, leave for funerals, and military leave. These nonproductive hours must be determined and added to personnel expenditures as replacement FTEs. An FTE is based on 2,080 hours per year. If the nonproductive FTE average is to be used for personnel budgeting, the human resource department payroll section will provide it. An example is as follows:

- Average vacation per FTE: 12.5 days
- Average holiday per FTE: 7.0 days
- Average sick days per FTE: 3.5 days
- Average training and education per FTE: 3.0 days
- Average other leave per FTE: 1.5 days
- Total: 27.5 days or 220.0 hours

As a general rule, the total work time for full-time employees is 2,080 hours annually less 220 hours; the actual work time is 1,860 hours. The percentage of nonworked to total hours paid is 10.6%. The percentage of nonworked to worked hours is 11.8%.

A cost center manager prepares the budget according to management rules. The budget should include a line item for replacement FTEs to cover nonproductive FTEs by assigning a fixed amount to each person's paid time off. An option is to determine the percentage of nonproductive FTEs and add this total to the budget. This information is then used for staffing determinations, as are seasonal fluctuations for vacations, census, and other pertinent factors.

SUPPLIES AND EQUIPMENT BUDGET

The supplies and equipment budget is part of the operating or cash budget. It includes all supplies and equipment used in the provision of services, except capital equipment and supplies charged directly to patients. Minor equipment, such as sphygmomanometers, otoscopes, and ophthalmoscopes, costs less than the base amount set for capital equipment. If the base amount is $500, all equipment under $500 appears as minor equipment in the supplies and equipment budget.

Generally, the director of materials management furnishes the total cost of supplies and equipment per cost center to the accounting office, which generates a cost per patient day. This cost is used for budgeting purposes, and increases for inflation are a decision of top management. Based on projected patient days and revenues, decisions can be made to increase or decrease the supplies and equipment budget. Controlling the amounts of supplies can decrease costs and equipment kept in inventory. Nurse managers should look at the inventories they control and reduce them according to usage.

CAPITAL BUDGET

A capital budget is usually separate from the operating budget (**Table 8-5**). A capital budget projects the planned costs of major purchases. Each capital budget item is defined in terms of dollar value and is an item of equipment that is used over a period of time. The budget provides for depreciation of each item in the capital budget, sets aside the amount of depreciation in an escrow account, and uses this account to finance new capital budgets. Depreciation records the declining value of a physical asset. In addition, department heads are required to justify and set priorities on capital budget items. The exact definition of what constitutes a capital budget item with regard to dollar amount and life expectancy varies among hospitals.

Capital budgets also deal with maintenance, renovations, remodeling, improvements, expansion, land acquisition, and new buildings. The financial manager for nursing is the nurse manager, who should evaluate past decisions and advise the nurse administrator whether they were good or bad.

All proposals for capital equipment must be fully evaluated for amount of use, method of payment, safety, replacement, duplication of service, and every other conceivable factor, including the need for space, personnel, and facility renovation (**Box 8-5**). The needs and desires of the medical staff should be considered. Staff involvement in planning helps ensure wise purchases of capital equipment.

A strategic capital budgeting method based on principles of decision analysis can help healthcare organizations allocate capital effectively when meeting requests for capital expenditures. There are eight steps in the strategic capital budgeting method:

1. Establish evaluation criteria.
2. Classify proposals by area of investment.
3. Ensure that proposals are complete and easy to understand.
4. Determine costs of proposals.
5. Rate proposals with respect to individual criteria.
6. Set priority weights for criteria.
7. Calculate weighted value scores for each proposal.
8. Rank proposals by cost–benefit ratios.

The results provide a reliable basis for optimal capital allocation (Finkler & Jones, 2013).

The capital budget must address increased forms of competition, dwindling financial resources, and regulatory constraints. Management should enhance conditions under which effective planning and capital budgeting increase the agency's chance of long-term survival. Capital budgeting is a part of the overall budget planning process for the organization, not an individual entity. When each entry or item in the capital budget list has been analyzed and reduced to the amount available, the budget is again tabulated. It is now ready to present to the board of directors. With the board's approval, the list is distributed to cost center managers, who prepare requisitions for purchase. The purchasing department prepares bid specifications, with input from cost center managers. Purchases are finalized based on results of bids submitted by vendors who meet the required specifications. Finally, purchases are entered into the depreciation budget schedule. The latter

TABLE 8-5   Capital Budget Requested Fiscal Year; Metropolitan Memorial Hospital

Dept.	Item	Quantity	Amount ($)
6th & 7th	Beds & misc. pat. furn.	85	$200,000.00
Admin	Pneumatic tube system	1	75,000.00
Anest	Capnograph—portable	1	4,200.00
Anest	Trans. Mon.–inc NIPB & O_2 Sat	1	9,200.00
Anest	Ventilators	2	5,050.00
ER Med	Pro Pac 106	1	13,790.00
Bio Med	Safety tester	1	1,695.00
Blood Bk	Table top centrifuge	1	2,000.00
Blood Bk	Automated cell washer	1	6,250.00
Cath Lab	Pulse oximetry	1	2,600.00
Cath Lab	Dynamap	1	3,800.00
Clin Lab	Miscellaneous equipment	1	250,000.00
Dialysis	Dialysis machine	1	25,000.00
Dietary	Refrigerator—bakery	1	3,500.00
Dietary	Refrigerator—bakery	1	6,950.00
Dietary	Refrigerator—cook area	1	3,500.00
Dietary	Refrigerator—PFS	1	3,100.00
Dietary	Meat slicer	1	3,500.00
ER	New monitoring system	1	160,000.00
ER	Propak monitor	1	3,500.00
Envir	High-speed burnisher	4	8,000.00
Envir	Slow-speed buffers	2	1,600.00
GI Lab	Video processor CV-100	1	20,000.00
CVStation	Blood pressure monitor	1	4,500.00
CVStation	Stress test system	1	20,000.00
CVStation	ECG management system	1	70,000.00
MICU/CCU	Faceplates—central monitors	12	4,920.00
Nursing	Medication carts	17	25,000.00
Nutri	Computer & printer	1	2,011.00
OR	Laparoscopic video system	1	30,165.00
OR	Electrosurgical cautery	2	17,200.00
PACU	RR stretchers	10	20,000.00
Plant Op	4,000-watt portable generator	1	1,495.00
Plant Op	8 ch. OPS card for telephone switch	1	1,337.00
Radio	Rebuilt film processor	1	12,000.00
Res Th	Sterile pass-through drier	1	12,567.00
SPD	Washer decontaminator	1	75,000.00
Staff Dev	Overhead projector	1	700.00
Staff Dev	CPR manikin	1	5,641.00
Total requested Metropolitan Memorial Hospital			$1,114,771.00

BOX 8-5 Capital Equipment Requisition Form

1. Project description: _____
2. Date: _____
3. Submitted by: _____
4. Department: _____
5. Equipment requested: _____
6. Useful life: _____
7. Justification for equipment:
   - Regulatory
   - New service
   - Replacement
   - Upgrade
8. How often will equipment be requested/utilized?
9. Equipment description: _____
10. Impact to other departments: _____
    - Plant operations (renovation, installation)
    - Bio-Med
    - ISD
    - Education department
    - Other
11. Costs:
    - Equipment costs: _____
    - Renovation/installation: _____
    - Service agreement: _____
    - Personnel: _____
    - Education/training: _____
    - Shipping: _____
    - Storage: _____
12. For any equipment $5,000 or over, an equipment evaluation must be completed.
    _____Yes   _____ No (attach evaluation form)
13. For any equipment $25,000 or over, a financial pro forma must be completed.
    _____Yes   _____ No (attach pro forma)
14. Approvals:
    Department Director: Date:
    Administrator: Date:

---

is published by American Hospital Publishing and is considered the standard for the industry. The following are a few examples of the composite estimated useful lives of depreciable hospital assets: boiler house, 30 years; masonry building with wood or metal frame, 25 years; electric bed, 12 years; and otoscope, 7 years. For budgetary purposes, the nurse manager should have access to the entire publication (Finkler & Jones, 2013).

When evaluating capital equipment, one should evaluate similar products one at a time. When purchasing capital equipment, one should determine whether it can be upgraded or must be replaced when the technology improves. One should consider construction, durability, modularity, warranty, availability of parts, and service agreements as part of the total cost of equipment. One should also consider leasing rather than buying (Penner, 2013).

CONTROLLING PROCESS

Now that we have seen the nursing budget from its planning and directing aspects, we can turn to its controlling or evaluating aspects. The budget establishes financial standards for the division of nursing and through the division's cost center for each nursing unit. Daily, weekly, monthly, and quarterly feedback provides information to compare managerial performance with the established standards. The results are used to make adjustments. You might ask yourself the kind of feedback nurses need relative to their budgets and cost control. Nurses need information to determine whether their goals are being met. Are they exceeding the budget? Is the excess both for costs and for revenues? Are the supplies and expenses of the quantity and quality planned? Is the equipment being purchased and installed as scheduled? Are employees being recruited and used effectively to produce the expected quality and quantity of nursing services? Is employee morale good? What adjustments need to be made? Where are the problems, and who is responsible for them?

Budget processes should be flexible to allow for increased and decreased volume of business. The hospital's finance department provides cost center managers with needed biometric information to make adjustments in staffing and in the use of supplies. The colossal mistakes of budgeting are made in the control area. Variations in budget should be used as a tool for decision making, not as an instance or reactionary intervention to make arbitrary cuts that result in unrealistic operating budgets for line managers (Penner, 2013).

MONITORING THE BUDGET

Various techniques have been described for monitoring the budget; however, all budget objectives should contain procedures for quality review, including identification of a team to perform such a review. If a program is not successful—that is, if it is not meeting objectives or is running above predicted costs and below predicted revenues—then a decision should be made about whether to rework or cancel it. Although it is very difficult, making this decision is essential to good control. The technique of canceling budgeted programs is sometimes referred to as sunsetting. A nurse manager should accept the responsibility for sunsetting programs that are costly and unprofitable.

In developing the nursing budget, it is necessary that the unit structures for nursing administration are comparable in type and quantity of workload. Developing and providing financial policies and guidelines are most successful when the top administrative team works with the budget monitor. The CNO is part of this team and brings to its meetings standards of service that are defensible (such as data on workload, including numbers and types of procedures, patients, surgical operations, and visits). These policies should reflect the long-term plans of the governing board.

Part of the information furnished to the CNO and managers is in the form of reports, which include statistical reports of revenues and expenditures for the current year. **Table 8-6** illustrates financial information needed by the cost center manager and the CNO.

TABLE 8-6	Accounting System Report						
Account: 2-7010 **Department: 7010**				**Fiscal Year Ending 20xx** **January–October (83% fiscal year elapsed)** **Medical–Surgical Unit—Expense**			
Subcode	**Description**	**Actual Budget Approved ($)**	**Current Month ($)**	**YTD ($)**	**Open Encumbrances**	**Remaining Budget ($)**	**Percent Used**
1000	Pool—Salary & Wages	1,008,559					
1100	Professional Salary	848,323	72,533	848,323			100
1200	Nursing Asst. Salary	55,032	4,085	55,032			100
1300	Unit Secretary Salary	57,515	4,347	57,515			100
1400	Patient Care Tech Salary	56,131	3,936	56,131			100
1500	Students	14,898	14,898	14,898			100
1600	Accrued Salaries	32,791	32,791	32,791			100
	Salaries	$1,064,690	132,590	1,064,690			103
2000	Pool—Empl Benefits	55,722					0
2100	FICA	112	112	112			100
2200	Health Insurance	59,973	5,887	59,973			100
2300	Retirement	62,158	5,591	62,158			100
2400	Disability	4,869	526	4,869			100
2500	Life Insurance	2,569	264	2,569			100
	Employee Benefits	129,681	12,380	129,681			100
3000	Pool—Med/Surg	10,000					0
3100	Med & Surg Supplies	185,000	22,000	185,000			100
3110	Drugs	2,317	1,100	2,317			100
3114	Solutions	44,000	10,000	44,000			100
	Med/Surg Supplies	231,317	33,100	231,317			100
4000	Pool—General Supply						0
4010	Office Supplies	1,010	220	1,009			100
4120	Forms	1,490	1,090	1490		400	100

(Continues)

TABLE 8-6	Accounting System Report (Continued)						
Account: 2-7010				**Fiscal Year Ending 20xx**			
Department: 7010				**January–October (83% fiscal year elapsed)**			
				Medical–Surgical Unit—Expense			
Subcode	**Description**	**Actual Budget Approved ($)**	**Current Month ($)**	**YTD ($)**	**Open Encumbrances**	**Remaining Budget ($)**	**Percent Used**
4134	Copying	35	30	36			100
4260	Dietary	620	50	620			100
4330	Linen Bedding	215	215	215			100
4440	Housekeeping Supply	2,880	350	2,880			100
	General Supplies	6,250	1,955	6,250		400	100
5000	Minor Equipment	450				450	0
	Total Expenses	1,432,388	180,025	1,431,938	400		100
	Account Total	**1,432,388**	**180,025**	**1,431,938**	**400**	**450**	**100**

OPEN ENCUMBRANCE STATUS

P.O. Account	P.O. Number	Date	Original Description	Liquidating Encum.	Current Expenditures	Last Act Adjusts Encum.	Date
2-7010-4120	D3333	4/10/14	Print-All	400.00	400.00		10/4/14

Note that the account number at the head of the table in Table 8-6 is 2-7010. The prefix 2 denotes that the account balance does not turn over at the end of the fiscal year. The cost center or department is 7010. Financial transactions, including purchase orders for supplies and minor equipment, and payroll are identified with this cost center number and are charged by the purchasing and accounting departments to this number and to the appropriate subcodes 1000 through 5000. The table columns indicate the operational budget, the actual expenditures for the current month and for the fiscal or budget year, open encumbrances, and the balance available. Because 83% of the fiscal year (which begins January 1) has elapsed, these figures have some relationship to the Percent Used column. Although 103% of the budgeted salary has been used, only 70% of employee benefits have been used, which indicates a use of overtime plus part-time employees working less than the 20 hours per week required to qualify for benefits. Zero percent of the budgeted money for minor equipment has been spent to date. The total budget expenses were 97%, indicating a variance of 10% overspending. This report serves as a control for nurse managers, but the expenditure of budgeted money for any one subcode could cause the total expenses to date to be greater than the percentage of fiscal year elapsed without creating an alarm. In this instance, overspending should be related to increased census and revenue.

CUTTING THE BUDGET

When the budget must be cut, planning is a vital aspect of the process. Budget cuts happen as hospital admissions and stays decrease and reimbursement changes. The form and process of nursing management can determine the course of events when the budget has to be cut.

A nursing administration that delegates decision making to the lowest level and encourages participative management is an effective administration. When clinical nurses are informed at the unit level and are invited to give their input, they can help with suggestions for cutting costs. They gladly implement and support the activities they recognize as resulting partly from their input. A nursing organization that promotes self-direction at the levels of clinical nurse, nurse manager, clinical consultant, and executive nurse supports direction to reduce costs and to increase productivity and profits. For example, when a hospital chief executive officer discovered that self-pay patient care was the only category not reviewed for use of resources, a clinical nurse established a review process. Physicians and other healthcare professionals supported this.

Nursing budgets are enormous, and budgets for a single unit can run into hundreds of thousands of dollars per year. Pay awards or increases must be offset by budget cuts (personnel cutbacks), use of less-expensive supplies and techniques, or increased productivity. The latter requires more paying patients, shorter stays, and increased sales of all paying services. When personnel cuts are to be made, nursing is vulnerable. Some cuts can come from all services, but nursing has greater numbers. Nurse managers who control these numbers daily, weekly, and yearly have greater credibility.

As workload data indicate shifts from one unit to another, resources also must be shifted. Asking for volunteers, moving vacated positions, and using as-needed pools can do this. Inpatient procedures in hospitals have shifted to outpatient procedures either in hospitals or at ambulatory surgery centers. New reimbursement rates, which are part of a system of ambulatory patient classifications, have been issued by CMS and affect revenues from ambulatory services. Many more diagnostic procedures are now being done on an outpatient basis; as a result, inpatients are often a sicker group, requiring more nursing care (Finkler & Jones, 2013).

Because CNOs control multimillion-dollar budgets, they are powerful people. They are also vulnerable to personnel cuts. Much of this vulnerability stems from external controls imposed by state and federal governments and health insurance companies. Power comes from the ability of CNOs to use knowledge and skills in defending, directing, and controlling their budgets. They learn to hold the line on staffing and overtime and monitor for the appropriate use of supplies and equipment.

REIMBURSEMENT BASED ON CLINICAL PERFORMANCE

With the continued escalation of healthcare costs, the healthcare system has evolved to emphasize patient outcomes, controlling costs, and rewarding organizations that can do both. It is important for the CNO, nurse leaders, and clinicians to beware of the changing environment of reimbursement based on clinical quality (Penner, 2013). Although traditional forms of reimbursement are still maintained, the amount reimbursed to an organization or the ability to be a hospital of choice for covered lives depends on required reporting and performance of evidence-based criteria, better known as pay for performance (Penner, 2013). Driven by the Institute of Medicine report *To Err Is Human: Building a Safer Health System* (Kohn, Corrigan, & Donaldson, 1999), which outlined the cost of poor quality in the form of medical errors, hospital-acquired infections, and medical errors resulting in patient harm, CMS and other payers are focusing on improving patient safety and outcomes. They are making improvements through financial penalties for lack of participation or poor performance compared with peer hospitals (Medicare.gov, 2015). Likewise, this information is also provided for skilled nursing facilities and home care agencies that first contributed data that became the foundation for hospital public reporting.

It is important in the budgeting process for the CNO to understand how these performance requirements affect the nursing department budget and the overall bottom line of their organization. While meeting or exceeding the targets for reimbursement is a desired state, many organizations are finding that additional resources, particularly process improvement specialists and analytic specialists, are needed to monitor and meet these performance requirements.

U.S. HEALTHCARE SYSTEM

The U.S. healthcare system has many components: patients, insurers, and employers; providers such as hospitals, ambulatory care services, home care services, long-term care facilities, physicians, nurses, allied health personnel, pharmacists and pharmacies, and providers of durable medical equipment; and federal, state, and local public health services. In an effort to reduce healthcare costs, new models of care delivery and shared risk contracts have emerged. As such, the implications for nurse leader proficiency in budgeting and the allocation of resources have taken greater prominence, particularly in care that is provided outside acute care settings.

The passage of the Patient Protection and Affordable Care Act will provide mechanisms for all U.S. citizens to have some form of health insurance coverage. To cover the cost of this expansion of coverage, more pressure will be placed on hospitals and other providers to produce cost savings through more efficient and coordinated care. Services once provided in the confines of an acute care hospital will be provided in skilled nursing facilities, clinics, outpatient centers, and homes. The emphasis on wellness and prevention will create opportunities for nurses to educate and empower the public through health education, but the delivery systems for this care are in their infancy, typically requiring significant financial support as they are initiated (Dunham-Taylor & Pinczuk, 2014). Once believed to be in the purview of hospital systems, new services supported by technology are being run by individuals outside the health sector (Penner, 2013).

Mechanisms such as value-based purchasing, bundled payments to providers, and continued payment reductions for poor clinical outcomes, including readmissions and hospital-acquired conditions, need to be translated into the budgeting process. Value-based purchasing provides a vehicle for incentive payments to hospitals based on the quality of care provided. Initiated in 2010 as part of the Affordable Care Act and the healthcare reform process, it provides payment incentives for demonstrated outcomes on select core measures for organizations that meet expected best practices or to those who improve their performance. In addition to clinical outcomes, the patient experience was added in 2013 to incorporate elements of patient satisfaction, healthcare team member communication, discharge information, and pain management. In 2015, an efficiency metric will be added (U.S. Department of Health and Human Services, 2011).

Bundled payments for all providers along the care continuum to share will become the norm, as opposed to the current payment model in which each location and individual provider receives reimbursement (Penner, 2013). As an example, a 70-year-old falls at home, fractures a hip, and presents to the emergency room for care by physicians. The patient is transferred to the operating room for surgical intervention and is then admitted to the orthopedic unit from the postanesthesia care unit. After 5 days on the inpatient unit, the patient is transferred to a skilled nursing facility for additional rehabilitation before returning home with home care. In a bundled payment environment, reimbursement for the episode of care starting in the emergency room and ending with home services will be shared by all involved providers, irrespective of the location of care and number of providers. Organizations that are able to manage costs and care coordination will be best positioned for longer-term viability.

In 2013, CMS initiated bundled payment pilot systems to align care coordination, clinical care outcomes, and reimbursement. The Bundled Payments for Care Improvement initiative required organizations to enter into payment arrangements whereby financial and performance accountability for specified diagnosis-related group (DRG) care episodes were selected. In one of four care delivery models, organizations committed to the provision of care across specialty and practice settings for payment arrangements that include financial and performance accountability for episodes of care. The foundational hypothesis of these pilots is that the new models may lead to higher-quality, more coordinated care at a lower cost. Although the results and outcomes are incomplete, they offer promise in informing future healthcare reform (Centers for Medicare and Medicaid Services [CMS], 2013).

Effective January 1, 2011, the Affordable Care Act included changes for certain preventive services, such as waiving patient cost-sharing requirements for most Medicare-covered preventive services; Medicare pays fully for these services. Currently, no coinsurance or deductible is required for personalized prevention plan services and any covered preventive service recommended with a grade of A or B by the U.S. Preventive Services Task Force. The Hospital Outpatient Prospective Payment System (OPPS) "applies to designated hospital outpatient services furnished in all classes of hospitals, with the exception of . . . hospitals that provide only Part B services to inpatients; Critical Access Hospitals (CAH); Indian Health Service (IHS) and Tribal hospitals, including IHS Tribal CAHs; hospitals located in American Samoa, Guam, and the Commonwealth of the Northern Mariana Islands; . . . hospitals located in the Virgin Islands; and hospitals in Maryland (that are paid under Maryland waiver provisions)" (CMS, 2014c, p. 4).

AMBULATORY PAYMENT CLASSIFICATIONS

For the most part, the unit of payment under the OPPS is Ambulatory Payment Classifications (APC). CMS assigns individual services (Healthcare Common Procedure Coding System [HCPCS] codes) to APCs based on similar clinical characteristics and similar costs. The payment rate and copayment calculated for an APC apply to each service within the APC.

Generally, new services are assigned to New Technology APCs, which are based on similarity of resource use only until cost data are available to permit assignment to a clinical APC. The payment rate for a New Technology APC is set at the midpoint of the applicable New Technology APC's cost range.

The payment rates for most separately payable medical and surgical services are determined by multiplying the prospectively established scaled relative weight for the service's clinical APC by a conversion factor to arrive at a national unadjusted payment rate for the APC. The scaled relative weight for an APC measures the resource requirements of the service and is based on the geometric mean cost of services in that APC. The conversion factor translates the scaled relative weights into dollar payment rates. For calendar year 2014, national unadjusted payment rates and copayments for each HCPCS code for which separate payment was made that applied to the date of service was published in the Addenda of the calendar year 2014 Hospital Outpatient Prospective Payment Final Rule with Comment (CMS, 2014c).

Nurse administrators need to understand the impact that changes both in care delivery systems and reimbursement will have on a healthcare system's fiscal viability and the demands placed on the nursing budget. Additionally, for care directly tied to clinical outcomes, nurses and nurse leaders will have greater responsibility and accountability in the provision of care and prevention of undesirable results. As such, they will need to demonstrate how requested nursing resources will make a difference at a cost that is not crippling to the organization.

SUMMARY

It is important for nurses to have a working knowledge of the objectives of budgeting and component costs. Every activity that takes place in a healthcare agency costs money. A standard must exist for assigning costs to departments. The nursing department should pay its share and no more. Knowledge of cost accounting systems provides accurate information for budgeting and for cost management.

The major elements of nursing budgets are personnel, supplies and equipment (minor), and capital equipment. Generally, equipment that costs less than a fixed dollar amount is included in the supplies and equipment budget. A product evaluation committee is useful for ensuring that supplies and equipment promote effective and efficient patient care. The capital equipment budget includes equipment that costs more than a fixed dollar amount; it is prepared separately from the supplies and equipment budget.

Evaluation is an administrative aspect of budgeting that in itself serves as a controlling process. Decentralization vests control at the lowest competent level of decision making. Good budget feedback is essential if the budget is to be an effective controlling process. Good feedback includes information about revenues and expenses as well as internal comparisons of projected and actual budgets. The budget can motivate professional nurses to facilitate their development of innovations.

The belief that budgets are beyond comprehension can sabotage a nurse's effectiveness. Spiraling healthcare costs, cost management efforts, and increasing accountability from individual cost centers should serve as an impetus for nurses to learn the fundamentals of budgets and the budgeting process. Assuming the responsibility for budget work increases the nurse's potential realm of planning, predicting, and reviewing programs within the nurse's jurisdiction. Like a nursing care plan, the budget is an activity guidance tool. It is a plan expressed in monetary terms and carried out within a time frame. To be an effective caregiver, the nurse must know how to develop and use a nursing care plan. Similarly, to be most effective as a manager, the nurse manager must know how to develop and use a budget.

One main competency the nurse manager must possess is understanding financial information and evolving payment for performance processes and measures. The objectives of this transformation are reduced costs, improved clinical quality, and increased efficiency. Although pay for performance continues to be developed, it is here to stay, and the nursing department must understand the implications of this reimbursement plan to play an active role in the organization's overall performance.

REFLECTIVE QUESTIONS

1. Locate and read five recent articles in nursing journals about pay for performance. Summarize the implications for the nursing profession.
2. Attend a marketing session given by an insurance company offering healthcare products. Analyze the presentation. What are the advantages and disadvantages for the patient?
3. You are having lunch with a nurse colleague who asks you about your current courses. She asks you what you think the three most important financial concerns are that face the nursing profession. Offer your three concerns and review the literature to find supportive evidence.

CASE STUDY 8-1   Budgeting to Enhance Professional Practice and Productivity

Lori Lioce and Kristen Herrin

Jennifer Broadwater is the director of women's health of a regional not-for-profit healthcare system. She has doctoral preparation in executive leadership. Prior to her current appointment, Jennifer served as a nurse manager at a small private hospital for 2 years after graduation.

Historically, Jennifer's department has run smoothly and efficiently and was one of the premier departments within the organization. Over the past 3 months, some of the nurses began requesting transfers to other departments, and some resigned to seek employment outside the organization. The CNO is concerned and would like Jennifer to make this her first priority.

The department consists of 175 full- and part-time employees: 88 BSN RNs, 61 ADN RNs, 24 patient care technicians, and 2 unit secretaries. In the past, the staff has worked well together. Recently, nonproductive turnover has increased and has resulted in additional stress among the staff, creating a negative, distrusting culture. Due to many seasoned nurses leaving and new nurses coming on board, the staff reports being overwhelmed with orienting new nurses and dealing with nursing students. In addition, the staff feels that the patients may not be getting the proper care.

CASE STUDY 8-1   Budgeting to Enhance Professional Practice and Productivity (Continued)

Staffing and Resource Management

An in-depth staff analysis reveals certain nurses with a pattern of callouts. Jennifer reports to her CNO that she will need to address productivity, accountability, and productive turnover versus nonproductive turnover. Jennifer considers the best use of her staffing mix to maximize efficiency and productivity. The hospital has Magnet designation and a shared governance model, using relationship-based care as their professional practice model. Jennifer is concerned that the shared governance model and the relationship-based care model may not be translating to the day-to-day operations of patient care delivery. Jennifer is considering an alternative nursing care delivery model that might be used with the current staffing mix to enhance productivity and better meet the needs of staff and patients.

Case Study Questions

1. Jennifer's department uses a decentralized budgeting process. Using the eight steps identified in the procedures for decentralized budgeting, identify how Jennifer would use her understanding of her staffing mix, patient care needs, and shared governance model to best address department problems.
2. Using the staffing mix, how might Jennifer maximize her professional nursing capacity, considering the need to increase her BSN RN pool?

REFERENCES

Advisory Board Company. (2012). Hospitals' Medicare cuts under sequester: $5.8 billion. Retrieved from http://www.advisory.com/daily-briefing/2012/09/17/how-much-medicare-money-will-hospitals-lose-to-sequestration

Aiken, L. H., Clarke, S. P., Sloane, D. M., Lake, E. T., & Chaney, T. (2008). Effects of hospital care environment on patient mortality and nurse outcomes. *Journal of Nursing Administration*, 38(5), 223–229.

Aiken, L. N., Havens, D. S., & Sloane, D. M. (2009). The Magnet nursing services recognition program. *Journal of Nursing Administration, 39*(7/8), S5–S14.

Aiken, L. H., Sermeus, W., Van den Heede, K., Sloane, D. M., Busse, R. McKee, M. . . . Kutney-Lee, Q (2012). Patient safety, satisfaction, and quality of hospital care: Cross sectional surveys of nurses and patients in 12 countries in Europe and the United States. *British Medical Journal, 344*, e1717.

American Nurses Association. (2014). Nurse staffing. Retrieved from http://nursingworld.org/MainMenuCategories/ThePracticeofProfessionalNursing/NurseStaffing

Budget. (n.d.). In *Merriam-Webster's online dictionary*. Retrieved from http://www.merriam-webster.com/dictionary/budget?show=0&t=1413311210

Centers for Medicare and Medicaid Services. (2013). Bundled payments for care improvement (BPCI) initiative: General information. Retrieved from http://innovation.cms.gov/initiatives/bundled-payments/

Centers for Medicare and Medicaid Services. (2014a). Cost report by fiscal year. Retrieved from: http://www.cms.gov/Research-Statistics-Data-and-Systems /Downloadable-Public-Use-Files/Cost-Reports/Cost-Reports-by-Fiscal-Year .html

Centers for Medicare and Medicaid Services. (2014b). Hospital outpatient prospective payment—final rule with comment. Retrieved from http://www.cms.gov /Medicare/Medicare-Fee-for-Service-Payment/HospitalOutpatientPPS /Hospital-Outpatient-Regulations-and-Notices-Items/CMS-1601-FC-.html

Centers for Medicare and Medicaid Services. (2014c). *Hospital outpatient prospective payment system.* Retrieved from http://www.cms.gov/Outreach -and-Education/Medicare-Learning-Network-MLN/MLNProducts /downloads/HospitalOutpaysysfctsht.pdf

Davis, P., Talaga, S., Binder, C., Hahn, J., Kirchhoff, S., Morgan, P., & Tilson, S. (2013). *Medicare primer.* Retrieved from http://fas.org/sgp/crs/misc/R40425 .pdf

Dunham-Taylor, T., & Pinczuk, J. Z. (2014). *Financial management for nurse managers: Merging the heart with the dollar* (3rd ed.). Burlington, MA: Jones & Bartlett Learning.

Ellerbe, S. (2013). What is driving the growing demand for consulting in hospital staffing, scheduling, and productivity? *Nursing Economics, 31*(5), 237–240.

Finkler, S. A., & Jones, B. C. (2013). *Financial management for nurse managers and executives* (4th ed.). St. Louis, MO: Elsevier Saunders.

Harper, K., & McCully, C. (2007). Acuity systems dialogue and patient classification system essentials. *Nursing Administration Quarterly, 31*(4), 284–299.

Lang, T. A., Hodge, M., Olson, V., Romano, P. S., & Kravitz, R. L. (2004). Nurse–patient ratios: A systematic review on the effects of nurse staffing on patient, nurse employee and hospital outcomes. *Journal of Nursing Administration, 34*(7–8), 326–337.

Mckesson. (2015). *Assignment and Workload Manager with Acuity Aggregator for ANSOS One-Staff.* Retrieved from http://www.mckesson.com/providers/health -systems/department-solutions/capacity-and-workforce-management /assignment-and-workload-manager-with-acuity-aggregator-for-ansos-one -staff/

Medicare.gov. (2015). Hospital compare. Retrieved from http://www.medicare .gov/hospitalcompare/search.html?AspxAutoDetectCookieSupport=1

National Database of Nursing Quality Indicators. (2012). Nursing hours per patient day. Retrieved from http://www.qualityforum.org/WorkArea/linkit.aspx ?LinkIdentifier=id&ItemID=70962

Needleman, J., Buerhaus, P., Pankratz, V. S., Leibson, C. L., Stevens, S. R., & Harris, M. (2011). Nurse staffing and inpatient hospital mortality. *New England Journal of Medicine, 364*(11), 1037–1045. doi:10.1056/NEJMsa1001025

Nelson, R. (2008). AJN reports: California's ratio law, four years later. *American Journal of Nursing, 108*(3), 25–26.

Patrician, P. A., Loan, L., McCarthy, M., Fridman, M., Donaldson, N., Bingham, M., & Brosch, L. R. (2011). The association of shift-level nurse staffing with adverse patient events. *Journal of Nursing Administration, 41*(2), 64–70. doi:10.1097/NNA.0b013e31820594bf

Penner, S. (2013). *Economics and financial management for nurses and nurse leaders* (2nd ed.). New York, NY: Springer.

U.S. Department of Health and Human Services. (2011). *Hospital value-based purchasing program*. Retrieved from http://www.cms.gov/Outreach-and -Education/Medicare-Learning-Network-MLN/MLNProducts/downloads /Hospital_VBPurchasing_Fact_Sheet_ICN907664.pdf

Maximizing Human Capital

Val Gokenbach

LEARNING OBJECTIVES

1. Explain how human capital affects staff satisfaction, turnover, patient satisfaction, and quality.
2. Define the concepts of emotional intelligence and emotional quotient as they apply to successful leadership approaches.
3. Define the term *empowerment* and describe its importance in a healthy work environment.
4. Develop a strategy for an effective communication infrastructure.
5. Discuss the management of difficult scenarios, including conducting crucial conversations, managing chaos, lateral violence, and bullying.
6. Discuss the management of a diverse work team, including gender, generational, and cultural differences.
7. Discuss strategies for renewing staff and reducing burnout.

AONE KEY COMPETENCIES

I. Communication and relationship building
II. Knowledge of the healthcare environment
III. Leadership
IV. Professionalism
V. Business skills

AONE KEY COMPETENCIES DISCUSSED IN THIS CHAPTER

I. Communication and relationship building
II. Knowledge of the healthcare environment
III. Leadership
IV. Professionalism
V. Business skills

I. **Communication and relationship building**
   - Effective communication
   - Relationship management
   - Influence of behaviors

- Ability to work with diversity
- Shared decision making
- Community involvement
- Medical staff relationships
- Academic relationships

II. Knowledge of the healthcare environment
- Clinical practice knowledge
- Patient care delivery models and work design knowledge
- Healthcare economics knowledge
- Healthcare policy knowledge
- Understanding of governance
- Understanding of evidence-based practice
- Outcomes measurement
- Knowledge of, and dedication to, patient safety
- Understanding of utilization and case management
- Knowledge of quality improvement and metrics
- Knowledge of risk management

III. Leadership
- Foundational thinking skills
- Personal journey disciplines
- Ability to use systems thinking
- Succession planning
- Change management

IV. Professionalism
- Personal and professional accountability
- Career planning
- Ethics
- Evidence-based clinical and management practices
- Advocacy for the clinical enterprise and for nursing practice
- Active membership in professional organizations

V. Business skills
- Understanding of healthcare financing
- Human resource management and development
- Strategic management
- Marketing
- Information management and technology

FUTURE OF NURSING: FOUR KEY MESSAGES

1. Nurses should practice to the full extent of their education and training.
2. Nurses should achieve higher levels of education and training through an improved education system that promotes seamless academic progression.
3. Nurses should be full partners with physicians and other health professionals in redesigning health care in the United States.
4. Effective workforce planning and policy making require better data collection and information infrastructure.

Introduction

Leadership theory in the United States has evolved over time, from the industrial era to the human resource era of today. Within the eras of discussion, various leadership strategies and approaches have evolved over time and have proven effective with management of the human being. Within the context of healthcare organizations, one must understand the nature of the individuals that choose healthcare careers and apply the leadership strategy that aligns with their preference for the optimal work environment.

A foundational understanding of human capital and strategies to effectively manage in a complex environment is essential to effective leading. Concepts of leadership approaches and operational strategies to maximize alignment, commitment, and effectiveness in the workplace with the goal of providing excellence in the quality of patient care will be addressed.

EVOLUTION OF LEADERSHIP IN THE UNITED STATES

Prior to understanding the current status of leadership theory in the United States, it is important to know how the current approaches evolved from the past to what they are today.

Prior to the Civil War, industry in the South was primarily farming, including cotton and consumable goods. Following the Civil War, there was a significant shift in the provision of goods and services from agriculture to manufacturing. The end of the war gave rise to capitalism. Businessmen from the North began to set up manufacturing facilities that utilized newly created technologies, such as the cotton gin, to help process crops for use in the textile industry. These machines needed people to run them, so local people were hired for wages to work in factories.

The increased demand for goods created a work environment that was less than acceptable for the workers. Long hours, unbearable heat, and a total lack of safety measures created dangerous work environments characterized by multiple cases of injury and death. There were no labor laws to protect workers, and oftentimes children were expected to work long hours in sweatshops. The general philosophy was that workers were a means to an end, and they were viewed as an extension of the equipment they were operating. The general leadership approach was autocratic, with managers pushing workers to continually do more at the expense of their health and for meager wages.

This abuse of labor continued for several decades until the early 1950s, when workers began to rebel by creating unions and using their collective power to pressure owners and leaders through work stoppages and strikes. Unions were formalized and provided a forum for the workers to be heard, ultimately leading to changes in leadership practices. These changes led to the birth of the human resource era of leadership.

Human Resource Era

The human resource era, which still exists today, changed the focus of leadership from using and abusing employees to recognizing employees for the value of their contributions to organizations. Competitive pay rates and benefits packages, including vacation time and health insurance, were becoming commonplace and were a way for companies to attract workers in an increasingly competitive marketplace. New styles of leadership began to arise that allowed employees to have more input about their work environment. Although autocratic leadership approaches continue to this day, the overall focus on safe work environments and care for employees has improved.

LEADERSHIP APPROACHES

There are many theoretical leadership approaches that have been identified over the years. It is important for nurse leaders to be aware of these approaches, as well as approaches that have been recognized as effective with certain populations and in certain circumstances. Based on the work of Bass (1990), the approaches discussed in the following sections have been identified.

Autocratic or Authoritarian

Autocratic leaders believe that employees need to be managed to achieve what the leader or the organization needs. These leaders have a tendency to dictate to the staff what they expect them to do based on their own perception of what is needed. If this approach is used consistently, it has the tendency to stifle creativity and sends a message to the staff that their opinions do not matter. Over time the staff will feel that they are not valued by the manager or the organization. This will lead to a loss of loyalty and increased turnover.

There is a situation, however, in which autocratic leadership is appropriate and effective. In cases of crisis or emergency there may not be time to discuss possible strategies in a group setting. In this scenario, the leader needs to be decisive and directive. Effective decision making in times of crisis will demonstrate leadership and strength and engender the trust of followers.

Democratic or Egalitarian

Democratic leaders engage staff in joint decision making by relying on the skills of the staff to help direct choices. In this approach, leaders focus on relationship building with the staff so they can work together for the greater good of the organization. The democratic approach is humanistic in nature and is more empowering for the staff, which is associated with a higher degree of staff satisfaction and trust in the leader.

Contingency Theory

In 1967, Fiedler proposed the contingency approach to leadership, which is transactional in nature and has two major tenets. First is the notion that in regard to the type of staff and the nature of the situation, the leader would choose the staff's approach, contingent on the current needs. For example, a leader that is working with unskilled labor may need to take a more autocratic approach because employees in this category may need more direction. When working with professional staff, the leader would change the approach depending on the needs of the staff. The second consideration is that staff members should be utilized in situations that best suit their education, skills, and capabilities.

Transactional Leadership

In transactional leadership, the leader motivates the staff with rewards or pay, which constitutes a transaction. An example in nursing is premium pay and rewards to entice the staff to help with organizational goals. The problem with this approach is that it does not engender staff loyalty to the leader but rather focuses on the next reward. Loyalty becomes associated with the reward, and when the reward is removed, so is interest in helping the organization. It is important to be extremely cautious when using transactional leadership by carefully crafting the guidelines and length of programming and to effectively communicate the program to the staff to solicit their support and understanding of the boundaries.

Transformational Leadership

Bass (1990) described transformational leadership as shared governance by the leader and the followers. This approach is empowering, and the experience transforms the staff, the leader, and the organization. The transformational approach to leadership is recognized as the most effective approach for professional staff members who are independent in their practice. The Magnet program recognizes transformational leadership as vital to successful healthcare organizations and has developed a review process to assess the presence of transformational leadership as a major component to achieve Magnet designation.

Followership

A leader cannot achieve anything without effective followership. Transformational leaders engage followers to work together for a common goal. Boatman defined followership as an important strategy for effective leaders and "the willingness to cooperate in working towards the accomplishment of the group mission, to demonstrate a high degree of teamwork and to build cohesion among the group" (1997). Although in followership the focus is on the staff members who are followers, it is the leader who creates the environment in which followers are engaged and willing to follow in a way that moves the organization forward.

Servant Leadership

Leaders should serve. The sole role of the leader is to focus on the growth of those around them and provide opportunities and resources for the staff to achieve their goals and to be successful in their work. The success of the staff translates into the success of the organization and ultimately the success of the leader. This approach stands in stark contrast to the philosophy of leaders who believe that the reverse is true and that the staff is there to serve them and the organization.

Greenleaf and Spears (2002) describe servant leaders as servants first who have a true desire to provide for others. This type of leadership approach can build a tremendous degree of trust and appreciation between the leader and the staff.

Coaching

Many philosophers and psychologists believe that all humans have within them all the components they need to make decisions and thrive. At times, however, individuals may need someone to support and coach them to think in new ways and to identify new strategies to achieve what they desire. Hillman (1996) relates these concepts to the acorn theory. Within the nucleus, an acorn is supplied with all the material it needs to grow into a beautiful oak tree. It simply needs support from the environment in the form of soil, water, and sun.

Coaching as a leadership approach is very similar. Employees are coached to success with the understanding that they already know what needs to be done and how to do it, yet they need the confidence and support of their leaders in a coaching and caring environment. Oftentimes people rebel when they are told what to do, but when they are coached into finding their own answers they are open to suggestions and opportunities. Wahl, Scriber, and Bloomfield (2013) described the concept of becoming and the psychological need for all human beings to become something. They further state that the coach has the ability to help people become through a holistic approach of caring and supporting.

A VOID OF LEADERSHIP

Many leadership theorists believe there is a true void of effective leadership in this country. This is partly due to the tremendous stressors faced by leaders and a reluctance of younger employees to seek leadership roles. Nurses are often chosen to move into formal leadership positions because they are recognized as the best clinical nurses who are worthy of recognition, not necessarily for their leadership skills and abilities. Without effective leadership in nursing, healthcare organizations will not be successful, and nursing as a profession will not be recognized for the value it provides to the greater good of the world population.

ACCOUNTABILITY CHAIN OF LEADERSHIP

Accountability can be simply defined as the willingness to accept responsibility and account for one's actions (Accountability, n.d.). Leaders must accept ultimate responsibility for their actions that result in the creation of the work environment and related outcomes. Schein (2004) attributes the creation of the culture, whether successful or not, to the leader. In other words, regardless of the environment and potential challenges in the organization, leaders must embrace their accountability and create a culture that nurtures and supports the staff. The culture encompasses shared values, rituals, artifacts, and core beliefs that must be espoused by the majority of the staff to be effectively inculcated and therefore leveraged. The culture also needs to be supported at all levels in the chain of leadership, from senior nursing executives to point-of-care leaders.

The role of leadership in healthcare organizations continues to become more complex and difficult with competing priorities and the need to reduce costs and improve quality. Nursing leaders must first of all realize the challenges inherent in such roles and accept accountability for the expectations. The following components are global responsibilities that align with the management of human capital in healthcare organizations:

- Create a nurturing culture of empowerment that supports the staff and allows them to function to their highest capacity.
- Accept responsibility for quality scores.
- Accept responsibility for patient satisfaction scores.

- Accept responsibility for nurse and staff satisfaction scores.
- Create a framework for empowerment, innovation, and communication.
- Develop successful relationships with physician and practitioner colleagues.
- Develop successful relationships with ancillary departments that aid in the delivery of care.
- Accept responsibility for effective budget management.
- Accept responsibility for turnover and vacancy rates.
- Serve as a liaison between the staff and senior administration.
- Maintain a high level of visibility with all staff.

CREATING A NURTURING CULTURE OF EMPOWERMENT

Price and Price (2012) describe the concept of empowerment as a function of allowing employees to make decisions about their own work. Transformational approaches to leadership most closely align with the inculcation of an effective culture of empowerment. The authors identified four major categories that are especially important to employees:

- How they work and the processes employed
- Where they work
- When they work
- How they complete their work

To develop an empowered workplace, there are several leadership strategies that must be employed by the leader:

- Set expectations: Since the leader is the one responsible for the organizational culture, the entire staff must understand what the expectations are in order to fulfill them. This should include operational issues; for example, if the staff will do self-scheduling, they need to understand the expectations surrounding budgets and staffing methodologies. The staff should also understand their responsibilities and the expectations surrounding satisfaction and quality scores and their ability to enact strategies to improve them at the point of service. Setting expectations provides the initial road map that serves as a basis for other decisions and strategies.
- Define responsibilities: Along with setting expectations, the staff needs to understand what their boundaries are related to what changes they can make in their work environment. For instance, a process change for care may need financial support or the support of other departments. The staff needs to understand who can reach out for financial support and who can help connect them with other departments. The staff may be interested in recommending changes to benefits packages and other human resources processes, but in absence of collective bargaining they will need to understand that this is not an area in which they can focus their efforts.
- Be open and approachable: As far back as the time of Abraham Lincoln, the leader's visibility and approachability is the key to developing the trust of the staff. In his book *Lincoln on Leadership*, Phillips related Lincoln's leadership success to his strategy of "leadership by walking around" (1993). Especially during turbulent times during his presidency, Lincoln felt that his presence provided a feeling of safety and support to his soldiers and staff members

and allowed for dialogue that helped him not only make better decisions, but also to also elicit the support of the staff for those decisions.

Studor, in his book *Hardwiring Excellence* (2004), supports visibility through structured and consistent rounding with the staff as a way to increase communication, improve the level of accountability at the point of service, and provide an opportunity for real-time support and recognition. Although leaders who feel overwhelmed with the responsibilities of their positions may find it difficult to commit to consistent rounding and a high degree of visibility to the staff, the evidence from Studor (2004) positively correlates both patient and staff satisfaction with these activities.

Another extremely effective way to increase visibility and trust with the staff is for leaders to wear scrubs and work with the staff on the units. This provides leaders with hands-on experience of the challenges of the work area and provides an opportunity for casual dialogue with the staff. The further away leaders are from the point of service, the less expert they are at processes that are taking place. The staff is the best resource for improvement recommendations.

- Understand the staff: To provide an effective and successful work environment for the staff, leaders must understand what the staff needs and wants. The only way to gain this understanding is to get to know the staff. Although leaders establish the underlying culture, it is important to craft an environment that allows for optimal staff satisfaction and effectiveness. Leaders need to get the know the staff in order to understand them. High visibility, an effective communication structure, staff meetings, and focus group meetings with two or three staff members at a time are strategies to increase connectivity.

- Encourage knowledge sharing: Clinical staff members have a high degree of academic preparation and the desire to learn and create. Sellman (2011) described several core values that are common to nurses across the globe, including care, compassion, altruism, and a desire for knowledge. Since nursing is a science-based profession, it makes sense that a thirst for knowledge is important. The utilization of an evidence-based approach to quality improvement provides the foundation for knowledge exploration and sharing.

- Encourage risk taking and innovation: After a foundation of trust has been built between the leader and the staff, a willingness to take risks can be encouraged. In a safe environment, staff will feel that their ideas and creativity can be shared and will be evaluated with an open mind. The leader needs to openly encourage this level of risk taking and help the staff think of process changes in new and different ways.

MAGNET DESIGNATION AND EMPOWERMENT

Magnet designation, created by the American Nurses Credentialing Center (ANCC), has become the gold standard for quality in nursing practice supported by a healthy work environment. The designation supports three particular goals for organizations:

1. To improve quality in a setting that supports professional practice
2. To identify excellence in the delivery of nursing care to patients

3. To disseminate best practices throughout nursing (Magnet Recognition Program Overview, 2014)

Over the years, more and more studies have been conducted that suggest the components upon which the Magnet culture is built directly correlates with superior patient care (Aiken, Havens, & Sloan, 2009). Magnet designation is now recognized for quality by *U.S. News & World Report* in its annual reviews of hospitals, the Best Hospitals Honor Roll and the Best Children's Hospitals Honor Roll.

The components that relate to this degree of quality are organized into five distinct categories:

- Transformational leadership: The ability of the nursing team, led by the chief nursing officer (CNO), to transform the work environment
- Structural empowerment: The evidence of a healthy work life supported by a philosophy of empowerment and inclusion of the staff in decisions for their practice
- Exemplary professional practice: Evidence that nurses are making a difference by being involved in strategies and programs to enhance the quality of care at the bedside and in the community in alignment with other care partners and colleagues
- New knowledge: Evidence that there is a consistent approach to innovation, improvement, and research and the sharing of that knowledge throughout the organization and beyond
- Empirical outcomes: Proof of quality measures as evidenced by scoring of nurse-sensitive indicators

The fact that ANCC has identified structural empowerment as a separate category for Magnet designation is evidence of the value it places on this component in the workplace. Although empowerment can be described as a philosophy of leaders who believe in the importance of reaching out to staff and including them in decision making, the most successful organizations hard wire the concept of empowerment through the establishment of a structure that suits the organization.

EMPOWERMENT MODEL STRUCTURES

Three criteria are necessary to support effective empowerment models:

- Supportive hospital administration: For nurses to feel truly empowered, they need to feel supported by the entire organization, including physicians and hospital departments that interface with them. Nursing leadership, in tandem with senior hospital administration, needs to build the case for the value of this structure and work with other departments to help them understand their roles in this structure. Some resources will need to be included in the budget, which will require support from senior leadership.
- Transformational nursing leaders: The entire nursing leadership team needs to align in total support of the empowerment philosophy. The staff will need time to work on projects and attend meetings, and managers need to provide this time. Nurse leaders also need to be open to recommendations and suggestions that are made by the staff and be willing to execute those that will benefit the organization.

- Formalized infrastructure: One of the best ways to align the organization and help communicate the approach to an empowered workplace is to create and share a comprehensive infrastructure that outlines a pictorial model, the vision and mission, and the bylaws. This infrastructure will depend on whether the organization stands alone or is part of a system and what type of general model is of interest to the leaders. Porter-O'Grady (1992) was the first to identify the importance of empowerment models in the nursing environment. His model was councilor in nature, with separate councils focusing on various categories of work and ultimately reporting to a leadership council. Later, Gokenbach (2007) experimented with a different approach, called the task force model, that proved to be productive and efficient. O'May and Buchan (1999) also identified unit-based, administrative, and congressional structures.

Councilor Empowerment Model Structures

The councilor structure requires the development of separate and independent counsels to manage particular genres of work, depending on the needs of the organization. Councils can focus on areas such as operations, education, administration, quality, policy, and procedure. One advantage of this structure is that the scope provides for the ability to accomplish a great deal of work. Some disadvantages include the potential for disconnect in the needs of the larger organization, depending on the breadth of including units and departments. Another disadvantage is the need to disperse members equally on each council, which possibly leads to appointments of staff members who do not have interests in the focus, leading to a decreased level of energy and productivity (Porter O'Grady, 1992).

Task Force Empowerment Model Structures

The task force model includes the same focus of work as the councilor model; however, rather than individual groups, the entire membership meets on a monthly basis to discuss issues throughout the organization. When a potential project or need is identified, members can volunteer to be on the task force to work on the project from inception to implementation, including an evaluation of the effectiveness of the work and revision, if necessary. The advantage of this approach is that there are enough projects for the staff to work on that they can find something that interests them, thus increasing the level of passion and commitment and therefore productivity (Gokenbach, 2008).

The model in **Figure 9-1** was created by Greenville Memorial Health System in Greenville, South Carolina. Under the leadership of Michelle Taylor, the organization utilized a ground-up approach to redesign their old councilor model and create a unique hybrid councilor and task force model that functions independently in the various organizations. The participants report to a system leadership council that monitors consistency across the system to ensure quality processes and care.

Choosing the Right Model for the Right Structure

There are many considerations when selecting the correct approach for an organization. The systems in many organizations will need to develop individual

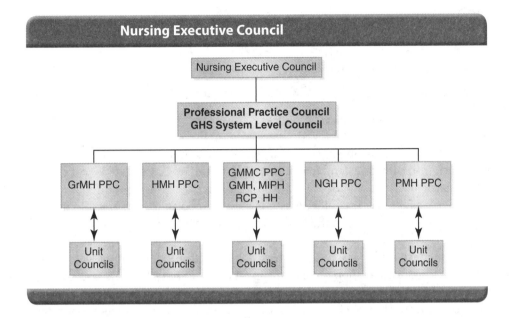

Nursing Executive Council

structures for each location, with a systems-based council that can ensure consistency and share ideas. In the case of one single organization, either a counselor or a task force approach is feasible, with representation from all areas of the organization. There will be a financial commitment regardless of the type of structure chosen, therefore the cost of the program may need to fit the budgeted dollars.

Regardless of the type of model to be applied in a given setting, unique changes will need to be made so it will fit the size and complexity of the organization, as well as the allocated resources. The best way to ensure buy in from the staff members and key nursing leaders is to include them in crafting a structure they feel suits the organization. This will be the beginning of a journey to empowerment.

Accept Responsibility for all Quality Scores

In Crossing the Quality Chasm: A New Health System for the 21st Century (2001), the Institute of Medicine defined quality as "the degree to which health services for individuals and populations increase the likelihood of desired health outcomes and are consistent with current professional knowledge" (1990, p. 232). The Agency for Healthcare Research and Quality later defined quality as consistently doing the right thing, at the right time, and in the right way for each patient, each time. For the purpose of this discussion, quality scores will include nurse-sensitive indicators, patient satisfaction, and staff satisfaction because these outcomes result from the quality of nursing leadership.

It is not uncommon to hear nurse leaders deflect responsibility for scores by blaming physician colleagues and other departments for poor service that negatively reflects on their unit scores. The literature suggests, however, that nursing care determines quality scores, and when nursing quality improves, so do the scores of all other departments (Hospital Consumer Assessment of Healthcare Providers and Systems, 2013). Blaming other departments for poor scores only reduces the focus away from point-of-care quality improvements. Nursing leaders must create the culture of quality on the units and focus their efforts on providing the resources for nurses to provide the best care possible.

DEVELOP SUCCESSFUL RELATIONSHIPS WITH PHYSICIANS, PRACTITIONER COLLEAGUES, AND OTHER DEPARTMENTS

The delivery of health care, especially with the advent of the Affordable Care Act, requires that healthcare organizations are accountable for the care provided at various levels of service, from outpatient to acute care to home care. This coordinated approach to health care can be achieved only through a team-based, coordinated effort. Such an effort will not occur without effective relationships and a laser focus on patients as the center of all efforts. There cannot be an us-versus-them mentality, or no one will be successful and patients will be the victims of this disjointed approach.

It is the responsibility of effective nurse leaders to reach out to physicians and other colleagues to develop a relationship wherein both parties can discuss issues and develop objectives together. Working with other department directors can improve teamwork and efficiency at the bedside and help to reduce errors and improve patient satisfaction.

RECRUITING NURSES

The recruitment of qualified nursing professionals is pivotal in the role of nurse executives and is paramount in ensuring safe and effective care delivery. The goal in recruiting is to attract the best and brightest talent. However, many nursing employers have settled for warm bodies to fill empty positions. Unfortunately, this often leaves the selection of new nurses to chance and may result in both unhappy employees and miserable employers.

Nursing employers must be willing to do what it takes to attract the best candidates. Today's workforce is not as complex as some believe. In fact, most nurses are looking for the basics: challenging assignments, opportunities to grow as professionals, authentic work–life balance, and economic rewards. The efforts to recruit nurses should be focused and intentional. Otherwise, recruitment efforts are left up to chance with disappointing results.

Successful recruitment efforts begin with a strategic plan. Without a plan, what do employers tell prospective employees about the organization's future? Bright people expect documented strategies and a game plan. One of the best ways to welcome developing nursing professionals into the workplace is to offer them a spot on a team. Generations X and Y—those born between 1965 and 1976, and 1977 and 1994, respectively—value the chance to be part of a group with a larger goal. However, if the prospective workplace has no goals, the potential employee may find a more attractive and exciting place to work.

Training and learning are no longer a benefit; they are an expectation. Today's nursing workforce expects more than just technical competence. They have been educated to insist on continuing education that will aid their professional development. Nursing leadership must commit to the investment. Additionally, the facility must provide up-to-date technology. The best employees expect the best tools.

Today's healthcare employers must be willing to offer nurses a work–life balance. One of the reasons many children of nurses shun the profession is the absence of work–life balance they witnessed while growing up. Today's nurses are no longer willing to work the long, arduous schedules that once dictated the lives of their professional predecessors. Successful employers who recognize that nurses need time to rejuvenate will maintain a healthy nursing workforce.

Finally, there must be room for advancement, or bright nurses will not stay. Facilities that are serious about recruiting will develop mechanisms that provide clear passageways for advancement. Examples are career ladders and clinical advancement programs. There are no magic formulas for recruiting nurses. A sound recruitment plan will clearly differentiate one healthcare facility from another and make it a strong contender in the fight for today's most talented nurses.

Turnover and Vacancy Rates

Every leader will experience staff turnover. Relocations, promotions, retirements, and pregnancies are considered good reasons for turnover, and they will constitute about 2% of the staff that leaves. When turnover rates begin to increase, the cause is a result of ineffective leadership. Efron (2014) identifies poor leadership as the number one reason for staff to leave and observes that staff members quit the leader, not the organization.

The highest turnover of nurses takes place within 1 year of employment. The cost of turnover for healthcare organizations is tremendous. The average cost of a replacement nurse is $75,000, which includes recruitment, replacement, temporary staff, overtime, and orientation. The remaining staff members are also affected. They often need to pick up heavier assignments or work overtime to cover for the vacancy, which contributes to burnout. If the vacancy rate remains high secondary to turnover levels, burnout will result in more turnover.

Efron identified six leadership failures that lead to turnover:

- Lack of vision: The leader needs to be able to articulate the vision to the staff so they understand why they are there and how they contribute to the fulfillment of the vision. Most organizations have a vision, but the leader needs to effectively communicate it to the staff.
- No connection to the bigger picture: Employees are the most important asset of any organization, and without their efforts it is impossible for the organization to achieve its mission and vision. An effective leader must be able to make the connection to the staff so they realize their importance and value to the organization.
- No empathy: Employees need to feel that they are cared for and cared about. Empathy can be defined as the ability to understand and share another person's feelings and experiences (Empathy, n.d.). An effective leader makes emotional connections with the staff members and make them feel valuable and important to the organization.
- No motivation: Although there continues to be a debate that employees are primarily intrinsically motivated, as opposed to extrinsically motivated, the leader is responsible for the creation of an environment of energy and purpose.
- No future: Not all staff members interpret the definition of *future* as a promotion. Nurses have a quest for knowledge and personal development. A skilled leader will know what the desires are of all the staff members

and help them achieve whatever their next level of success is: an advanced degree, a certification, a promotion, or an opportunity to be involved in the unit.

- No fun: Employees need to enjoy the environment that they work in along with their colleagues. If there is intense stress, poor inter-professional relationships to the point where the environment is toxic, employees will leave to find an environment that they believe will be more fun. It is important for the leader to allow for some stress release through fun activities.

Liaisons between staff and senior leadership predicated on trust within the organization: To have trust in the organization, staff members need to feel comfortable with their senior leaders. Nursing leaders represent senior leadership, and in many situations they are the only connection between the staff and senior leaders. There is usually a great deal of tension in any organization related to performance and financial stability, especially given the current economic pressures on healthcare organizations. These forces can lead to mergers, acquisitions, changes in service offerings, layoffs, and other scenarios that can create a great degree of stress and fear. The nursing leader needs to be the buffer for these fears by being honest and positive. If the nursing leadership is not supportive of senior leadership and does not share their feelings, neither will the staff. All effective leaders control their emotions and present an honest but positive front to the staff.

High level of visibility: It is not uncommon for staff to say they never see their leaders on their work units. One of the most effective ways to connect with the staff is to be visible. Spending time with the staff in meaningful ways provides several advantages: the staff becomes familiar with the personal side of the leader; and the leader learns about the staff and has the opportunity to learn about processes and problems that the staff faces daily. This exchange builds a foundation of trust and allows the nursing leader to make important improvements that were identified by the staff and to identify problems that need to be conveyed to senior leadership.

One way to achieve a high level of visibility for nursing leadership is to set criteria for the various management levels. For example, nurse managers should work a certain number of days on the off shifts, and directors should visit the off shifts. The best leaders spend time working shifts with the staff.

Marketing

An organization that is perceived to be an employer of choice retains its employees and is more capable of replacing its losses than less sought-after employers. A variety of recruitment methods may be used for communicating nursing vacancies and reaching potential employees. Some popular options are internal job postings; newspaper, radio, and television advertisements; trade magazine advertisements; Internet job sites; college campus interviews; and employee referrals. The choice of option depends on the number of positions to be filled and the cost.

In considering marketing and recruiting materials, it is important to remember that image matters. Recruitment brochures, pamphlets, and written materials should be enticing and make applicants want to work for the organization. Websites in particular should be professionally designed and easy to navigate. Efforts should be directed toward providing applicants with information that directly influences their desire to pursue employment (Costello & Vercler, 2006).

Interview

Llarena (2013) describes an interview as a face-to-face discussion between a job seeker and a person with full authority to fill the position under discussion. Nurses, as job seekers, want a face-to-face discussion with the person who has hiring authority. Applicants may be considering several jobs and have narrowed the field down to those that specifically fit their career goals.

The nurse recruiter or a human resources specialist will compile a personnel file that contains a completed application form, a resume or curriculum vitae, references, and any documents that are required by policy or law, such as a current, valid license to practice nursing and school transcripts. The interviewer should prepare for the interview by reading the information in the applicant's file. The interviewer should make notes of questions to ask the applicant about the information contained in the file. Adequate time should be set aside for the interview, which should take place in a private office where there will be no interruptions. An interview guide is helpful in conducting an interview that is satisfactory to both the nurse manager and the applicant (**Box 9-1**).

All candidates for nursing jobs should be treated as professionals. It is illegal to ask candidates certain questions, such as those listed in **Box 9-2**. Information

---

BOX 9-1   Interview Guide

Candidate:

Date and time of interview:

1. Arrange seating.
2. Make introductions and establish rapport.
3. Ask prepared questions:
   a. Tell me about yourself.
   b. What is your present job?
   c. What are your three most outstanding accomplishments?
   d. What is the extent of your formal education?
   e. What three things are most important to you in your job?
   f. What is your strongest qualification for this job?
   g. What other jobs have you held in this or a similar field?
   h. What were your responsibilities?
   i. Do you mind irregular working hours? Explain.
   j. Would you be willing to relocate? To travel?
   k. What minimum salary are you willing to accept?
   l. Ask about any gaps in the work history on provided resume.
4. Answer candidate's questions.
5. Note the following: Candidate was
   a. On time
   b. Well dressed
   c. Well mannered
   d. Positive about self
6. Maintain eye contact.
7. Note candidate's personal values.
8. Close the interview:
   a. Make an offer
   b. Obtain acceptance
   c. Set timetable for making offer or receiving response to offer

---

BOX 9-2 Illegal Questions

Employment interviewers are forbidden by law to ask the following questions:

- Age
- Date of birth
- The length of time residing at present address
- Previous address
- Religion; church attended; spiritual adviser's name
- Father's surname
- Maiden name (of women)
- Marital status
- Residence mates

- Number and ages of children; who will care for them while applicant works
- Transportation to work, unless a car is a job requirement
- Residence of spouse or parent
- Whether residence is owned or rented
- Name of bank; information on outstanding loans
- Whether wages were ever garnished
- Whether bankruptcy was ever declared
- Whether ever arrested
- Hobbies, off-duty interests, clubs

---

about age and date of birth that may be necessary for insurance or other benefits can be obtained after the candidate is hired. Also, consider that many candidates have questions. When complete information cannot be given, the interviewer should make a note, get the information, and communicate it to the candidate as quickly as possible. **Box 9-3** lists questions that candidates may ask and that the interviewer should be prepared to answer. Eye contact, rapport, and follow-up after the interview are important strategies to incorporate into the interview process. **Box 9-4** outlines the nurse executive's responsibilities as well as those of the candidate.

MODERN LEADERSHIP COMPETENCIES

Lombardo and Eichinger (2004) identified several competencies that are necessary for skilled leaders in the current environment. Once mastered, these competencies contribute to the leaders' success in the management of human capital.

For the most part, leaders have an instinct to repair problems with ordered thinking and a rational decision-making model, which has serious limitations in a rapidly changing environment. Leaders face problems that are multifaceted and more complex than ever before. Answers to these dilemmas do not fit old thought patterns. To be effective, modern leaders need to quickly scope out a situation and anticipate potential unknowns and other forces, then react quickly and decisively. This requires innovation leadership.

In a white paper released by the Center for Creative Leadership, Horth and Buchner (2014) identified six vital skills for innovation leaders:

- Pay attention: Stay alert for subtle changes and anticipate problems. O'Hara-Devereaux (2004), a well-known futurist, says that great leaders watch for trends that may become mainstream and react on their instincts with courage and decisiveness. It is critical to continually think differently about the

BOX 9-3   Candidate's Questions and Interviewing Tips

- How much job security does this job have?
- What previous experience does this type of job require?
- What is the future of this type of job?
- What is the growth potential for this particular job?
- Where will the most significant growth for this type of job in the healthcare industry occur?
- What is the starting salary for this job?
- How do pay raises occur?
- How does one find out when other job openings occur?
- What are the fringe benefits of this job?
- What are the requirements for working shifts and weekends?
- What is the floating policy?
- What are the opportunities for continuing education?
- What are the opportunities for promotion?
- What child care facilities are available?
- What are the staffing and scheduling policies?

Tips

- Keep the atmosphere positive, pleasant, and businesslike.
- Focus on the essential goals.
- Provide answers in a brief, factual, and friendly manner; use a soft and clear tone of voice; maintain a relaxed posture; keep hands still.
- Do not attempt to bluff answers to questions.
- Review information sent to you before the interview.
- Be prepared for questions related to personal philosophy and style, community relations, professional goals, clinical and administrative style, decision-making ability, flexibility in working with diverse groups, fiscal issues, personnel management, and group relationships.
- Avoid controversial issues of religion, abortion, and politics; do not discuss confidential matters.

meaning of the leadership role and challenges in the environment and in the organization.

- Personalizing: Become the customer and see things through his or her eyes. In a healthcare organization, put yourself in the place of the patient and honestly assess the situation. Focus on service improvement based on what is best for patients, not what is best for the organization. Patients are the reason that healthcare organizations exist, not the reverse.
- Imaging: Forget thinking in words, which can be limiting. Think in pictures, which open the mind and allow for another venue of thought. Picture what you would like the outcome to be and what that would look like to you.

BOX 9-4 What Happens During An Interview?

The Hiring Executive	The Candidate
1. Gives accurate information about job and institution.	1. Gives information about self.
2. Assesses the competencies the candidate possesses in relation to the job opening.	2. Assesses the opportunity for developing and using competencies on the job.
3. Evaluates the candidate's personal characteristics in relation to the staff members with whom candidate will work (fit to staff).	3. Assesses ability to relate to the employees with whom candidate will work.
4. Assesses candidate's potential to move organization toward its goals.	4. Assesses potential for achieving personal career goals.
5. Assesses candidate's enthusiasm and state of health.	5. Assesses the institution's climate and the morale of the employees.
6. Forms impressions about candidate based on behavior, appearance, ability to communicate, confidence, intelligence, personality.	6. Assesses opportunities for promotion and success.
7. Assesses candidate's ability to do the job.	7. Assesses own ability to do the job.
8. Determines facts about candidate.	8. Determines facts about the organization and working conditions.

- Serious play: Children learn through play, and leaders can too. Take the liberty to see things in new and creative ways, the way children do. Give yourself permission to explore, improvise, and experiment.
- Collaborative inquiry: It has been said that synergistic creativity produces more innovation than one person making decisions from a single point of view. Especially in an empowered environment, reach out to the staff and stakeholders for ideas and insights, and act on those recommendations.
- Crafting: Innovation requires the ability to let go of the past and craft a new future. Comments like "we have never done that before" or "in this organization we do things this way" should be stricken from the vocabulary in exchange for a culture of inquiry. Along with willingness to explore creative alternatives is the ability to be agile in the absence of information and to take risks. Ambiguity in this context is an opportunity that allows for innovation; it is not an anchor that stifles change. The best question that can be asked is "what if?"

Fearlessness

Risk taking, creativity, and innovation require strength and fearlessness. Change is not easy, and innovation requires change. Leaders need to be willing to face fears and continue to move into the unknown, soliciting support along the way. Day-to-day pressures create difficult scenarios that require strength of conviction to handle. The management of budgets and budget cuts, board presentations, layoffs, and adversity are common occurrences that create tension and fear in the staff. The leader needs to demonstrate strength so the staff will feel supported.

Emotional Intelligence

Goleman (2004) defines emotional intelligence as the ability to sense and appreciate others' perspectives in a nonjudgmental way. In other words, there are three sides to every story: mine, yours, and what really happened based on an individual perception of the situation. Complex individuals with various backgrounds, experiences, and values assess the world through their own sets of lenses, which often-times are contrary to the perceptions of those around them.

Goleman also described that successful management of human capital requires leaders to connect with their employees on an emotional level, which triggers hormones in the limbic system that either make them feel good about themselves or feel frustrated or fearful. For instance, if a superior called an employee on Friday afternoon and simply told him or her to report to the office on Monday morning, it would trigger a negative emotional response and create fear and probably anxiety for the entire weekend. Conversely, if a superior called an employee on Friday afternoon and asked if he or she could meet early Monday morning to discuss a project they were working on, the emotional response would be neutral and not trigger fear. Effective leaders who master the skill of emotional intelligence achieve success by eliciting positive feelings in their staff, thus gaining their support and trust.

Social Intelligence

Human beings are social and are wired to connect to the larger environment through relationships with others. Goleman (2006) identified a neural bridge that exists in the brain that creates brain-to-brain linkages with others when it is engaged. This then creates a "dance of feelings" (p.3, 2006). In other words, social relationships mold not only our perception of the experience, but also our biology. Humans need to be social and to fit in to the larger context of their environment.

Work environments are social environments with both positive and negative neurological exchanges happening constantly. Early studies of neuroplasticity conducted by Cacioppo and Berntson in the 1990s suggested that negative emotions in social situations damage genes and lower activity of the T cells, thus reducing resistance to disease and ultimately reshaping the brain. Positive emotions have the opposite effect, thus increasing the activity of the T cells. These findings have powerful ramifications in the management of human capital. For employees to be satisfied with their work environment, the leader needs to first be aware of the application of this science to social situations then create an atmosphere to reduce negative interactions. This includes the elimination of negative forces such as lateral violence, abusive relationships, poor performers, and negative interdepartmental relationships.

Change Agency

Successfully managing human capital requires the successful implementation of change because change is the only constant in a turbulent environment such as health care. Leaders are responsible for effective change and the management of such. Understanding the fundamentals of change agency and the change process is vital to instituting and maintaining change.

Probably the most well-known theorist on the subject of change is Kurt Lewin. Lewin identified three district components of change processes (Kritsonis, 2005):

1. Unfreezing: This stage is described as the institution of an idea presented in a way that others begin to let go of their old patterns and begin to accept the notion of change. It is important for leaders to understand employees' emotional status and present the change proposition in a way that makes sense to them. During this stage it is advantageous to include employees whenever possible to help craft the change and further ensure acceptance. Oftentimes crisis or emergency situations present great opportunities for change. Leaders need to be able to identify those situations.

2. Moving: This stage represents the emotional movement toward acceptance following the implementation of a change. At this point it is critical to support the staff and be willing to make subtle changes based on their recommendations and the successful rollout of the new process.

3. Refreezing: This stage of change represents acceptance of the new model as the way to do business. Maintaining the change, however, requires leaders to consistently evaluate the outcome to make sure the processes are not reverting to old practices. It is not uncommon for well-intended changes to migrate back to old patterns in the absence of a postchange evaluation.

Within the context of effective change, Lewin also identified three forces that affect the change process. Leaders must understand and manage these forces, which are as follows:

1. Driving forces: Driving forces are those that create the impetus for change and help move the change forward by creating a scenario of need. Savvy leaders can identify these forces and use them to their advantage to implement change.

2. Restraining forces: Restraining forces oppose driving forces and can allay or inhibit change. A proactive understanding of these forces is vital for leaders to prepare for them and to develop strategies to handle them.

3. Equilibrium: Equilibrium is the point at which driving forces equal restraining forces, and thus no change can take place. To move forward, leaders need to create strength in the driving forces, which may include increasing communication to promote the positive outcomes of the change or modifying the change to an acceptable level for the staff. If restraining forces take over, the change will not occur.

One of the major reasons for restraining forces in the change process is the notion of organizational culture, which must be understood and managed. Schein (1999) defined culture as a pattern of shared basic assumptions that the group learned as it solved problems of external adaptation and internal integration; the assumptions worked well enough to be considered valid and, therefore, are taught to new members as the correct way to perceive, think, and feel in relation to those problems. Humans as social beings support a culture wherein their environment is safe and supportive. Change disrupts this perception of safety and represents a restraining force in an attempt to re-create the security of the past. Effective leaders understand the power of culture and work within the boundaries to successfully move change forward.

Five Characteristics of a Change Agent

Couros (2014) identified five characteristics of an effective change agent:

1. Have a clear vision: To move any change forward, leaders must be able to articulate the vision in a way that employees can understand and begin to embrace the concepts. A strong understanding of the underlying organizational culture is an advantage to leaders who can then craft a message that resonates with those who will be affected by the change.

2. Be patient yet persistent: It is a fact that all change will be resisted in some manner. One positive factor is that it takes only 20% of the staff to begin to move change in the right direction. Leaders needs to be patient with the fact that employees are going to be fearful of any change, which will result in resistance; however, leaders need to be persistent in continually moving the change forward. Including the staff in crafting the change is an effective way to increase the likelihood that the change will be accepted. It is also acceptable to make changes to the process along the way to help mold the change in a way that will be accepted and then inculcated.

3. Ask tough questions: There is a greater likelihood that change will be accepted if people have an emotional connection to the change. In a healthcare setting, the common denominator for all work is patient outcomes. Placing patients at the center of all an organization does can help align employees behind common goals. Leaders need to continually ask the tough questions: How can we improve patient care? What will that look like to the patient? It is not uncommon for staff to think of change in terms of how it will affect their work environment or themselves instead of how it will affect patients.

4. Be knowledgeable and lead by example: Prior to any change, leaders must make sure they have done their research and have an intimate knowledge of the environment in which the change will take place. As leaders continue to move into higher positions, they begin to lose touch with the staff and the processes at the bedside or point of service, although some of them think they still have an understanding. Leaders can maintain credibility with the staff by working with them to understand the situation and the potential outcomes of the change. Change creates anxiety for all involved, including the leader. During times of change, leaders must continue to

focus on the importance of the change and lead by example. This level of commitment to the change helps the staff build trust.

5. Build strong relationships on trust: Employees should never be afraid to communicate to their leaders. The best change agents are those who have built a foundation of trust through inclusion and consistency, which enhances the staff's perception of safety and security during times of change.

Political Savvy

One critical skill of effective leaders is to understand the political landscape of the organization. DeLuca (1999) defines political savvy as the ability of a leader to cut across organizational, cultural, and geographic lines to pull together strategic alliances to accomplish work. He further defines this ability as "invisible" leadership that functions behind the scenes, as opposed to "limelight leadership" that focuses on visible functions such as meetings and management processes (p. 5). Real leaders must be effective behind the scenes and understand factors such as delicate egos, power struggles, vested interests, turf wars, relationships, financial tensions, and influences beyond appearances.

Behaviors of politically savvy leaders include the following:

- The ability to accept differences at face value
- Do not take things personally or defensively
- Be aware of land minds or tenuous scenarios
- Be approachable and consistent in leadership style and behavior
- Be open to new ideas and new approaches
- Be willing to compromise
- Be grateful to those who are helpful
- Continuously deliver on promises

Role Modeling

Erickson (2006) identified modeling and role modeling as critical motivators to improve the health of patients in clinical settings based on the holistic needs of individuals and helping them find meaning for themselves. This is the key to establishing a trusting relationship between the nurse and the patient, and it is also an important skill for leaders to help build trusting relationships with their staff members. Leaders who follow their own rules are more effective than those who say one thing but demonstrate something else. It has been said that whatever you tolerate, you endorse, so leaders need to be consistent in their messaging and in their follow through of expectations. For instance, it is not appropriate for a nurse manager to set the expectation that all staff members are to report to work on time, then ignore it when some people report late. It is also important that leaders make sure they are on time for staff meetings or other important events that are visible to the staff.

Role models do not have to be perfect; in fact, leaders who are not perfect are more real to the staff and are viewed as more human. It is important for leaders to admit their mistakes, accept accountability for those mistakes, and apologize if necessary. Mistakes are part of the human experience, and the important issue is to learn from them.

Strong role models have inherent respect for others and treat them accordingly without favoritism. This kind of respect requires quick follow through on issues and questions and a willingness to be open and available to the staff.

Assertiveness

There is a fine line between assertive and aggressive. Strong, effective leaders have constancy of purpose and therefore are not afraid to be assertive in their approach to problem solving.

Honesty

It is important to share all the information you can with the staff, in the most complete and honest way possible, especially in times of rapid change. The quickest way to destroy any type of trusting relationship is to be caught in a lie. Employees deal with the truth more effectively than unknowns—even if the truth is difficult—when there is trust between the leader and the staff.

Decisiveness

Especially in times of change and turbulence, leaders need to make decisions quickly and decisively. Not all decisions lend themselves to planning and collaboration. Decisiveness requires leaders to make good decisions quickly using a mixture of analysis, wisdom and experience, judgment, and input. When an analysis of a leader's past decisions demonstrates that the solutions and suggestions turned out to be correct, that leader is often sought out by others for advice because this skill is easy to identify in an organizational context.

TEAM MANAGEMENT

Effective team management continues to grow in importance as the movement grows toward accountable care organizations as an important approach to manage the needs of patients with complex chronic conditions in acute and outpatient settings. Shortages of physicians and other healthcare providers will require a team approach to ensure safety and a seamless transition throughout all aspects of health management (Taplin, Foster, & Shortell, 2013). Apart from the management of patient care, the high degree of change in the healthcare industry requires the use of effective teams to craft new programs and processes.

As early as 1965, Tuckman realized the importance of effective team leadership and developed his theory of the evolution of teams. He identified five stages of team development: forming, storming, norming, performing, and adjourning. Effective team leaders understand the various stages and the leadership actions that are acquired at each phase to keep the team moving forward. Descriptions of the stages are as follows (Tuckman, 1965):

1. Forming: This first stage is the most critical because since it sets the tone and charter for the expectations of the team. Leadership behaviors in this stage include clear articulation of the vision along with the desired outcomes and goals, ground rules for the way the team will be organized and behave, time lines, and expectations. Members of the team should be

introduced and individual responsibilities identified. The leader can expect to answer many questions during this time to help clarify the charter.

2. Storming: This stage is one of tension. The team members understand the goals and begin to exert their power and influence. This step is important because tension, if managed well by the leader, ultimately leads to increased trust among the members and increased sharing of ideas. An effective leader will harness this energy, embrace the ideas, and keep the team on track until the struggles subside. It may be important at this time to remove members that consistently demonstrate behaviors that risk the success of the team.

3. Norming: At this stage the team has settled into an operational rhythm that allows for great progress. Ideas are shared, strategies are discussed, and work is accomplished. At this stage the leader is responsible for encouraging the team and recognizing the good work to date.

4. Performing: This is the stage in which the true work is accomplished. The focus is on strategy and achievement, and there is a great deal of excitement. The role of the leader in this phase is to support the members and their accomplishments, provide direction, and effectively delegate work. The increased sophistication of the members at this time allows for delegation so individuals can work on tasks independently.

5. Adjourning: Tuckman later added this fifth phase to his model. Adjourning is recognized as a period of mourning for many team members, who feel a loss as the team is dissolved. Teamwork is an opportunity to develop strong relationships, and the initial loss of structure can be difficult at times. The leader needs to focus on positive outcomes and gratitude for the team's work. Celebration is appropriate to recognize the accomplishments of the team. The leader can keep the team engaged to follow-up on the status of the change and any revisions that may be needed.

Virtuoso Teams

There has been increased attention in the literature about team processes for virtuoso teams. At times of great need for change, some organizations engaged the concept of virtuoso teams to achieve rapid change and unparalleled innovation. Virtuoso teams are comprised of members who are elite experts in a particular discipline, and they are utilized for very ambitious projects. These teams are characterized by high levels of energy, ambitious goals, and relentless commitment to the project to produce extraordinary results. An example of a virtuoso team is Microsoft's Xbox team, which developed a gaming system that literally overtook the Sony PlayStation2 (Fischer & Boynton, 2005). It appears that the pressure on healthcare organizations could potentially warrant the utilization of such teams, which are very different from the usual team structure that is utilized today. Fischer and Boynton, though supportive of using virtuoso teams, recognize their limitations, including burnout due to the high level of energy and team members who have a tendency to be difficult to work with due to their egocentric and elite perceptions of themselves. If virtuoso teams are engaged from outside the organization, there may be insensitivity to the organizational culture, which may lead to a lack of acceptance by employees who need to buy in to the changes.

COMMUNICATION

One of the most important leadership skills is the ability to connect with staff members through effective communication, which is vital for understanding others, disseminating information, soliciting suggestions and ideas, and gaining support for change initiatives and increased productivity. Effective communication is far more than just speaking to another person; it includes understanding the emotions and motivations behind the exchange. It is only with this understanding that true dialogue can occur. Patterson, Grenny, McMillan, and Switzler (2012) described effective communication as persuasive, not abrasive, and identified several important strategies for leaders to improve communication.

- Effective listening: Leaders must be good listeners in order to be good communicators. When they are engaged in a discussion with a staff member, the most important focus is on the staff member. The environment needs to be conducive to a successful exchange, which means turning off the phone, preventing interruptions, and ignoring emails. Employees should feel that leaders care about what they say; this can be conveyed with eye contact, asking appropriate questions, and rephrasing statements to ensure understanding.
- Nonverbal communication: Nonverbal cues comprise 80% of communication. Effective communicators can read the body language of the person they are speaking to; more important, they have insight into their own body language and can control it accordingly.
- Managing stress: It is not uncommon for staff members to feel fearful or uncomfortable when they are engaged in conversations with their superiors, especially in a one-on-one format.

   Realizing that this is common is the first step in reducing stress and increasing comfort during the interaction. This can be achieved by beginning the discussion with small talk or questions that focus on the other person to help them relax and set the stage for a productive exchange.
- Emotional awareness: Regardless of how effective leaders are with communication, there are situations that test one's patience and result in a potential visceral response. To control these responses and the associated body language, self-awareness of emotions is important. It is also critical to identify the staff's emotional stressors during the exchange and take steps to prevent escalation and minimize stress.

Communication Infrastructure

There are many barriers to effective communication, including the size of the organization, the reporting structure, shift issues, and the amount of information to be shared. The most effective way to ensure effective communication is to organize a strategy in the infrastructure that clearly outlines expectations for the leaders. The structure example outlined in the following sections has been utilized by Gokenbach throughout her leadership career to strengthen communication and build accountability.

Vision

A vision statement sets the tone and charter for where the organization sees itself in the future. It can also be used for effective programs and processes. The vision statement for the communication infrastructure discussed in this example is as follows: All staff members will feel valuable in their role as it relates to the provision of high-quality care. All staff members will feel that they are expected to participate in the creation and maintenance of a successful work environment.

Mission

The mission statement is related to the vision statement. Its purpose is to provide a standardized process of communication throughout the organization. The goal is to inform, include, align, and empower all staff members.

Objectives

The objectives of the communication infrastructure are as follows:

- Provide a consistent methodology for the management of communication throughout the organization.
- Provide a template for meeting agendas and minutes.
- Provide education for various aspects of communication.

Information Flow to Staff

There are several directions from which communication and information can flow from various levels in the organization to the staff. The following diagram (**Figure 9-2**) identifies the various levels of leadership and the subsequent sources and routes of information. This model may change slightly from organization to organization, so it is important to customize it for variations.

Chain of Command

The following diagram (**Figure 9-3**) depicts the appropriate chain of command for the information flow between staff members and their manager. The titles may be different in various departments and organizations; however, the chain of command must be consistent. Leaders should replace the titles with those that are used in their department.

It is always advisable to use the chain of command, but there are situations when the next-level person should be contacted. If there are concerns that your direct supervisor is involved in a questionable issue, if your supervisor is not readily available and the issue is urgent, or if the judgment of your supervisor is in question, advancing through the chain of command is appropriate.

Communication Standards

To ensure effective communication, standards are developed and the responsible parties are held accountable. The following is an example of communication standards that may be modified to meet the needs of various organizations:

- Conduct monthly staff meetings, take minutes, and place the minutes in staff members' mailboxes and email them to all staff members.
- Conduct monthly professional nurse council or staff council meetings, and take and distribute minutes.

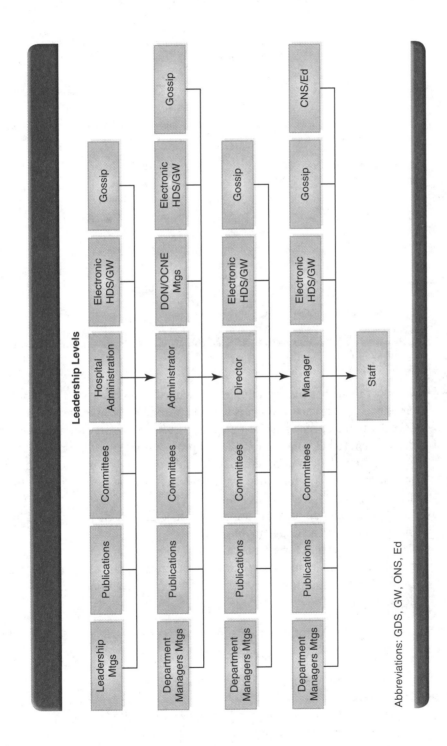

Abbreviations: GDS, GW, ONS, Ed

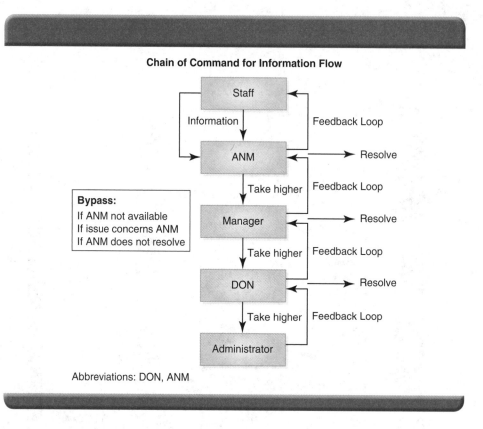

Chain of Command for Information Flow

Abbreviations: DON, ANM

- Conduct regular focus group meetings with three or four staff members so employees can discuss problems with their director or manager.
- Directors, managers, assistant managers, and supervisors work shifts in the department to help them identify with problems that staff members experience in the work environment. This should be done quarterly and include off shifts. Leaders cannot take assignments if they are not oriented to the area.
- Create and maintain process improvement, staff council, and general information boards in all departments.
- Designate a location for staff members to receive mail.
- Conduct town hall meetings, with directors in attendance, at least quarterly.
- Define and communicate the appropriate chain of command for the unit or department.

The following are recommendations for the types of information that could be communicated to the staff on a regular basis:

- Information from department manager meetings
- Service scores
- Department metrics, including operations and quality
- Information from service line meetings
- Recognitions
- Policy and practice changes, such as safety, process, and equipment

- Corporate plans, such as building projects, new services, benefits, and salaries
- Objectives and progress toward department or unit goals
- Committee meeting minutes
- Input exchange prior to making a decision
- Professional council information at both the unit and hospital levels
- Department leadership meeting information
- Compliance information

Feedback Standards

Feedback is a critical factor in successful communication. Ignoring a staff member's request or delaying a response may send the message that the staff member's concern is not important to the manager. The following are recommendations for managing feedback standards:

- Feedback must be given when a staff member requests it.
- Feedback will be given within 24 hours or as agreed by the two parties.
- Feedback will be verbal unless another communication method is agreed upon.
- The feedback must be confidential.
- The feedback must convey respect for all persons involved.
- The feedback should be provided by the appropriate person according to the chain of command unless the manager informs the staff member that feedback will be given by another person.

Tools

There are many tools and strategies that can enhance the effectiveness of communication:

- Agenda format: Develop a consistent format for agendas to be used at all meetings. Logos and models can be included to help increase familiarity.
- Meeting minutes format: Develop and share a consistent format for publishing information. This will help new or inexperienced leaders organize their thoughts and collect the appropriate information. Standard processes also help in data retrieval for quality reviews, such as The Joint Commission and Magnet.
- Meeting effectiveness tool: Not all meetings are effective, and not all leaders run good meetings. One way to evaluate the effectiveness of a meeting is to ask the members what they thought of the outcomes.

MANAGEMENT OF CRUCIAL CONVERSATIONS

Another critical skill for effective leaders is to handle crucial conversations. Complex organizations, a diverse staff, and rapidly changing environments continually present scenarios that require crucial conversations. Patterson and colleagues (2012) define crucial conversations as those that address tough issues and require positive outcomes when the stakes are high. They also recognize that humans prefer nonconfrontational environments and therefore either try to avoid them or handle them poorly. The key to managing crucial conversations is mastering dialogue, versus monologue. Dialogue is the exploration of options and understanding the perspectives of others (Gerzon, 2006). Many of the strategies previously discussed contribute to effective management of crucial conversations; however, Patterson and colleagues (2012) also include the importance of starting with the heart and approaching such dialogues in a compassionate way. They also recommend beginning any crucial conversation with the leader's understanding of the desired outcome and the ability to steer the discussion along a path that will move in the right direction.

MANAGING A DIVERSE WORKFORCE

A diverse workforce is an advantage for organizations, especially in the current turbulent healthcare environment, because diversity allows for a variety of opinions and experiences that lead to innovation. Diversity includes differences in age, gender, ethnicity, and religion, all of which the savvy leader needs to manage.

Age Differences

As new generations enter the workforce, challenges among generations increase. A leader in such an environment will manage as many as four generations at a time. With employees retiring later, older members of the workforce are staying longer.
Tulgan (2006) categorized and characterized generational periods as follows:

- Senior or silent generation: This generation was born before 1946. Most people in this generation are currently leaving the workforce, taking with them a great deal of wisdom, knowledge, and expertise. They are hard workers and are committed to their careers and employers.
- Baby boomers: Baby boomers were born between 1946 and 1964 and are currently becoming the aging generation. They perceive that they are change agents, but they remain in the status quo. This is the first generation to experience layoffs and downsizing in their organizations, as well as the realization that employers are not necessarily committed to the workforce.
- Generation X: This generation was born between 1965 and 1977. This is the generation that watched their parents' work long hours result in the need for day care and after school care. Often termed the latchkey generation, they were forced to care for themselves and are therefore very independent. Because of their family experiences, they lack commitment to their jobs and want to leave at 5:00 to be with their families.
- Generation Y: This generation was born between 1978 and 1989. People in this generation are referred to as trophy kids who have an unrealistic sense of entitlement that carries into their jobs. This is the most challenging group to work with due to their impatience and personal needs.

The term Millennials is often used to describe those born between the 1980s and 2000. People in this generation have characteristics common to Generation X and Y.

Tulgan (2006) further described the workforce revolution that is the result of technology, the expected need for speed, and changes in organizations that increase employee free agency. Because of free agency, employers can expect employees to move from job to job and not necessarily be committed to any one organization. This will result in additional challenges to maintain adequate staffing levels at the bedside.

Nursing leaders need to be fair in their approach to the various generations. It is therefore important to understand the communication preferences of each generation (**Table 9-1**).

Gender Differences

Gender differences are an inherent part of society that define behaviors and expectations of males and females. Gender differences carry into the workplace with concerns of inequality in pay and the ability of women to be promoted as quickly as their male counterparts. For years female nurses have questioned fairness in the healthcare workplace in regards to perceived advantages of males over females in pay, promotional opportunities, and preferential treatment of men by physicians and other colleagues (Davies, 1995).

Carless (1998) studied the differences between men and women in their ability to be transformational leaders. In this study, superiors identified that women were more transformational in their leadership styles, especially in the area of interpersonal relationships. Conversely, staff members indicated that male and female leaders were equal in their ability to be transformational.

Gender differences will never go away in society and the workplace. Effective leaders need to manage fairly, understand the perceptions among the workforce, and handle the issues appropriately.

TABLE 9-1   Communication Preferences across Generations

Generation	Spoken Preference	Written Preference
Silent generation (Born between 1927 and 1945)	Formal linear thinkers, polite, to the point, direct, respectful, proper grammar, no foul language, no small talk, follows chain of command	Well organized, sequential, proper grammar and punctuation, direct and to the point, likes written communication to refer to later
Baby boomers (Born between 1946 and 1964)	Like small talk to build camaraderie and consensus, values teamwork	Prefers written word for later reference, creates a paper trail
Generation X (Born between the 1960s and 1980s)	Informal, direct, does not enjoy small talk, focus is on what it means for them, believes chain of command is a waste of time	Less emphasis on reading, prefers concise and to the point, bullets and clear delineation of outcomes, not focused on grammar and punctuation
Generation Y (Millennials born between the 1980s and 2000)	Informal, does not understand need for chain of command, needs immediate gratification and to know what this will do for them, needs help seeing the bigger picture, has a sense of entitlement	Prefers electronic communication, bullets and short statements, no emphasis on grammar and punctuation, may need direction about how to communicate in written format

Data from Tulgan, B. (2006). *Managing the generation mix: From urgency to opportunity.* Amherst, MA: HRD Press.

Ethnic Differences

There is no question that the world continues to become more diverse. The care of diverse populations creates challenges, such as patient teaching, language, and the written word. Most organizations have developed systems to handle these challenges, including translators and providing materials in several languages. In ethnically diverse situations, leaders should role-model their acceptance of diversity and support the appropriate systems that support quality patient care.

Ethnic differences among staff members can be more challenging and require strong, sophisticated team leadership skills. The best approach to lead diverse teams has been studied for many years. Homan and Greer (2013), in a study based on the categorization–elaboration model, found that leaders who practiced considerate leadership were the most effective with diverse teams. Considerate leadership is defined as a process wherein the leader focuses on relationships and the intent to meet the goals and needs of individuals (Homan & Greer 2013). This is especially important in tense situations that are often found in diverse environments. When working with diverse teams, leaders should consider the thoughts and needs of all members and care for them as individuals, with a focus on patients as the center of the work.

PERFORMANCE MANAGEMENT

It has been said that whatever you tolerate, you endorse. The appropriate management of performance is critical to an effective workforce and the perceived strength and character of the leader. Leaders who allow staff members to underperform are considered weak and unable to manage problematic staff members. Such staff members cause increased pressure on their peers because others have to work harder and pick up the slack for those who underperform, whether the cause is absenteeism or lack of skill. Leaders needs to set expectations and deal with every situation of nonperformance, even if it may lead to elimination of staff members. The elimination of staff members for poor performance provides an opportunity to hire high performers in their place and improve the efficiency and integrity of the group.

Setting Expectations

The initial step in effective performance management is setting expectations of the staff. Healthcare organizations have expectations that are described in job descriptions and other performance policies; however, they are usually not enough, especially in the case of poor performers. Schein (2004), in his studies on corporate culture, says leaders create the culture and expectations of the staff. An example is the expectation that all staff members come to work on time, but there are always some that show up late. If the leader does not uphold the expectation, more and more staff members will arrive late because it will be perceived as an acceptable behavior that the leader does not care about. In the spirit of empowerment and with a goal of inclusion, an effective leader can utilize the staff to develop a code of conduct that is acceptable to the unit, then address the fact that some staff members are not in line with the mutually developed code. After the leader shares the expectations, the staff will know what is needed for compliance and can be successful in their roles.

Performance Evaluations

Performance evaluations are a valuable tool for leaders to manage staff effectiveness, but if they are not used appropriately, they can be useless. Most organizations have robust infrastructures for performance evaluations; however, it is important for performance to be measured more often than annually. Oftentimes leaders think performance appraisals are time consuming and, especially when raises are small, staff members do not respond to them. The best leaders address performance continually by taking time to meet with staff members midyear to discuss their status. It is also important to bring poor performance to the forefront rather than waiting. Blanchard and Johnson (2003) said the most effective way to change behavior is to address issues immediately rather than wait until the behaviors are forgotten. This applies to both problems and recognition for a job well done.

Peer Review

In 1989 the American Nurses Association established a definition for the process of peer review:

> Peer review in nursing is the process by which practicing registered nurses systematically access, monitor, and make judgments about the quality of nursing care provided by peers as measured against professional standards of practice . . . Peer review implies that the nursing care delivered by a group of nurses or an individual nurse is evaluated by individuals of the same rank or standing according to established standards of practice. (Haag-Heitman & George, 2010, para. 4)

Boehm and Bonnell (2010) identified peer review as an advanced tool to use in the development of both students and staff. Peers view one another through a different lens than the leader, and they learn more effectively through sharing stories and experiences. Magnet designation requires that organizations demonstrate evidence of a formalized peer-review process that is well articulated by the staff. Peer review is housed within the Exemplary Professional Practice component of the Magnet model.

There are two categories of peer review, and effective leaders utilize both approaches. The first approach is the improvement of clinical care through the systematic process of case review, identifying best practices, and improvement opportunities. The second approach is through the inclusion of peers and colleagues in performance evaluations. It is important to consider both options to develop a comprehensive approach.

Discipline

When performance expectations have been set and communicated to the staff, it is critical for leaders to address staff members that are not complying. After counseling has taken place, the next step is to begin the progressive discipline process, which begins the journey to termination. Employees are not comfortable with the disciplinary process; at times, neither are leaders. Regardless, astute management of the disciplinary process protects the organization legally and helps ensure safety at the bedside. Unless the infraction is so egregious that the employee is immediately terminated, most poor-performing employees work very hard at getting themselves fired. There are five strategies to help leaders manage the discipline process with fairness and integrity:

- Know the human resource policy for discipline so the steps can be followed consistently and the progression continues.
- Develop a relationship with the human resources department and call on them for advice. They are there to help and are a valuable asset.
- Maintain consistency throughout the disciplinary process. Reacting to one incident but not reacting to another will slow down the process and send mixed messages to the staff member.
- Disciplinary action should always be given in a private office to protect the integrity of the staff member and allow for recommendations for improvement.
- All disciplinary action should be confidential. Oftentimes staff members will complain about their colleagues and may expect feedback about their concerns. Sharing information about staff members can cause the staff to mistrust the leader.

Lateral Violence

Lateral violence is a serious problem among nurses. The lack of attention to this issue can create dysfunction among staff members and potentially dangerous situations for both patients and the staff. The Institute for Safe Medication Practices (2004) reported that 48% of nurses and pharmacists identified incidents of serious verbal abuse, and 43% identified incidents of threatening body language. Longo (2007), in a study of student nurses in clinical environments, reported that 53% had been put down by a professional nurse. A study by the American Nurses Association (2011) reported that 56.9% of nurses have experienced some type of abuse at work.

One concern is fear that is associated with bullying and lateral violence and the resulting refusal of staff members to report an individual for fear of reprisal. Incidents that are not reported can create an unsafe work environment for patients because the staff may similarly not report breaches in practice if the bullying nurse is involved.

There is no place for this type of behavior in the workplace, and leaders must be alert to potential signs of these problems. Many organizations have adopted a zero-tolerance approach to bullying and lateral violence; however, leaders must effectively manage these problems.

Collective Bargaining

Collective bargaining began with the industrial era of manufacturing in this country, with the goal of protecting workers from their tyrant supervisors. Collective bargaining began with the attempt to create a safe work environment by addressing issues of pay, burnout, staffing workload, and mandatory overtime. Many organizations that have collective bargaining restrict the power of unions to contract negotiations for payroll and benefits; staffing levels are excluded.

Pittman (2007) conducted a study of staff satisfaction levels in union and nonunion organizations to discover any differences. The results revealed that the unionized staff were more satisfied with pay and benefits and were not satisfied with leadership. The nonunionized staff were more happy with their supervisors than with pay and benefits. The concern is that unions drive a wedge between leaders and the staff, making trusting relationships difficult. Leaders in unionized organizations report an increase in bureaucracy, which slows down decision making, reduces the leader's ability to exert authority, incurs higher costs due to negotiations and lawyer involvement, and increases polarization among staff members.

Regardless of whether an organization is union or nonunion, nurse leaders must apply the tenets of transformational leadership and care for the staff in a fair and consistent manner. Trust between a nursing leader and the staff is important regardless of union involvement.

EMPLOYEE SUPPORT

The most valuable asset in any organization is the staff. Effective leaders understand that and work to care for the staff in a holistic manner, including body, mind, and spirit. Especially given the competition for good staff and the increased pressure and acuity in healthcare organizations, it is important to create or identify systems to help the staff care for themselves. Employee assistance programs and creative approaches to wellness in the workplace can help reduce stress and renew the staff.

Employee Assistance Programs

The U.S. Office of Personnel Management defines an employee assistance program (EAP) as

> a voluntary, work-based program that offers free and confidential assessments, short-term counseling, referrals, and follow-up services to employees who have personal and/or work-related problems. EAPs address a broad and complex body of issues affecting mental and emotional well-being, such as alcohol and other substance abuse, stress, grief, family problems, and psychological disorders. (U.S. Office of Personnel Management, 2014, para. 1)

EAPs are underutilized due to a lack of awareness on the part of leaders and staff members. After a trusting relationship is established between leaders and staff members, accessing the EAP can be suggested for a variety of needs.

Wellness Initiatives

Many categories fall under the blanket of wellness initiatives, including healthy eating, stress reduction, and exercise. Busy work schedules and long shifts leave nurses tired and limit their time for extra wellness activities.

Exercise

Countless studies over the years demonstrate the value of exercise for physical fitness, strength, mental clarity, and personal well-being. On-site exercise options for employees increase the possibility that they will partake in an exercise program. In the absence of an on-site exercise and wellness facility, creative and low-cost options have been developed by hospitals across the country. Iowa University Hospital, under the direction of Dr. Sharon Tucker, developed a series of exercise videos called *Well Me in Three* that staff members can access through the intranet during lunch and break times. Staff members are the stars of the vignettes, and the program was well received and utilized. Other organizations encourage the staff to take the stairs and have posted graphics and music in stairwells to help motivate them. Walking paths and walking teams are options for exercise during breaks and lunches. Leaders can also utilize walking meetings and increased rounding to encourage exercise. Staff involvement in the creation of such programs is vital to the development of strategies they think will work.

Healthy Dietary Options

Along with exercise, nutrition contributes to increased wellness. Many organizations have developed healthy dietary options in their cafeterias and vending machines, along with educational programs. Some organizations have on-site weight loss programs that may be commercially available or created by the organization.

Stress Reduction

There is no question that there is stress in the healthcare workplace. Employees vary widely in their ability to control and handle stress. Adequate staffing ratios, an empowered work environment, and receptive leaders can help minimize the stress level. However, additional strategies can help the staff when needed. Many organizations have holistic care centers for oncology patients that employ massage therapists, Reiki specialists, and meditation coaches. These options can be made available to the staff.

Renewal Activities

A wide range of renewal activities are available depending on individual preferences. Reading, meditating, hiking, kayaking, walking, nature, music, and many more activities have the potential to renew. Apart from activities that individuals can choose in their personal lives, the organization can offer meditation and yoga classes, healing gardens, and chapels.

Whether it is exercise, healthy eating, or renewal, the intent of the leadership to supply wellness options sends a clear message that the organization cares about the staff and their well-being. This caring builds a healthy relationship and improves the work environment. A cared-for staff is a productive staff.

CAREER PLANNING

Employees tend to stay longer in organizations when they experience personal and professional growth. Employers who share their vision for the organization, including the growth plan, foster a climate of organizational connectedness and reduce employees' intent to leave. When employees feel challenged and cared for, they are more likely to stay on the job longer. Nurse leaders must learn ways to help professional nurses have satisfaction in their careers if they are to retain them. To be successful in their careers, professional nurses need a sense of personal fulfillment and job significance.

Career Ladders and Career Development Programs

A career ladder can be used to depict vertical job promotion. In business and human resources management, the ladder typically describes the progression from entry-level positions to higher levels of pay, skill, responsibility, or authority.

Moving up the career ladder should be a function of three factors: time, performance, and skill set attainment. Advancing in a career development program should not be so easy that it becomes automatic simply because of seniority. Most experts agree that employees should demonstrate a commitment to the organization before being considered for advancement. An employee should put in a designated amount of time before being eligible to climb to the next rung of a career ladder (Gaffney, 2005).

A good employee development program must be based on performance over an extended time period. Documentation typically includes the annual performance appraisal and more informal items, such as written commendations for outstanding service.

Continuing education is a critical component in an effective employee development program and career ladder. To climb the career ladder, the employee should participate in a specified amount of continuing education. This education can be in the form of advanced college credits or continuing education units acquired through workshops or seminars that are related to the nurse's area of expertise, thus enhancing the existing skill set.

When properly administered, a career ladder should result in a win–win situation for both employers and employees. When progressing up a career ladder, nurses may receive recognition, salary increases, or prestige; the organization benefits from a more stable and better educated workforce.

However, there is one caveat that nurse leaders should consider: not every nurse will be interested in career ladder advancement. Some employees are comfortable and function well at a lower level of responsibility and still meet the requirements of the job. Advancement on the career ladder should never be mandatory.

A clinical career ladder should do the following:

1. Improve the quality of patient care.
2. Motivate staff in the following areas:
    a. Job proficiency and expertise, that is, motivate nurses to reach their highest level of professional competence.
    b. Pursuit of education, which is an important factor in mobility.
    c. Development of career goals.
3. Provide methods of objective and measurable performance evaluation, and reward clinical competence for the purpose of advancement.
4. Promote retention within the clinical area and reduce the turnover rate (Noe, 2005).

Performance criteria in any clinical ladder system should be clearly differentiated and specific at each level. The evaluation process must be measurable, and salary differentials must be significant enough to provide motivation. Any system should involve evaluation of educational and leadership criteria as well as skill performance. **Box 9-5** is an example of a basic clinical career ladder.

Job Variety and Job Sharing

Rotating employees through different jobs has many advantages, such as keeping employees stimulated and productive and eliminating boredom and burnout. It also lets employees gain other useful skills, which can increase organizational

BOX 9-5   Basic Clinical Ladder Model

A. Clinical/Staff Nurse I (beginner/novice)
   1. Experience and Education
      Current state licensure with less than 1 year of experience.
   2. Description
      a. Needs close supervision.
      b. Performs basic nursing skills/routine patient care.
      c. Begins to develop patient assessment skills/communication skills.
B. Clinical/Staff Nurse II (advanced beginner)
   1. Experience and Education
      a. Current state licensure with more than 1 year of experience.
      b. BSN with more than 6 months of experience.
      c. MSN without experience.
   2. Description
      a. Demonstrates adequate/acceptable performance.
      b. Can differentiate importance of situations and set priorities.
      c. Requires less supervision.
      d. Demonstrates interest in continuing education.
C. Clinical/Staff Nurse III (competent)
   1. Experience and Education
      a. Current licensure with 2 or more years of experience.
      b. BSN with more than 1 year of experience.
      c. MSN with more than 6 months of experience.
   2. Description
      a. Demonstrates unsupervised competency using the nursing process.
      b. Is able to plan and organize in terms of short-range and long-range goals.
      c. Demonstrates direction in actions.
      d. Accepts leadership responsibility readily.
      e. Demonstrates well-developed communication skills.
      f. Shares ideas and knowledge with peers.
D. Clinical/Staff Nurse IV (proficient)
   1. Experience and Education
      a. Current licensure with 3 years of clinical experience and pursuit of BSN.
      b. BSN with more than 2 years of experience.
      c. MSN with more than 1 year of experience.
   2. Description
      a. Demonstrates specialized knowledge and skills.
      b. Continues professional education.
      c. Assumes leadership/supervisory responsibility.
      d. Recognizes and adjusts to situations that vary from the norm.
      e. Delegates responsibility appropriately; uses wide range of alternatives in solving problems.

(continues)

BOX 9-5   Basic Clinical Ladder Model (Continued)

    E. Clinical/Staff Nurse V (expert)
        1. Experience and Education
            a. MSN with more than 2 years of appropriate clinical experience.
            b. BSN required with more than 3 years of experience; pursuing MSN.
        2. Description
            a. Demonstrates expertise in clinical practice.
            b. Assumes/delegates personnel and management responsibility.

---

productivity. Job rotation can be used for entry-level employees as well as employees with more work experience. It could even be used for employees nearing retirement; they can teach newer employees valuable knowledge that is useful within the company.

Job rotation can be tailored to fit the organization by rotating employees through special projects, partial week rotations, internships, or temporary assignments. The outcome of a properly run job rotation program includes retaining, motivating, and educating employees.

However, nurse leaders should not confuse job rotation programs with shift reassignment (pulling) to another unit. The chronic reassignment of nursing personnel to cover vacancies is always viewed by nurses as a negative and has been the cause of a great deal of disgruntlement. One sure way to negate any positive recruitment and retention efforts is to allow perpetual shift reassignment within the healthcare agency.

Another option for nursing is job sharing, that is, two persons filling one full-time equivalent job at a ratio of work agreed on by them. This option is convenient for nurses who want and can afford to work part time and need time off. Less acceptable to nurses is mandatory sharing of work in organizations when technology and restructuring have reduced staffing levels (Erenstein & McCaffrey, 2007).

SUMMARY

Nurse leaders are challenged to create work environments that address the needs and respond to the opportunities of a diverse workforce. Transformational leaders move beyond their own cultural frame of reference to promote strong intercultural communication and create cultural synergy in the workplace. They recognize and take full advantage of the productivity potential that is inherent in a diverse population. Experts caution organization leaders that developing an effective diversity management strategy is a long, challenging process that cannot be solved simply by attending a few half-day workshops. Managing a culturally diverse workforce does not happen haphazardly. Instead, it requires a deliberate and proactive approach.

REFLECTIVE QUESTIONS

1. Describe how human capital affects staffing, scheduling, patient satisfaction, and quality.
2. For nurse leaders who are responsible for empowering teams, what strategies foster healthy work environments and a culture of quality?
3. Develop a strategy for an effective communication infrastructure.
4. Describe the management of difficult scenarios, including conducting crucial conversations, managing chaos, and preventing lateral violence and bullying.
5. Discuss the management of a diverse work team, including gender, generational, and cultural differences.
6. Identify best strategic practices for staff renewal and reduction of burnout.

CASE STUDY 9-1   Healthy Work Environments

Sergül Duygulu

After having worked in a private eye hospital following her graduation from her bachelor's degree program in nursing, Pelin has been working in the emergency unit of a university hospital for the past 4 years. With her energy and desire to exercise her profession, Pelin attends the surgical nursing doctoral program in the nursing school of another university in addition to working. Since she is attending doctoral courses during the day, she works night shifts during the week and on weekends. The charge nurse of the Emergency Unit continually supports Pelin's development and considers her needs when preparing the work schedules.

The Emergency Unit has a resuscitation room with 7 beds, an examination room with 12 beds, and a trauma room with 4 beds. Patient interventions are also performed on 10 stretchers in the corridors. There is a total of 23 nurses and 14 physicians, and there are 12 auxiliary staff (janitors). Nurses work two shifts: 08:00–16:00 (day shift) and 16:00–08:00 (night shift). There are four nurses with the unit charge nurse during the day shift, and there are generally three nurses during the night shift. Sometimes there are three senior nurses working the night shifts. Some nurses work 24-hour shifts on the weekends due to family demands. Also, there are trainee nurses and doctors continuing their education.

In the Emergency Unit there is a locked medicine cabinet, a locked emergency cart, and four cabinets in which disposable supplies are stored. Although there is no written protocol, the key to the locked medicine cabinet is with the unit charge nurse and another nurse during the day shift. It is handed over to a qualified nurse during the night shift. The key is handed over to the next nurse during the shift change. Nurses attend to patients under the supervision of a senior shift nurse.

One day, when Pelin takes over the night shift with two other nurses, she, being the most senior nurse on the shift, has organized the patient care duties and assigned them to other nurses. About 4 hours after she took over the shift, the phone rings, and Pelin talks to a police officer who is calling from the police station. The officer says they received a warning about a bomb left in the Emergency Unit and that a team, including bomb disposal experts, is on their way and will arrive at the hospital soon. The officer says steps should be taken in the Emergency Unit and hangs up. Despite being an experienced nurse, Pelin realizes that she doesn't know what to do in this situation and immediately calls hospital security to report the situation.

There are 3 patients in the resuscitation room, 12 patients in the examination room, and 3 patients in the trauma room. A patient is receiving an active intervention in the resuscitation room. Pelin immediately calls the hospital duty administrative director and the duty physician to report the situation. Meanwhile, in the absence of instructions for what to do in case of a bomb threat, Pelin, three duty doctors, and two other nurses decide to send the patients to other clinics or home, depending on their conditions. They call the hospital supervisor to ask for support, and three nurses, three physicians, and three janitors are sent to the Emergency Unit to transfer patients to the clinics. Meanwhile, the police come to the Emergency Unit to start searching the entire department for a bomb. Five patients in the examination room are in good condition, so they are sent home. The other seven patients in the examination room and the patients in the trauma room are transferred to other clinics. The three intubated patients in the resuscitation room are left in the Emergency Unit to continue receiving care.

Two hours after the bomb threat, the search in the Emergency Unit has been completed and the threat was found to be a hoax. During the rest of the shift, Pelin and the Emergency Unit team ensure that the unit resumes services and continues to care for patients. There is a good chance that during the ordeal, the conditions of the patients in the Emergency Unit did not deteriorate.

During the shift change the patients are handed over to the newly arrived nurses who work the 08:00–16:00 shift. During the shift change, it is discovered that a box of 10 dolantines, as well as 5 dolantines from another box, are missing from the locked medicine cabinet. Dolantine is a synthetic opioid analgesic belonging to the phenylpiperidine class. The Emergency Unit charge nurse speaks with the nurses and other team members who worked the night shift. Everyone says they know nothing about the issue. According to what one nurse remembers, the most recent time dolantine was dispensed was in the resuscitation room during an intervention, and the medicine cabinet was not locked due to the panic and rush caused by the bomb threat. The hospital management reports the situation to the police, and the entire Emergency Unit team who worked the night shift is under suspicion. The investigators inspect the hospital security records for the night of the event, but they find that there is no record of what happened during the bomb threat.

The investigation remains inconclusive, and it cannot be determined who took the dolantine. Fifteen days after the incident, Pelin and the other Emergency Unit team members receive an admonition and are warned to be more careful. A procedural change was made on the Emergency Unit so the key to the locked medicine cabinet, which was previously given to a qualified nurse during the night shift, will now be given to the most experienced nurse.

Case Study Questions

1. Considering the principles of healthy work environments (effective leadership, staffing, human resources planning, risk planning, communication, interpersonal relations, decision making, etc.), describe the various issues that complicate the case.
2. What factors caused the problems?
3. How are these problems interrelated?
4. If you were Pelin, how would you have handled the situation?

REFERENCES

Accountability. (n.d.). In *Merriam-Webster's online dictionary*. Retrieved from http://www.merriam-webster.com/dictionary/accountability

Aiken, L., Havens, D., & Sloane, D. (2009). The Magnet Nursing Services Recognition Program: A Comparison of Two Groups of Magnet Hospitals. *Journal of Nursing Administration, 39*(7/8), S5-15.

American Nurses Association. (2011). Lateral violence and bullying in nursing. Retrieved from http://www.nursingworld.org/Mobile/Nursing-Factsheets /lateral-violence-and-bullying-in-nursing.html

Bass, B. M. (1990). *Bass and Stogdill's handbook of leadership: Theory, research and managerial applications* (3rd ed.). New York, NY: Free Press.

Blanchard, K., & Johnson, S. (2003). *The one minute manager*. New York, NY: William Morrow.

Boatman, S. A. (1997). The role of followers in the charismatic leadership process: Relationships and their consequences. Retrieved from http://prezi.com /behlqfrmbra2/copy-of-the-role-of-followers-in-the-charismatic-leadership -process-relationships-and-their-consequences/

Boehm, H., & Bonnell, W. (2010). The use of peer review in nursing education and clinical practice. *Journal of Nurses Staff Development, 26*(3), 108–115.

Carless, S. (1998). Gender differences in transformational leaders: An examination of superior, leader and subordinate perspectives. *Sex Roles, 39*(11/12). 887–902.

Costello, D., & Vercler, M. A. (2006). Are your recruitment strategies up to date? *NursingHomes, 6*(1), 26–34.

Couros, G. (2014). 5 characteristics of a change agent. Retrieved from http:// georgecouros.ca/blog/archives/3615

Davies, C. (1995). *Gender and the professional predicament in nursing*. Philadelphia, PA: Open University Press.

DeLuca, J. R. (1999). *Political savvy: Systematic approaches to leadership behind the scenes*. Berwn, PA: EBG.

Efron, L. (2014). Six reasons your best employees quit you. Retrieved from http://www.forbes.com/sites/louisefron/2013/06/24/six-reasons-your-best -employees-quit-you/

Empathy. (n.d.). In *Merriam-Webster's online dictionary*. Retrieved from http:// www.merriam-webster.com/dictionary/empathy

Erenstein, C. F., & McCaffrey, R. (2007). How healthcare work environments influence nurse retention. *Holistic Nursing Practice, 21*, 303–307.

Erickson, H. (2006). *Modeling and role-modeling: A view from the client's world*. Cedar Park, TX: Unicorns Unlimited.

Fischer, B., & Boynton, A. (2005). Virtuoso teams. Retrieved from http://hbr .org/2005/07/virtuoso-teams/ar/1

Gaffney, S. (2005). Career development as a retention and succession planning tool. *Journal for Quality and Participation, 28*, 7–10.

Gerzon, M. (2006). Moving beyond debate: Start a dialogue. Retrieved from http:// hbswk.hbs.edu/archive/5351.html

Gokenbach, V. (2007). Professional Nurse Councils: A new model to create excitement and improve value and productivity. Journal of Nursing Adminis

Goleman, D. (2004). *Primal leadership*. New York, NY: Bantam Dell.

Goleman, D. (2006). *Social intelligence: The new science of human relationships.* New York, NY: Bantam Dell.

Greenleaf, R., & Spears, L. (2002). *Servant leadership: A journey into the nature of legitimate power and greatness.* New York, NY: Paulist Press.

Haag-Heitman, B., & George, V. (2011). Nursing peer review: Principles and practice. Retrieved from http://www.americannursetoday.com/nursing-peer-review-principles-and-practice/

Hillman, J. (1996). *The soul's code: In search of calling and character.* New York, NY: Warner Books.

Homan, A., & Greer, L. (2013). Considering diversity: The positive effects of considerate leadership in diverse teams. *Group Processes & Intergroup Relations, 16*(1), 105–125.

Horth, D., & Buchner, D. (2014). Innovation leadership. Retrieved from http://www.ccl.org/leadership/pdf/research/InnovationLeadership.pdf

Hospital Consumer Assessment of Healthcare Providers and Systems. (2013). HCAHPS patient-level correlations. Retrieved from http://www.hcahpsonline.org/Files/Report_HEI_April_2013_Corrs.pdf

Institute for Safe Medication Practices. (2004). Intimidation: Practitioners speak up about this unresolved problem (Part I). Retrieved from http://www.ismp.org/Newsletters/acutecare/articles/20040311_2.asp

Kritsonis, A. (2005). Comparison of change theories. *International Journal of Scholarly Academic Intellectual Diversity, 8*(1), 2004–2005, p 1–7

Llarena, M. (2013). What to expect during an HR interview? Five questions you'll be asked during a screening interview. Retrieved from http://www.forbes.com/sites/85broads/2013/10/18/what-to-expect-during-an-hr-interview-five-questions-youll-be-asked-during-a-screening-interview/

Lombardo, M., & Eichinger, R. (2004). *FYI: For your improvement* (4th ed.). Minneapolis, MN: Lominger.

Longo, J. (2007). Horizontal violence among nursing students. *Archives of Psychiatric Nursing, 21,* 177–178.

Magnet Recognition Program Overview (2014). Retrieved from: http://www.nursecredentialing.org/Magnet/ProgramOverview

Noe, R. A. (2005). *Employee training and development.* New York, NY: McGraw-Hill.

O'Hara-Devereaux, M. (2004). *Navigating the badlands: Thriving in the decade of radical transformation.* San Francisco, CA: Jossey-Bass.

O'May, F., & Buchan, J. (1999). Shared governance: A literature review. *International Journal of Nursing Studies, 36,* 281–300.

Patterson, K., Grenny, J., McMillan, R., & Switzler, A. (2012). *Crucial conversations: Tools for talking when stakes are high* (2nd ed.). New York, NY: McGraw Hill.

Phillips, D. T. (1993). *Lincoln on leadership: Executive strategies for tough times.* New York, NY: Warner Books.

Pittman, J. (2007). Registered nurse job satisfaction and collective bargaining member status. *Journal of Nursing Administration, 37*(10), 471–476.

Porter O'Grady, T. (1992). *Implementing shared governance.* USA: Mosby Year Book.

Price, D., & Price, A. (2012). Introducing *Management: A practical guide.* UK: Icon Book.

Sellman, D. (2011). Professional values and nursing. *Medicine, Health Care and Philosophy*, *14*(2), 203–208. doi:10.1007/s11019-010-9295-7

Studor, Q. (2004). *Hardwiring excellence: Purpose, worthwhile work, making a difference*. Gulf Breeze, FL: Firestarter.

Taplin, S., Foster, M., & Shortell, S. (2013). Organizational leadership for building effective health care teams. *Annals of Family Medicine*, *11*(3), 279–281. Retrieved from http://www.annfammed.org/content/11/3/279.full

Tuckman, B. (1965). Developmental sequence in small groups. *Psychological Bulletin*, *63*, 384–389.

Tulgan, B. (2006). *Managing the generation mix: From urgency to opportunity*. Amherst, MA: HRD Press.

U.S. Office of Personnel Management. (2014). What is an employee assistance program? Retrieved from http://www.opm.gov/faqs/QA.aspx?fid=4313c618 -a96e-4c8e-b078-1f76912a10d9&pid=2c2b1e5b-6ff1-4940-b478-34039a1e1174

Wahl, C., Scriber, C., & Bloomfield, B. (2013). *On becoming a leadership coach: A holistic approach to coaching excellence*. New York, NY: Palgrave MacMillan.

CHAPTER 10

Managing Performance

Kathryn M. Ward-Presson

LEARNING OBJECTIVES

1. Differentiate among standards for performance appraisals.
2. Distinguish among the major types, designs, and criteria for pay for performance.
3. Utilize techniques that foster individual development.
4. Illustrate the value of a portfolio for professional development.

AONE KEY COMPETENCIES

I. Communication and relationship building
II. Knowledge of the healthcare environment
III. Leadership
IV. Professionalism
V. Business skills

AONE KEY COMPETENCIES DISCUSSED IN THIS CHAPTER

I. Communication and relationship building
II. Knowledge of the healthcare environment
III. Leadership
IV. Professionalism
V. Business skills

I. **Communication and relationship building**
- Effective communication
- Relationship management
- Influence of behaviors
- Ability to work with diversity
- Shared decision making
- Community involvement

- Medical staff relationships
- Academic relationships

II. Knowledge of the healthcare environment
- Clinical practice knowledge
- Patient care delivery models and work design knowledge
- Healthcare economics knowledge
- Healthcare policy knowledge
- Understanding of governance
- Understanding of evidence-based practice
- Outcomes measurement
- Knowledge of, and dedication to, patient safety
- Understanding of utilization and case management
- Knowledge of quality improvement and metrics
- Knowledge of risk management

III. Leadership
- Foundational thinking skills
- Personal journey disciplines
- Ability to use systems thinking
- Succession planning
- Change management

IV. Professionalism
- Personal and professional accountability
- Career planning
- Ethics
- Evidence-based clinical and management practices
- Advocacy for the clinical enterprise and for nursing practice
- Active membership in professional organizations

V. Business skills
- Understanding of healthcare financing
- Human resource management and development
- Strategic management
- Marketing
- Information management and technology

FUTURE OF NURSING: FOUR KEY MESSAGES

1. Nurses should practice to the full extent of their education and training.
2. Nurses should achieve higher levels of education and training through an improved education system that promotes seamless academic progression.
3. Nurses should be full partners with physicians and other health professionals in redesigning health care in the United States.
4. Effective workforce planning and policy making require better data collection and information infrastructure.

Introduction

Why is managing performance a critical activity for healthcare and nursing leaders? The primary answer can be found in the Institute of Medicine report *The Future of Nursing: Leading Change, Advancing Health* (2011). This report identified concerns about increasing healthcare costs and suboptimal patient outcomes, as well as challenges with healthcare complexity, gaps in evidence-based performance activities, and diminishing resources (Weberg, 2012). The report identified the nursing profession as the largest component of the healthcare workforce that works in close proximity to patients and understands the complexities of patient care delivery in a variety of healthcare settings. Other Institute of Medicine reports (1999, 2001, 2004) also described quality and safety deficiencies in healthcare organizations and discussed the need to manage performance to achieve improvements that reduce waste, eliminate errors, and improve clinical patient outcomes. Individual-, unit-, or system-based performance management allows healthcare system leaders to utilize reliability principles to reduce errors and improve patient outcomes (Riley, 2009).

The 2010 Patient Protection and Affordable Care Act established reforms to the Medicare reimbursement system that are designed to improve efficiency by moving from a fee-for-service payment system to bundled payments for hospitals and providers (Centers for Medicare and Medicaid Services, 2010). When organizations fail to meet benchmark targets related to unanticipated complications or infections, Medicare reimbursement to facilities is reduced. The Centers for Medicare and Medicaid Services (2013a, 2013b) is considering additional quality measures to assess acute care and long-term care hospitals, as well as accountable care organizations' compliance with Medicare standards (Gordon, 2014). Healthcare reform initiatives directed toward improving care and decreasing costs requires the engagement of nurse leaders who are able to balance business objectives and relevant clinical practice standards to manage units or health systems effectively (Welton, 2014). This need obliges leaders to balance business acumen skills and a strong understanding of professional practice standards. For example, personnel cost analyses that explore unit and overall facility cost improvement initiatives may be helpful to provide a road map for balanced cost containment decision making. Jenkins and Welton (2014) conducted a study in a Magnet hospital in which they evaluated direct nursing care time and costs for similar patients over a 2-year time frame. They concluded that nursing costs per patient could be benchmarked across the facility and provided valuable data to inform nursing administrative decisions.

The need for performance management activities is further supported by Provision 7 of the American Nurses Association *Code of Ethics for Nurses with Interpretive Statements* (2001). This provision requires nurses to create, implement, sustain, and improve nursing practice standards and patient care delivery models. All nurses have a responsibility to maintain acceptable standards of care while reviewing those practices to ensure that a safe environment (free from error) exists for all patients and coworkers. Nurse leaders have an additional responsibility to create and foster work environments to support staff engagement, which is necessary to evaluate standards of care and care delivery processes that promote safe practice environments. Creating autonomous work environments enables staff to demonstrate clinical leadership behaviors when functioning in direct care roles (Patrick, Laschinger, Wong, & Finegan, 2011). Through the coordinated delivery of respectful, compassionate care that is provided in collaboration with other disciplines, nurses support patient-centered environments and health care, which reduces errors and injuries and improves patient satisfaction (Letcher & Nelson, 2014). Nurse leaders can serve as advocates for performance management in their roles as change agents when they work with staff to establish collaborative interprofessional partnerships that improve efficiencies and patient care delivery processes. Creating a culture of safety that promotes daily improvement in patient care delivery and transparency should be an ongoing leadership process during reporting and the provision of feedback (Blouin & McDonagh, 2011). Such collaborative activities represent examples of performance improvement initiatives that support a culture of safety.

Managing performance enables leaders to implement performance improvement initiatives that provide the foundation to redesign patient care processes, enhance data management, and influence healthcare policy. Revised processes are needed to improve efficiency (reduce waste), support a safe environment (eliminate errors), enhance patient outcomes (reduce infections), and provide new models for patient-centered care. Improvement plans and revised processes must be evaluated and adjusted to meet the desired objectives after they are developed and implemented.

Transforming care delivery also requires robust data management related to a broad range of performance measures and healthcare delivery processes. Data obtained from performance management activities may also provide valuable information for nurse scientists engaged in scientific inquiry. Such inquiry is necessary to provide new evidence-based recommendations that enhance nursing knowledge, improve nursing practice, and promote a collaborative agenda for healthcare reform in practice and policy development. Challenges for staff occur when data management systems are inaccessible, not easy to use, and generate untimely reports. To mitigate these obstacles, nurse leaders must advocate for adequate data management systems that are accessible, generate reports in a timely manner, and are user friendly. They must also share patient outcomes and performance improvement results with staff and all other key stakeholders.

Transparency is critical in establishing a trusting and ethical work environment that fosters a sustained culture of safety embraced by all levels of staff and key stakeholders. Transparency also provides healthcare organizations with a complete view of operational performance that compares an organization's performance with like facilities (Kerfoot, 2009). The publication of nursing outcomes and program evaluation reports is an example of transparent information sharing about organizational performance management activities. This will be discussed in more detail later in this chapter.

Avoidance leadership behaviors include indecisiveness, ambivalence, or hostility when responding to staff suggestions or concerns (Jackson, Hutchinson, Peters, Luck, & Saltman, 2013). Such behaviors should not be used because they undermine the principles of transparency and staff empowerment.

With the evident need for continual innovation, today's healthcare environment is vastly different from previous years. Programs such as the Magnet Recognition

Program (American Nurses Credentialing Center, 2014) provide a framework for transformative efforts that utilize performance management activities to create autonomous, high-functioning units capable of addressing transformational needs. Such units develop and implement interventions that address existing and future challenges with patient care delivery (Wolf, Finlayson, Hayden, Hoolahan, & Mazzoccoli, 2014). Participation in the Magnet Recognition Program requires data management, benchmarking, and strong evidence of an organization's performance management and sustained improvement of nurse-sensitive indicators (pressure ulcers, catheter-associated urinary tract infections, assault rates, etc.) compared to national benchmarks. Improvement in nurse-sensitive indicators has been linked to shorter lengths of stay, increased patient and staff satisfaction, and decreased morbidity and mortality rates. These activities represent opportunities for nurse leaders and staff to actively participate in the healthcare organization's performance management program.

Because healthcare performance measurement criteria are continually evolving, in 2014 a Magnet Recognition Program task force created a new set of ambulatory care nurse-sensitive indicators (medication reconciliation, controlling high blood pressure, depression assessment, pain assessment and follow-up, and pain) (Lewis, 2014). The development of these measures serves as an example of proactive performance measurements during transitions that previously occurred in acute care settings and now are practiced in ambulatory care.

HIGH-PERFORMANCE ORGANIZATIONS

High-performance work systems are established by leaders who create a culture guided by performance management and improvement principles. Davis and colleagues (2014) conducted a case study review of 10 healthcare agencies that conducted early quality improvement activities. Those that conducted informal quality improvement initiatives did so primarily to meet accreditation standards; those that established a quality improvement culture were more likely to demonstrate evidence-based decision making, lower rates of staff turnover, and the use of performance improvement tools to deal with issues as they arose. A qualitative study of 28 clinicians and managers (Leggat, 2013) demonstrated that effective clinical leadership does not involve simply providing staff with leadership skills; rather, it ensures that the staff understands and fully embraces the distribution of power and control among disciplines involved in patient care delivery. Leggat (2013) also identified four important leadership areas—"emotional intelligence, resilience, self-awareness and an understanding of other health care professions" (p. 312)—as being supportive of interdisciplinary collaboration.

Healthcare leadership support and guidance are essential in achieving cultural transformation and staff acceptance of a quality culture. To that end, leaders must provide staff with time and resources (including accessible data management and analytical systems) to sustain a culture that embraces quality. Leaders who function as champions of performance improvement are critical for managing performance and developing new standards and care delivery processes. A mixed-methods study by Dixon-Woods and others (2014) found that unclear and overlapping organizational goals create staff distractions from operational duties, and a bureaucratized culture causes staff to struggle with providing efficient, safe care. This study further highlighted the need for leaders to provide an innovative, patient-centered environment with clearly established goals that are embraced by the staff. When the staff is motivated to change, the leader's ability to provide expert guidance and knowledge greatly augments their performance (Hamstra, Orehek, & Holleman, 2014).

Highly reliable organizations may exist within environments at great risk for error or untoward events because they operate in a manner that addresses issues proactively in an organized manner. Doing so mitigates and reduces errors, waste, and unfavorable patient outcomes. Nurse leaders who monitor and manage performance to enhance safety and proactively address challenges provide the opportunity for creating highly reliable healthcare organizations. The adage "what gets monitored gets managed" seems to perfectly describe the advantages of establishing a performance management culture. Reducing errors and violations in nursing practice can be achieved using team education and system redesign principles (Riley, 2009). Riley further recommends that nursing leaders purposefully design key care processes, conduct interdisciplinary team education, ensure team members' understanding of care processes, error proof the organization, and standardize care delivery mechanisms.

Historically, patient care processes (steps used to achieve goals) have not been designed with patients at the center or with safety and error reduction in mind. Managing performance using performance improvement tools (flowcharts, fish bone diagrams, and clinical bundles) enables nursing leaders and staff to proactively identify issues and develop corrective action plans that prevent harm and enhance the work environment. The use of evidence-based standards, clinical bundles, and models of care provide the best prospects to improve patient outcomes and care delivery processes. Outcomes improvements and safer work environments are promoted by the creation of "tightly synergized teams" (Kerfoot, 2009, p. 245). Leadership modeling that demonstrates a real commitment to clinical excellence and high standards helps organizations avoid mediocrity, which stifles innovation and performance management efforts. Nurse leaders may use innovative team-building exercises or new roles, such as clinical nurse leader, to address interdisciplinary collaboration and improved patient outcomes at the microsystem level. In 2007, the American Association of Colleges of Nursing (2007) published a clinical nurse leader white paper that proposed the use of a master's-prepared generalist who utilizes evidence-based practice innovations and partners with unit nursing staff and interprofessional colleagues to improve unit-based patient outcomes and efficiencies. A revision of the white paper in 2013 underscored the quality and safety initiatives at the point of care, reinforcing clinical leadership (American Association of Colleges of Nursing, 2014). Leaders must also be aware of the need to evaluate any new roles (clinical nurse leader, clinical nurse specialist, nurse educator, etc.) to determine their impact and the value for the organization when investing resources in those roles (Bleich, 2011).

Communicating the organization's values and ethical expectations clearly and often provides the greatest potential for sustained staff engagement. Regularly scheduled interactive staff meetings, frequent rounding in patient care and work areas, employee email communication, widely distributed newsletters, and an open-door policy are examples of how leaders can model such behavior. Email makes it possible to provide information to employees quickly and often.

Communication should occur in both directions between leaders and staff and provide ongoing opportunities for staff interaction and feedback. Quarterly small-group meetings with a representative sample of staff members can also provide opportunities for open-ended dialogue, staff input, and clarification of goals and expected performance outcomes.

COMPLEXITY SCIENCE

Considering current and future healthcare system challenges, traditional leadership principles that promote linear thinking and minimal innovation are no longer adequate to address the highly complex environments of health systems. Today's nurse leaders must embrace the principles of complexity science and understand that a state of constant change and the interdependence of processes and interprofessional relationships are requisite competencies (Weberg, 2012). These leaders must review their biases, their commitment to professional standards, and their organizations' values to minimize acceptance of the status quo and guide staff in the exploration of evidence-based innovations that reduce costs and improve care delivery and patient outcomes. True leader accountability should result in new innovations and models of patient care delivery that reduce errors and place patients at the center of decision making (Allen & Dennis, 2010). When plans to implement innovations are being devised, adequate time should be provided for staff to attain knowledge, new competencies to be validated, and work processes to be redesigned (Malloch, 2010). This is especially true when new technology-based systems are introduced (such as electronic health records and bar code medication administration).

All nurse leaders (managers, directors, and senior executives) play critical roles in influencing excellence in patient care delivery. Establishing shared decision making and leader–staff partnerships are key components to creating cultures of nursing care excellence. Shared governance structures, with corresponding nursing unit and system-wide councils, provide for information sharing and staff engagement in performance improvement activities. Authentic leadership principles provide the road map to engage and support leaders and staff (McSherry, Pearce, Grimwood, & McSherry, 2012).

AUTHENTIC LEADERSHIP

Authentic leaders create empowering work environments that increase staff satisfaction and overall performance (Bamford, Wong, & Laschinger, 2013; Leigh, 2014). Trust in nurse leaders also promotes staff engagement and perceptions of the quality of care that is delivered. Nurse leaders are poised to positively influence staff performance, satisfaction, and patient care outcomes by creating positive staff relationships, allowing for different points of view, providing honest feedback and information, and demonstrating ethical conduct in all actions (Wong, Spence Laschinger, & Cummings, 2010). Authentic nurse leaders are patient advocates who do not hesitate to step back and reassess progress toward their own professional and organizational goals on an ongoing basis. Demonstrating a sense of gratitude, respect for others, and humility enables authentic leaders to sustain trust (Kerfoot, 2010). Acknowledging and celebrating the contributions and successes of others will also convey leaders' appreciation and recognition of others as opposed to focusing on themselves. Active introspection provides leaders with insights about what works well in a variety of situations and what might be better accomplished using different approaches. Authentic leadership highlights a genuine, open, self-aware, and change-oriented style that is committed to improving performance and embracing collegial relationships to improve patient outcomes (Murphy, 2012). Projecting a sense of self-assurance and leadership confidence is also important, which can be achieved by presenting a polished, well-groomed professional image in dress and appearance (Wocial, Sego, Rager, Laubersheimer, & Everett, 2014). Leader self-awareness provides another catalyst for staff engagement and team member ownership in the success of performance management processes.

Compromising professional standards and ethics is not consistent with authentic leadership principles. Most healthcare organizations are undergoing efforts to reduce costs. These transformations provide an ideal opportunity to use authentic leadership skills to appropriately address the fiscal challenges encountered by most nurse leaders today. Because nursing personnel costs comprise a large component of any healthcare organization's budget, nurse staffing levels are often under scrutiny. Using evidence-based data related to staffing models can help leaders determine the appropriate skill mix and number of staff members needed to provide quality care on a given unit. Adequate staffing and an appropriate mix of professional and nonprofessional staff members have been associated with positive patient outcomes. However, competing financial agendas in most healthcare facilities will require the use of evidence-based calculations to determine what nursing staff is needed. Some elements that should be included in staffing need calculations are a transparent staffing methodology that incorporates such elements as scientific references, professional organization standards, unit workload and turbulence, staff education levels, student preceptor activities, staff vacancies, time for performance improvement activities, time for nursing research inquiries, and staff development activities. Obtaining senior-level buy-in of the proposed staffing methodology before sharing it with the line staff can facilitate a more positive outcome during budget negotiations. Asking staff members to calculate the unit's staffing needs and to actively participate in managing the fiscal performance metrics for their unit can create a sense of shared accountability for resource utilization. In this age of monetary performance awards and pay-for-performance compensation plans that reward the achievement of fiscal and clinical goals, it is very important that leaders are ethically mindful of their duty to protect patients first and provide a safe practice environment for the staff. Compromising professional standards to obtain a bonus or financial reward is inconsistent with the American Nurses Association *Code of Ethics for Nurses with Interpretive Statements* (2001), specifically Provision 2, which addresses the need for professional nurses to be patient advocates and maintain a distance from any activities (including financial) that may be considered conflicts of interest. Nurse leaders and staff members must declare any concerns related to potential conflicts of interest through appropriate mechanisms.

Unit nurse managers are in a unique position to influence staff safety behaviors and the overall culture of safety on a given unit, such as nurse managers who regularly round on their units to observe staff practices and evaluate the unit's potential for regulatory violations (crowded hallways, blocked fire escapes, slip and fall hazards, unlocked medication carts, outdated drugs and supplies, etc.).

The staff's compliance with safety standards can be favorably influenced by the leadership of nurse managers (Lievens & Vlerick, 2014) as they model concern for safety risks and hazards and convey that such behavior is expected. Rounding is an example of a performance management activity that promotes a culture of safety and communication.

EVIDENCE OF PERFORMANCE MANAGEMENT

Assessments of authentic leadership should include evaluating the leader's self-awareness, ethical conduct, and balanced decision making that is reflective of business, clinical knowledge, and skills. Because nurse managers have direct contact with unit staff members, they are in a prime positon to influence staff behaviors and attitudes in the work environment (Bamford et al., 2013). Obtaining feedback from staff, peers, and supervisors, as well as a self-evaluation, provides a 360-degree or global perspective of a leader's performance. Similar principles can apply to other leadership roles, such as those held by nursing directors and nurse executives. Because input is obtained from key stakeholders, a 360-degree evaluation provides a more objective and complete view of a leader's strengths and opportunities for improvement. The feedback provided in such a review can be used to formulate more robust career development and improvement plans designed to facilitate leader growth.

Trust and respect for their leader promotes teamwork among staff members and prevents untoward safety events (Blouin & McDonagh, 2011). The opportunity to provide staff feedback for 360-degree leader evaluations supports a culture of transparency and honest dialogue between management and staff members about the perceived existing state, and it offers suggestions for leader improvement. Initially leaders may find this exercise awkward and painful. Comments from others about your performance may be difficult to accept, but authentic leaders who understand and actively promote a culture of safety and performance management seek opportunities for feedback, introspection, renewal, and growth. Their willingness to participate in this process provides a model for staff members to emulate.

LEADERSHIP DEVELOPMENT

Authentic and transformational nurse leaders do not magically appear in healthcare settings. Academic, professional, and clinical organizations are poised to provide a variety of leadership development programs to support existing and future nurse leaders. Academic nursing institutions that offer graduate degrees at the master's and doctoral levels may provide formal learning environments for emerging leaders. A newer academic option is the pursuit of a doctor of nursing practice (DNP) degree (American Association of Colleges of Nursing, 2004). The DNP degree was designed to address gaps in advanced practice nursing knowledge and leadership skills for chief nursing officers (CNOs). A capstone project published by Swanson and Stanton (2013) described the perceptions of CNOs regarding the applicability of the DNP degree to their practice. The authors found that acute care CNOs (especially those with more tenure) believe the DNP degree is an appropriate option to enhance executive knowledge and skills. Beyond formal education, participation in other programs—military leadership development courses, on-the-job experiences, mentoring relationships, and so forth—provide growth and development opportunities for emerging leaders.

Additionally, formal and informal education can provide nurse leaders with tools to use evidence-based practice principles, conduct nursing research, implement performance improvement projects, and advocate for quality patient care delivery. Feedback from nurse leadership development program participants has found that such programs improve managers' levels of professionalism, consistency in exercising leadership behavior, and awareness of a broader view of an organization's overall goals and decision-making processes (Abraham, 2011; Patton et al., 2013). Leadership development programs that emphasize the importance of evidence-based practice principles and research methods are necessary to improve the delivery of high-quality care and improve patient satisfaction (Johansson, Fogelberg-Dahm, & Wadenstein, 2010). The implementation and ongoing use of evidence-based practice principles is necessary to improve delivery and patient outcomes and is further dependent on leadership advocacy and support.

Before leaders can influence others, they need to possess a clear vison of the nursing profession and demonstrate requisite skills to drive excellence in patient care delivery in their organizations (Graham, 2010). The psychological competence of leaders should also be addressed as a component of any leadership development program. Authentic leaders who are psychologically competent are more likely to exhibit strong empowering competencies that energize staff. Energized staff generally experience stronger ties to the organization's goals and mission (Havaei, Dahinten, & MacPhee, 2014).

Career development programs may also serve as recruitment mechanisms that assist with identifying potential leaders within the existing staff. Such programs may offer tools for self-assessment, career development, networking, targeted assignments to enhance skills, executive leadership programs, annual evaluations (including 360-degree reviews), and internal job advancement (Lynas, 2012). Leadership development plans should include experiences that enhance psychological competencies and staff empowerment and should also be guided by formalized organizational and system-wide succession planning strategies.

SUCCESSION PLANNING

Succession planning strategies that are readily available to all levels of staff are necessary to provide healthcare organizations with an adequate supply of qualified internal leadership candidates. The primary component of successful succession planning programs is senior leadership support (Bargininere, Franco, & Wallace, 2013). The development of internal talent requires planning and contributes to maintaining corporate knowledge and improved employee morale. Current and projected nursing shortages highlight the need for ongoing succession planning strategies designed to address future nursing leadership gaps (Carriere, Muise, Cummings, & Newburn-Cook, 2009). Cooperation among healthcare facilities and academic institutions in creating succession planning programs is recommended (Griffith, 2012).

Preparing for known and unknown leadership vacancies at all levels is vital at a time when capable nurse administrators are needed to lead staff in the use of evidence-based decision making and collaborative teamwork. Only proactive succession planning can ensure that healthcare organizations will have a pipeline of nurse leaders to meet these objectives. Without such planning, the shortage of prepared nurse leaders will be exacerbated. The increasing age and anticipated retirements of many in the nursing workforce (along with the expected shortage of qualitied nurse leaders) requires the use of carefully structured succession planning strategies that target and recruit talent and identify and evaluate leadership competencies that are needed for future healthcare environments (Titzer, Shirey, & Hauck, 2014). Particular attention should be focused on unit nurse manager succession planning. Unit nurse manager positions are particularly important because these leaders work closely with nursing staff and collaborate with other disciplines that provide direct care. Because nurse managers lead staff members who are closest to patient care delivery, they provide the greatest influence on engagement and the improvement of patient care process and outcomes.

MENTORING

The American Organization of Nurse Executives (2014) identified communication and relationship building, knowledge of the healthcare environment, leadership, professionalism, and business skills as requisite competencies for nurse executives to help CNOs function effectively in today's chaotic healthcare environment. Now more than ever, nurse leaders are challenged with increasing complexity and the implementation of new care delivery models. Today's aging nursing workforce, with large numbers of nurses eligible to retire at any time, also stresses nurse leadership capacity. For many years, the need to recruit and retain talented nursing leaders who can lead staff to deliver and improve patient care has been a major concern for healthcare organizations. Successful mentoring of internal staff members who have leadership potential may address many of these concerns.

Nurse managers implement the facility's organizational strategies and goals at the unit level, and nurse executives provide the vision to achieve the organization's overall clinical and fiscal objectives. The knowledge, competencies, and skills needed for various roles in the nursing leadership hierarchy differ in scope, complexity, span of control, and capability (Thompson, Wolf, & Sabatine, 2012).

How do we prepare and support novice nurse leaders for the variety of first-line management and executive roles that are needed to address today's complex healthcare environments? Mentoring provided by an experienced and competent role model who can serve as an advisor and resource is an effective way to provide growth and development for new nurse leaders. Coaching focuses on specific goals, whereas mentoring transfers expertise to enhance a person's relationships and overall professional development (McKinley, 2004). Mentors may be internal or external to the organization; when possible, mentees may seek a relationship with one or both types of mentors during their careers. Internal mentors have organizational knowledge and a greater understanding of an organization's or system's culture, but external mentors may provide more objective guidance that is free of institutional bias and offer different viewpoints. Both types of mentors offer benefits to prospective mentees.

Similar to the nursing process, mentor–mentee relationships should be guided by planning for meetings, learning opportunities, competency observations and skills demonstrations, and evaluation and feedback. Ground rules should be established so plans and expectations are clear (McKinley, 2004). During these encounters the mentee should be observed, and constructive assessments of progress and planned opportunities for improvement should be outlined (Greene & Puetzer, 2002). A qualitative study of novice nurse self-evaluations following mentorship found that their self-confidence and interest in maintaining high-quality standards was directly linked to mentoring. This was especially true when the mentor exhibited trust (confirming mentorship) in them and reinforced that perspective (Ronsten, Anderson, & Gustafsson, 2005). A qualitative study that focused on individual participants in a national clinical leadership development program for Irish nurse midwives found that participants, their managers, and their mentors could articulate observed examples of clinical growth and development over the course of their 6-month program (Patton et al., 2013). These examples provide evidence of real-world applications of clinical nursing leadership in practice.

More than an orientation process, mentoring invests in the ongoing success of the organization or healthcare system and considers the needs and capabilities of the mentors and mentees involved (Block, Claffey, Korow, & McCaffery, 2005). Administrative support for mentorships is critical to sustain these relationships on a long-term basis. Selecting the right mentors and pairing them with the right mentees is an important element of a successful mentor–mentee relationship. Mentors should be selected based on their availability, knowledge, interpersonal skills, experience, and teaching ability. Mentors who commit to mentoring must be capable of listening, guiding, and empathizing with a mentee while offering sage counsel and solutions derived from tested experiences (Kanaskie, 2006).

For the mentor–mentee relationship to be successful, mentees must willingly commit to mutually agreed upon goals, follow outlined plans, and seek and positively accept feedback. They should be clear about what they expect from the mentorship experience. Is their need based on a new role or the desire to achieve upward mobility? Does the mentee wish to have broader professional experiences or assistance with obtaining new work challenges and growth opportunities? Being forthright, grateful, and motivated will provide mentees with better opportunities for positive mentoring experiences (Jones, 2004).

Mentors must understand that they will work beyond their traditional roles, and they need to be given adequate time to develop and foster a relationship with the mentee, whether the relationship is internal or external to the organization. Exemplar mentors demonstrate caring behaviors and expertise in the relevant field and display good critical thinking skills. A mentor's sense of self-confidence can impart a sense of strength and knowledge to the mentee, and this fosters the needed mutuality in a successful mentor–mentee relationship. The mentor–mentee relationship may go through various phases, including closure of the relationship to promote independence, but an ongoing relationship may exist for any number of years (Hayes, 2005; Owens & Patton, 2003). Depending on the position and experiences of the mentor, the relationship may become reactivated when the mentee is promoted to another role, and it may even evolve until and after the mentee becomes a mentor to others.

Owens and Patton offered 10 strategies to foster nursing mentorships:

1. Take a chance on others and be willing to engage.
2. Take advantage of the excitement a mentor–mentee relationship can provide.

3. Be creative in communication to ensure ongoing interaction.
4. Keep all formal and informal commitments.
5. Evaluate progress periodically to maintain the right course.
6. Use adult learning principles when engaging the mentee, and foster an eventual peer relationship.
7. Be open. Don't promote or mandate objectives. Allow for mentee mistakes and input.
8. Push boundaries and welcome new learning experiences.
9. Be thankful for the caring and supportive feedback or praise.
10. Spend time enjoying the collegiality of the relationship and be open to a new friendship. (Owens & Patton, 2003, p. 203)

Mentors may use 360-degree evaluations (especially in conjunction with structured career development programs) to provide a baseline assessment of a mentee's strengths, competencies, and opportunities for improvement (Karsten, 2010). From this information, further growth-oriented plans, stretch goals, and new learning experiences that are consistent with the mentee's overall career objectives (and those of the organization) can be designed.

Because feedback is an important evaluation tool, mentees' impressions of their mentorship experiences may be captured to provide mentors and mentees with qualitative insight regarding the value of such experiences. Such feedback can help mentors and senior nursing leaders to improve methodologies to provide mentor guidance. Examples of such reflections can be found in Case Studies 10-4, 10-5, and 10-6. The mentee in Case Study 10-4 is a first-time CNO who obtained a DNP degree in 2014. The mentee in Case Study 10-5 recently assumed an associate chief nurse leadership role and completed a DNP degree in 2014. The mentee in Case Study 10-6 earned a PhD with postdoctoral nursing education several years ago and recently transitioned from an associate chief nurse leadership role to a high-level performance management and policy development role within a national healthcare system. Depending on the educational preparation of the mentor and mentee, role reversals may occur if the mentor enrolls in academic programs of higher learning that were already completed by the mentee. Each of the mentees in the case studies continue to engage in mentorship relationships. They also provide mentor guidance to subordinate novice nurse leaders and peers.

Generational Mentorship

Effective mentoring depends on understanding the values and perspectives of others. Because today's healthcare workforce represents several distinctly different generations, understanding the characteristics of those generations is critical to establishing successful mentoring relationships (Chung & Fitzsimons, 2013; Jobe, 2014; Kanaskie, 2006; Stewart, 2006). According to Jobe (2014), baby boomers were born from 1946 to 1964; generation X was born from 1965 to 1979; and millennials were born from 1980 to 1999. Due to different socioeconomic and cultural life experiences, each generational group has different values about work ethics, work–life balance, and professional reward and success expectations. Because empowering staff members and providing an adequate supply of new nurse leaders is important to meet healthcare organizations' performance management goals, creating a work environment that engages all staff members requires generation-specific leadership development strategies. As subsequent groups emerge, their motivations and expectations will also need to be considered.

Tension among staff members due to generational differences impacts unit and facility performance, practice patterns, employee morale and satisfaction, and recruitment and retention efforts (Stewart, 2006). The results of a qualitative, quasi-experimental cross-sectional study (Jobe, 2014) found that the 285 completed surveys of nurses in two teaching hospitals in the southern United States showed similarities among the three generations, but there were differences in hard work, leisure, and delay of gratification. In this study, nurses from the generation X and millennial generations placed greater emphasis on leisure time, future plans, delay of gratification, and hard work when compared to baby boomers. Because baby boomers are closer to retirement than the other two groups, the emphasis on future plans is probably less important to them. Younger groups also tend to place higher importance on hard work, with expectations for related success, advancement, and affirmation.

Creating generationally dependent leadership development strategies may also assist nurse leaders in resolving staff conflicts. Leaders may use a variety of tactics to minimize differences. These include discussions during staff meetings, focus groups, and role playing to promote staff understanding of generational differences and a culture of acceptance (Stewart, 2006). Leaders should also recognize that all staff do not share the same motivation to work long hours whenever the manager requests it. Work schedule choices and the flexibility to accommodate family and school plans are usually more important to people in the generation X and millennial generations. Other generations frequently view baby boomers as workaholics.

If mentors are from the baby boomer generation, they must recognize that mentees from other generations will very likely be motivated by other values and expectations. Generation Xers need new growth experiences, opportunities for teamwork, and formal feedback sessions. Because self-reliance is highly valued by this group, an occasional redirection of their energy may be necessary (Stewart, 2006). On the other hand, millennials need personal attention and opportunities to use technology-based solutions and innovations. Texting, emails, and social networking are major avenues for communication among members of this group. They also possess high self-esteem and believe they can accomplish anything, but they are skeptical of job security. As a result, they focus on skills development and networking to establish future professional prospects (Chung & Fitzsimons, 2013). Their mentors should support lifelong learning and cross training, provide rationale and evidence for recommendations, and solicit opportunities for input and innovation (Stewart, 2006). Capitalizing on millennial staff members' interest in innovation, technology, and inquiry can greatly support the performance management efforts of nurse leaders at all levels in healthcare organizations.

CRUCIAL CONVERSATIONS

At times it is necessary for leaders to help staff become more aware of their behaviors and the impact of those behaviors on others and in unit operations. Having the courage to confront others is a skill that requires development and practice, and it is often leaders' least favorite activity. Improving performance requires leaders to demonstrate courage and the ability to question the status quo so new models of care can be explored (Malloch, 2010). Doing so may require crucial conversations with team members.

Crucial conversations between leaders and staff usually occur when emotions are high, different points of view emerge, and stakeholders are not able to resolve differences among themselves. These differences may manifest in negative non-verbal behavior and may even escalate into loud verbal exchanges, refusals to work together, and other undermining behaviors or even physical violence (Major, Abderrahman, & Sweeney, 2013). Such behaviors should never be tolerated. Effective management of these situations rests with leaders.

When individuals are working together and making decisions with others, threats to a person's competence may emerge. Reactive behaviors, such as defensiveness and competiveness, may emerge as protective mechanisms, and mediation may be required (Sommet et al., 2014). Prior to engaging staff members in crucial conversations, leaders should pause and identify the best approach to provide staff with performance-related feedback. Keeping focused and being clear about the expected outcome helps leaders and staff members chart a course of resolution based on common goals. If union representation is requested by a staff member, the leader should honor the request, assuming it is consistent with any negotiated contracts and approved agreements, or explain why such representation would be counterproductive. Arbitrary refusals to allow union participation can undermine good faith working agreements that have been established between management and labor partners. Avoiding power struggles promotes an environment of transparency and collaboration. Innovative, authentic leaders need to keep their emotions in check and leave their egos at home, and they must help other staff members do the same. Modeling a willingness to listen to all sides promotes a culture of safety and collegiality.

Staff conflict is a natural by-product of working in complex healthcare environments, and developing skills in conflict management is essential to foster teamwork and collaborative care delivery (Pines et al., 2014). Although many studies have described the deficits created in healthcare organizations due to lack of teamwork and poor communication and interdisciplinary collaboration, creating positive environments in which communication establishes a culture of performance improvement and mutual trust among coworkers can minimize or eliminate poor outcomes (Polito, 2013). Several theories (Stone's five-step process, Leebov's caring feedback model, Ury's breakthrough strategies, and Crawford's workplace issues discussions) provide similar themes to assist leaders in dealing with conflict (Polito, 2013). These themes include collecting complete facts, eliminating emotional interpretations, understanding the purpose of the crucial conversation, practicing and role-playing a variety of conflict conversations with peers or mentors, keeping emotions in line, listening and asking probing questions, setting expectations in advance, and being prompt in providing decisions and feedback as promised (Polito, 2013). In other words, leaders must be professional, objective (there are two sides to every conflict), fair but firm, and timely in addressing disruptive behaviors (Elder, 2014). Doing so will foster a climate of performance management that also promotes staff engagement, mutual respect, and improved patient care delivery processes and outcomes.

When unresolved problematic behaviors and unprofessional conduct persist, leaders may be in a position that warrants termination of an employee. Hopefully these situations are rare, but when necessary the leader has a moral and professional obligation to take such action. Necessary terminations provide another opportunity for leaders to deal effectively with conflict in the workplace. In facilities represented by bargaining units, union representation that is consistent with negotiated contracts should be supported. Termination conversations are often the most contentious and difficult for leaders to encounter. As with other conflict-based conversations, leaders should have engaged the staff member in progressive disciplinary processes and provided opportunities for improvement that are clearly documented and communicated. Unless the circumstances necessitating termination are so egregious that immediate action is indicated, such discussions with the employee should not be a surprise. Only validated facts should drive the decision to terminate an employee. Leaders should also understand that the documents related to the facts in their case will be important if the employee decides to exercise any number of legal actions to appeal the termination (Young, 2014).

PROFESSIONAL PORTFOLIOS

Because professional development is necessary to support the growth of current nurse leaders and educate new nurse leaders, the creation of a professional portfolio to demonstrate individual accomplishments or a prospective leader's potential for advancement provides a foundation for improvement and career planning (Tofade, Abate, & Fu, 2014). A portfolio also provides a level of transparency in outlining a leader's performance management activities and outcomes. Mentors may use a mentee's portfolio in concert with other assessment results (such as 360-degree evaluations) to plan appropriate learning experiences and identify stretch goals.

Garrett, McPhee, and Jackson (2013) conducted a study to evaluate the use of electronic portfolios for the assessment of bachelor of science in nursing students' progress. They found that electronic portfolios created a convenient and accessible tool that improved transparency and tracking of student competencies. However, student and faculty concerns about possible privacy breaches were also found, so it is important to maintain the confidentiality of student information. The identification of further student learning needs, made possible through access to a student's electronic portfolio, was strengthened by student reflection and active engagement in the learning process. It is notable that many graduate nursing program admission procedures require applicants to submit paper or electronic portfolios as evidence of a candidate's potential for success in pursuing advanced nursing education.

Quality portfolios among physician academics are an increasingly common way to demonstrate evidence of quality performance and safety activities. The portfolios may also include examples of scholarly research efforts, teaching activities and preceptorships, publications, honors, awards, grant funding, and so forth (Taylor, Parekh, Estrada, Schleyer, & Sharpe, 2014). In addition to quality improvement, a culture of safety and improved efficiencies is needed in all areas of healthcare delivery; nurse leaders can adopt a similar model for demonstrating engagement in quality and patient safety efforts.

Portfolio-based assessment tools are a way to collect, organize, and evaluate achievements, accomplishments, and potential learning and career development needs. Portfolios should contain a variety of items that demonstrate the broad accomplishments of the individual. Such accomplishments should include statements of the individuals' professional philosophy and career goals, evidence of educational achievements, certifications, awards, continuing education, mentorship activities, faculty appointments, activities in professional organizations, system committees and task force memberships, peer-reviewed publications, paper and poster presentations, research and grants, reference letters, and any other relevant professional accomplishments.

In addition to other assessment tools, such as annual evaluations and references, the orderly consolidation of evidence-based individual accomplishments enables mentors to collaboratively identify development plans that are consistent with the mentee's future career goals and opportunities for improvement. Portfolios also provide managers with information about a job candidate's capabilities and potential contributions to the team (McMillian, Parker, & Sport, 2014). Job applications and resumes alone do not provide an evidence-based picture of candidates' past accomplishments and future team member potential. E-portfolios in particular provide leaders with easily accessible insight into the specific performance-based contributions of a nurse over time. This information is especially important in the selection of new nurse leaders at any level in an organization because it provides information about the candidate's adherence to professional standards and embrace of performance management principles. Current leaders may create portfolios to document ongoing achievements that may be used to evaluate performance, productivity, future goal setting, and career planning. Having a readily available current portfolio may also be very beneficial when unforeseen opportunities for additional professional experiences arise.

NURSING PERFORMANCE IMPROVEMENT STRUCTURE, DASHBOARDS, AND OUTCOMES REPORTS

Establishing a facility-wide nursing performance improvement structure with a designated senior nurse leader builds the best foundation for active nursing participation in any healthcare organization's performance management activities. Presenting data that is usable and easy to interpret is facilitated by advances in technology. For example, technology may be used to develop clinical and administrative dashboards that enable nurse leaders to use evidence-based performance improvement practices to support decision making (Chorpita, Bernstein, & Daleiden, 2008). Dashboards may assist in presenting data for multiple units or systems, and they provide leaders with the ability to communicate large amounts of information, track progress regarding results and program outcomes, and identify needed improvements. They also provide executive leaders with a mechanism to visualize the progress of individual units and the organization's overall performance toward strategic goals (Harrison, 2012). To be useful, data must be presented in a format that engages all staff members, including those working at the bedside and those in executive or corporate positons. Linking data reporting to an organization's strategic plan promotes staff buy-in and stakeholder awareness. Doing so promotes an organizational culture of safety and quality (Heenan, DiEmanuele, Hayward-Murray, & Dadgar, 2012).

Creating regular reporting mechanisms, including publishing monthly, quarterly, and annual benchmarked nursing outcomes reports, establishes a transparent method to communicate performance improvement activities and results with board members, staff, patients, interdisciplinary colleagues, regulatory agencies, and affiliation partners. An annual nursing outcomes report may be produced in print and electronic form, and it should be widely distributed to key stakeholders. At a minimum, the report should contain the following:

1. Provide the CNO's statement of the philosophy and vision for nursing care delivery and performance management.
2. Provide the nursing services mission statement.
3. Describe all monitored, trended, and benchmarked nurse-sensitive indicators, and all performance improvement strategies and results. The results should be displayed in line and bar graphs, run charts, and so forth. Examples of topics to cover include the following: fall rates with and without injuries, restraint usage, seclusion and assault rates for mental health units, critical care unit ventilator-acquired pneumonia rates, central line blood stream infection rates, catheter-associated urinary tract infection rates, hospital-acquired pressure ulcer rates, high-alert medication errors, prn effectiveness compliance, verbal order usage rates, patient and staff satisfaction rates, rapid response team and code rate comparisons, and ambulatory care access and discharge callback rates.
4. Provide a description and the outcomes of special program initiatives, such as infection control bundle implementation, new role (such as clinical nurse leader, clinical nurse specialist, etc.) impact evaluations, nurse-led health promotion and disease prevention clinics, health screening and influenza campaigns, and safe patient handling programs.
5. Provide an analysis of the effectiveness of budgetary considerations and staffing methodologies. Include graphs demonstrating nursing hours per patient day by unit with targets and applicable benchmarks. The trended RN turnover, vacancy rates, and nursing staff terminations should also be graphically displayed and discussed. A discussion of the impact of nurse staffing on specific nurse-sensitive outcomes should be included and shown on graphs with applicable targets and benchmarks.
6. Describe the activity and outcomes of all shared governance and leadership committees or councils. Examples of shared leadership groups include clinical professional practice councils, administrative operations councils, advanced-practice councils, evidence-based practice councils, and performance improvement councils.
7. Describe staff professional practice activities and awards. Include all publications, podium and poster presentations, nursing research and grant activities, participation in regional and national system committees and professional organizations, and so forth.
8. Describe career ladder and nurse staff promotions, national certifications, and educational achievements (including degrees obtained).
9. Describe affiliations with academic partners, including the number and education level of student experiences, and provide the results of student evaluations.
10. Describe and evaluate any internal (fires, facility floods, power outages, etc.) or external (community-based fires, floods, hurricanes, tornadoes,

snowstorms, etc.) disaster response activities. Include any staff deployments to assist other facilities with their disaster responses. Also include any collaborative partnerships with other healthcare facilities that provided expertise or additional support. Postdisaster evaluations should be completed and communicated (as a part of after-action briefing sessions) close to the time of the event. The annual report evaluation component should include assessments of what worked well and what changes were recommended to improve responsiveness and effectiveness in future disaster scenarios.

SUMMARY

Managing performance in healthcare systems is necessary to reduce errors, eliminate waste, and improve clinical patient outcomes. Nurses have an ethical and professional responsibility to improve standards of care and patient care delivery models. Nurse leaders have a responsibility to create work environments that support staff empowerment to address organizational deficiencies and transform patient care delivery.

Authentic leadership, high-performance organizations, and complexity science principles provide a foundation for the development of transformational strategies that are necessary to guide nurse leaders' performance management and improvement initiatives in healthcare organizations. The pursuit of higher academic education, informal career development programs, and mentoring relationships provide leaders with opportunities to gain new knowledge and competencies to meet these evolving challenges.

Succession planning strategies that include opportunities for novices to engage in mentoring relationships provide organizations with a pipeline of new nurse leaders. Ongoing leader evaluations, including 360-degree assessments, provide a framework for defining individual leader needs and development plans. Evidence of nursing performance management, which supports the principles of transparency and ongoing monitoring and improvement, include developing individual professional portfolios and establishing organizational nurse-driven performance improvement programs. The activities of a robust nursing performance improvement infrastructure enable nurse leaders to monitor progress, communicate and engage staff in improvement activities, and generate a variety of dashboards and nursing outcomes reports that can be used to communicate progress to key stakeholders. Engagement in these performance management activities contributes to a healthcare organization's reduction of errors, elimination of waste, and improvement in clinical patient outcomes.

REFLECTIVE QUESTIONS

1. Identify the requisite skill sets necessary for managing individuals and teams.
2. The workforce is aging at an alarming rate. What are the essential skills needed by transformative leaders in the future to manage a changing workforce mix?

3. What evidence supports high-performance organizations' success?
4. What is the value of developing a portfolio as an individual healthcare leader?

CASE STUDY 10-1   Conflict Management

Sergül Duygulu

Nurse Pinar completed her bachelor's program in nursing and has started working in a physical therapy and rehabilitation unit in a clinic with 50 beds. Most patients who are diagnosed with paraplegia, quadriplegia, and hemiplegia have relatives who stay with them. The length of stay varies depending on the diagnosis; it can be as long as 8 to 10 months.

There are seven nurses and a unit charge nurse at the clinic. The unit charge nurse and four nurses provide care to 50 patients during the day shift, from 08:00–16:00, and one nurse provides care during 24-hour shifts on holidays. The clinic has a shortage of nurses. Services are provided in compliance with the healthcare quality standards that were developed by the Ministry of Health, with a focus on patient and employee safety. However, there are issues in fulfilling the quality standards, which causes the employees to be unsettled.

Pinar, as a new nurse graduate, adapts quickly to the clinic, which pleases the unit charge nurse and the other nurses. At the end of her first month, Pinar worked the 16:00–08:00 shift by herself. She took over the shift from the day nurses and performed routine nursing care. While she was checking on the patients at 20:00, Pinar was approached by the wife of a patient who has quadriplegia and is staying in room 20. The wife said her husband suddenly began to breathe with difficulty. Pinar immediately went to the patient's room and found that he has difficulty breathing and is in poor condition. Pinar immediately went to the nurses' desk to report the situation to the duty physician. She could not reach the physician and had to make several phone calls.

In the meantime, the son of a patient who has hemiplegia and is staying in a private room came to the nurses' desk and told Pinar that his father's blood pressure was not measured at 20:00. The son added that his father doesn't look good, and he asked Pinar to come and take his father's blood pressure. Pinar told the son that another patient's condition has worsened, and she will measure his father's blood pressure when she is free. The intervention with the patient in room 20 takes longer than expected. He needs to be admitted to an intensive care unit and must be transferred to a facility that can accommodate his needs. Pinar informed the night supervisor about the transfer.

Finally, an hour later, Pinar attended to the patient in the private room. When she entered the room, the patient's son accused Pinar of not fulfilling her duty and angrily tells her that his father is not receiving proper nursing care at the hospital and that they have been waiting for a blood pressure measurement for an hour. He also said that since his father is in a private room, he is entitled to special care. The son said he will file a complaint with the authorities about the situation. Pinar tried to explain what happened, but the son is not convinced, and the atmosphere remained tense. At the shift change in the morning, Pinar told the unit charge nurse what happened. The unit charge nurse told Pinar that similar incidents happen from time to time and that she should get used to them and not be upset.

The next day, the chief doctor angrily told the nurse manager that he had received a call from the Ministry of Health because a patient had not received proper care at night. He asked the nurse manager to investigate the situation. The nurse manager called the unit charge nurse and said there is a complaint about Pinar and she will be investigated, and that her own reputation as the nurse manager is at stake. The nurse manager accused the unit charge nurse of assigning Pinar to a shift alone before she was ready for the responsibility. Although the unit charge nurse tried to explain the situation, the nurse manager wouldn't listen, and she hung up. The unit charge nurse called Pinar and told her to come to the hospital right away. Pinar arrived at the hospital and told the nurse manager what happened. However,

CASE STUDY 10-1   Conflict Management (Continued)

she received a written admonishment because of the complaint that had been filed with the Ministry of Health, and she was being held responsible.

After the incident, Pinar started to work in another clinic at the hospital, and 15 days later the unit charge nurse was assigned to the outpatient clinic as nurse. Six months later, Pinar resigned and started to work as a nurse in a private hospital.

Case Study Questions

1. What were the sources and possible causes of the conflict?
2. What kinds of system problems caused the conflict?
3. What is the level of conflict?
4. How do you assess the behaviors of Pinar, the unit charge nurse, and the nurse manager?
5. What would your strategy be to manage this situation?
6. What actions you would take?
7. What management and leadership skills are needed to manage this conflict?

CASE STUDY 10-2   The 360-Degree Change

Debbie R. Faulk and Arlene H. Morris

Jane has been the manager of a 40-bed medical–surgical unit in a large urban hospital for 15 years. She has worked very hard over those years to create a just culture and a healthy work environment. Her leadership style is primarily democratic, but she is aware of and does not hesitate to use other styles when situations dictate. Jane is well liked and respected as a person and professional by all her staff members and other healthcare professionals on the unit. Three days ago, her immediate supervisor informed Jane that a new performance appraisal process would begin in 1 month. The new process will be used for evaluation of all upper- and midlevel managers.

The Department of Human Resources held around-the-clock training sessions for staff who will be impacted by the new process. During the training sessions, Jane learned that a 360-degree feedback process will be used for performance appraisals. She learned that this feedback process is a multirater, multisource assessment and that an employee's immediate work group will provide feedback on the managers' performance. In other words, patients, subordinates, peers, and supervisors will provide performance feedback. In addition, the employee will complete a self-evaluation. Jane is open to this new process, but she expressed some reservations related to the use of external sources, such as patients, for the evaluations.

Jane decided to research the literature regarding the 360-degree feedback process. She was troubled when she found titles such as *360: The Good, Bad and Ugly, 7 Reasons Why 360-Degree Assessment Doesn't Work, The Fatal Flaw of 360 Survey*, and so forth (Heathfield, 2001). However, Jane was determined to keep an open mind about this new process. She learned that the process is more accurate if the rater has known the individual being evaluated for 1 to 3 years. The least accuracy was reported in the literature if the rater had known the individual for 5 or more years. To Jane, this meant that a rater who has known the person being evaluated for at least 1 year has had time to get past first impressions, but if they have known the individual for longer than 5 years, the nuances of the person's characteristics can interfere with an objective evaluation. The literature also reported that self-ratings are generally higher than ratings from others.

(continues)

CASE STUDY 10-2   The 360-Degree Change (Continued)

Jane presented her findings from the literature to her immediate supervisor and expressed concern about using the new process. The supervisor informed Jane that the new process would begin and that Jane would be evaluated using the established procedure within 1 month. Although Jane was skeptical, she was determined to ensure that the process was used effectively.

A month later, when Jane was presented with her evaluation, she was told that her peer scores were low. However, her subordinate scores were very high. Unfortunately, the focus of the face-to-face evaluation was about Jane's low scores. Jane was told she was not a team player. She remembered several incidents that had happened over the past few months and expressed concerns that her peers may have been responding based on those issues. For example, Jane remembered a particular incident when she was busy helping her staff take care of a critically ill patient. There were a number of nurses, physicians, and other providers in the patient's room when a manager from the maintenance department came in to the room to investigate a problem with an air vent. He knew Jane well and shouted out that he was there to fix the vent problem. Jane told him the time was not appropriate and that he must return later. He insisted that he would do the job now. Jane stopped what she was doing and walked over to the individual; she calmly but sternly told him that he could not check on the air vent at that moment. The maintenance manager was furious and said he would not come back and that the air vent could stay inoperable as far as he was concerned.

Jane also remembered an incident that occurred during a huddle meeting. Another unit manager told Jane that she was always late or often did not bother to come to huddles because she was too busy. The manager expressed to Jane, in front of other managers, that she was more concerned with doing patient care than being a manager.

Jane believed those events directly influenced her peer 360-degree evaluation, and she expressed this to her supervisor. Her supervisor told Jane that perhaps she really was not manager material. Jane was shocked and hurt.

Case Study Questions

1. How would you have responded to the initial announcement of the imminent change in evaluation procedures? What is the rationale for your answer?
2. What do you think that Jane should have done, based on the evidence she found in the literature?
3. If you were the administrator, what would you have done if Jane had shared her findings from the literature? What is the rationale for your answer?
4. How could a 360-degree evaluation foster or hinder an individual's development?

CASE STUDY 10-3   Celebrating Generational Differences

Debbie R. Faulk and Arlene H. Morris

F. P. is celebrating her new appointment as the director of nursing (DON) at a 200-bed long-term care facility by having dinner with a longtime friend who is also a nurse. F. P. admits that she is very concerned about her leadership role in creating a value-based work environment where generational differences are supported. F. P. tells her friend that it is important for her as the DON to recognize and act on generational differences in values and behaviors. F. P.'s friend tells her that she recently read a research study that would help F. P. structure the work environment to accommodate generational differences. F. P. is excited to hear

CASE STUDY 10-3   Celebrating Generational Differences (Continued)

about the study and begins using the findings to facilitate the growth and development of her staff. F. P. realizes this task is not going to be easy, but she knows that using the best evidence can help her be a leader in creating a long-term care workforce that will thrive and meet future healthcare challenges.

Case Study Questions

1. How can F. P. accommodate generational differences in attitudes, values, and behaviors?
2. To effectively coach and motivate her staff, what generation-sensitive styles will F. P. need?
3. When generation conflicts occur, how can F. P. resolve or minimize the issues to build an effective work team?
4. Do you believe the generational differences in a long-term care environment are different from those in other healthcare settings? If yes, describe; if no, why not?
5. How can F. P. capitalize on generational differences to enhance staff performance?

CASE STUDY 10-4   Mentee Reflections from the Field

Jennifer Melvin Pifer

A mentoring relationship can be either spontaneous or sought out and intentional. I believe great leaders mentor naturally because they are internally centered with a strong desire to see others grow in their roles and succeed. They hold a belief that by giving of themselves, others can benefit. A leader is not a position or a title but rather an internal drive to impact others around you in a positive way.

In my career I have had the good fortune to have many mentors who have been both spontaneous and intentional. As a brand new staff nurse many years ago, my nurse manager understood the art of mentorship in a way that was genuine and heartfelt. She pushed me daily to grow as a strong, clinically gifted nurse, and through her steadfast pace and tireless dedication she showed me how to fend for myself in a large system that was full of complex challenges and diverse personalities. I quickly learned that timely feedback was a gift to be cherished and that, if I would listen, I could grow and outpace even seasoned nurses who had long ago closed themselves off to feedback.

Later in my career I had the good fortune to be mentored by the first doctorally prepared nurse I had ever known. This was an intentional mentoring relationship; I requested to be his mentee, and we formalized the structure of the relationship. This mentoring relationship proved to be the biggest growth opportunity in my nursing career. He encouraged me in so many ways. Here are just a few: return to school, open up major hospital programs, build networks within the community, be a lifelong learner, laugh at myself, be meticulous, do not believe all that I hear, and publish my accomplishments. He still remains a valuable resource to me today. It was because of this mentoring relationship that I was able to seek out a good mentor when I moved to another state.

After I moved, I knew the value of having a mentor who believed in me and wanted my best. I knew that making a move to another state would be a huge stressor. I needed to have someone to bounce ideas off of and who would help me grow in my new role. During the initial job interview I requested to have the nurse executive be my mentor, and I clearly articulated my goals, dreams, and fears. Thankfully she accepted this humble request.

Recalling several mentoring events with my nurse executive, one stands out clearly, and I will never forget the impact it had on me both personally and professionally. As a new associate chief nurse in

(continues)

CASE STUDY 10-4   Mentee Reflections from the Field (Continued)

the system, my first challenge kept me awake at night and was highly complex. The legalities of human resources matters in the situation were more than I had ever dealt with as a nurse manager. Dealing with such a weighty issue and being new to an organization created a great deal of scrutiny from my peers, subordinates, and superiors. I felt as if my every move was under the spotlight. As I continued with my nurse executive, I learned several valuable lessons about a mentoring relationship. First, you can be a mentor and still feel inadequate to deal with the situation and not always have the answers. For example, there were many times I would bring issues to the nurse executive and she would say she was not certain; she suggested that we call the regional council or some other resource that would help. Second, I learned that some of the best growing opportunities are from great pain, struggles, and difficulty—mentoring is not always pretty. Finally, a mentoring relationship never fails, regardless of a situation's outcomes. My nurse executive's ability to mentor me through this troubling experience was remarkable, and I will forever tuck it away as a precious event that I draw from.

Mentoring is giving of yourself at all costs and never turning back—always pressing onward. Mutual respect lays a firm foundation for the mentoring relationship. I will be forever grateful for the mentors in my life and thank them for teaching me to give to others. In a way, I see mentoring as a way to pay it forward, and I choose to do this today.

Case Study Questions

1. Reflecting on the author's experience, what lessons did you learn that you could use to seek out mentors during your professional development as a leader?
2. How would you use this reflected experience to provide coaching and mentoring for those who seek you out as a role model for leadership development?

CASE STUDY 10-5   Lifelong Learning and Professional Development

Jennifer Melvin Pifer

After recently graduating with my doctoral degree in nursing, I am about to transition to a new role as an associate chief nurse leader at a large teaching hospital. As I recover from several hectic, full years of both educational and professional growth, I am excited and appreciative of the journey of lifelong learning, encouraged by my unofficial mentor. My mentor and I never had an official contract, plan, or even discussion about our mentor–mentee relationship. Yet, unofficially, I knew my mentor was always there for me.

My mentor was a true leader in every sense of the word. She had the presence, experience, and wisdom to recognize potential pitfalls. She would delicately guide me with her probing questions, setting me up to come to the conclusions that I needed to know. Initially, I even thought I was the brainchild of some of her teaching moments. This is the brilliance of true teachers; they have the patience and foresight to lead their students to beneficial discoveries. My mentor always preached evidenced-based practice and data-driven decisions as she advocated for quality, safe patient care. Her expectations were high, but everyone would profess that they learned so much from this individual. I cannot claim her as only mine because our mentor grew so many of us.

As a leader, my mentor demonstrated solid decision-making skills and always shared the underpinning ideologies to encourage best practices. When I was discouraged, my mentor would offer support and encouragement. When I screwed up royally, my mentor offered protection. I recognize the key to

CASE STUDY 10-5   Lifelong Learning and Professional Development (Continued)

ensure patient quality is to promote an environment of shared learning. When people are fearful of repri-sal, they are less likely to come forward with mistakes that could be prevented by sharing information with others. This does not mean that my mentor did not hold me and others accountable for our deci-sions. My mentor absolutely did as any mentor should; she coached me and provided more guidance and oversight when needed.

As I grew and became better in my role, my mentor sent me for executive leadership training and encouraged me to seek out my doctoral training. She even gave me wings to fly and was a proponent of an offer I received for an executive nurse position.

In writing these pages, I remember that it was my mentor who taught me the importance of self-reflection. My mentor has since left our organization, but our relationship has transitioned from supervisor–employee to friendship. If my mentor reads this, I hope she recognizes her impact on many people; with the growth of many nurses, that mentor's wisdom has a domino effect. I routinely pay forward the wisdom my mentor shared. My mentor's résumé could never clearly define the true stature of this fine person, leader, teacher, advisor, coach, mentor, and friend. When we met for lunch not too long ago, she lauded my improved leader confidence. I left reassured and cognizant of the fact that my mentor will always be in the background promoting my professional development. My hope is that every nurse will have a special mentor relationship.

Case Study Questions

1. Describe the benefits of self-reflection within a mentoring relationship.
2. Discuss lifelong learning and how mentoring relationships can be developed as new skills and experiences are encountered.

CASE STUDY 10-6   Professional Career Development: Planning for Success

Kathryn G. Sapnas

When we begin a professional career, we often do not know where that journey will take us. The trajectory of a professional career begins with hopes and aspirations, a dream, a vision. Education provides a structure and the process for professional development, yet it is the quality of the mentor–mentee dyad in the education process and in the professional setting that produces exceptional outcomes for both the mentee and the mentor. These exceptional outcomes are achieved when there is synergy between the mentor and mentee. It is irrelevant how the dyad is created, whether the mentor is selected by the mentee, or whether the mentor selected the mentee.

I've been blessed and privileged to have had extraordinarily diverse professional and educational experiences that have been shaped by gifted mentors. In both of these phases of my career, I have either chosen a mentor or have been chosen as a mentee. In each of these experiences there was tremendous electricity, a chemical reaction. There is a formula for successful mentor–mentee dyads—perhaps a chemistry of understanding, caring, respect, intellect, values, trust, confidentiality, humility, engagement, tolerance, patience, advocacy, energy, negotiation, and risk taking; the mixture of each of these ingredients is context and volume dependent. Various mixtures and compounds yielded different levels of achievement and success and supported me during disappointments and failures. I've had varied experiences with mentors: one on one, groups and networks, face to face, and virtual.

(continues)

CASE STUDY 10-6   Professional Career Development: Planning for Success (Continued)

Reflecting on my 38-year nursing career, I would never have imagined all the peaks and valleys and the keen navigation needed to stay on course while keeping focused on learning, achieving, and, most of all, contributing to society. This vignette acknowledges that I was gifted with exceptional mentors. I can remember a conversation with one of my early graduate faculty mentors. She said, "You are the vanguard, the world is your oyster and you are the pearl." That was my beginning! She launched my curiosity and prepared me for the world of academe and practice. The wisdom and guidance and exquisite caring that I experienced with my doctoral mentor has developed into a 20-year friendship and sharing of families. The transition was seamless as my mentor became my peer and my friend. She helped prepare me for the realities, joys, and challenges of professional nursing in executive roles that I would come to experience.

Ten years ago I began a journey into executive management in a national enterprise organization. I was in an executive nursing role in nonoperational clinical support. My chief nurse executive was a seasoned leader, an exemplar in creating a learning environment for her nursing leadership team. She was my mentor and was truly gifted; she was truly a visionary, had passion for high expectations, and provided a high level of engagement and independence. She was a transformational leader who was hired to restore an underperforming nursing division in an urban tertiary academic medical center that had been serially deconstructed over the years to an effective, efficient nursing care delivery team. She was a caring and creative leader and was also electric, known as the "the rocket" by her peers. We shared equal levels of professionalism, caring, energy, passion, and enthusiasm for our work, as well as a shared commitment to service. The transparency with which she led and her openness to share her knowledge were hallmarks of this mentoring experience. This executive, while she was not doctorally prepared at that time, respected and celebrated my education and professional achievements. Our mentor–mentee relationship had just the right amount of chemistry for navigating the challenges of rebuilding a nursing division on a Magnet journey with a caring nursing philosophy and model. In my orientation, she discussed her expectations and ground rules, and she shared her vision for the nursing division. I clearly remember what she said as she shared her vision: "This is the outcome that we need to achieve, what I'm looking for, you get to paint the picture from the vision that I've shared, you can write the story, and I've given you the ending. The ground rules are that everything is fair game, just nothing illegal, nothing immoral, and nothing XXX!"

Over a 5-year period our nursing service collaborated to coauthor more than 44 professional peer-reviewed presentations, posters, and papers. Much of this work occurred during off-duty hours and was a labor of collective engagement. I remember that at 10 p.m. one evening, I was mentoring one of my colleagues on a phone call for the preparation of a poster. We were discussing a theoretical model. We both remarked that it was so unreal—we were collaborating and working on something we loved on our own time, and it was with joy! We commented that our experience on this team, with this executive as our mentor, was a once in a lifetime experience and that we'd ride the wave as long as it lasted.

Our team won national recognition and awards for the work we did. There was amazing energy because, as nursing leaders on the team grew and succeeded, their staffs grew and succeeded. The empowerment was contagious! Ultimately, our successful engagement was directly related to shared goals, beliefs, and values—a shared work ethic. There was a mutual respect, give and take, and an ability to respectfully agree to disagree. How remarkable to have an executive like that as my supervisor.

I was given creative license to operationalize that vision and achieve the outcomes that were jointly negotiated. Under her supervision and tutelage, she provided me opportunities for participating in leadership experiences outside of nursing in the facility. I was nominated to represent our nursing division in national enterprise committees, which led to a position as a national committee cochair. Subsequently, I

CASE STUDY 10-6   Professional Career Development: Planning for Success (Continued)

received national funding to work with a strategic planning project in an evidence-based nursing health information technology implementation and led virtual teams of 60 staff members, including national leaders across disciplines in enterprises across the United States, and delivered the project. My executive was an active collaborator in this work.

My executive saw promise in my work and supported my desire to advance in the organization. Each of these experiences helped me learn about the complex inner workings and executive management of the national healthcare enterprise, a complex adaptive system. Recognizing my capacity and motivation to grow in an executive role and advance in the organization, my mentor encouraged me and marketed me by giving me a national platform. The wisdom and guidance and exquisite caring I experienced with my executive mentor has developed into a 10-year friendship and sharing of family that continues to this day. A most interesting note is that this executive allowed and encouraged me to be an academic mentor to her during my employment. In the years that followed, the executive completed her doctoral degree. The former mentee was a mentor, the former mentor, a mentee.

I spent almost 4 years in my next executive position in the same enterprise, again in another urban tertiary academic medical center. This role focused on day-to-day operations, patient experience, and staff satisfaction. I had an executive nursing leadership role in clinical operations, again in an underperforming and historically deconstructed nursing service. My previous position, supporting and leading our Magnet journey, prepared me for the challenges in an underperforming facility. My executive recognized my interest for challenge beyond clinical operations.

My executive mentor was an expert at labor relations and negotiation. We spent lots of time discussing approaches and reviewing cases; she shared her experiences in human resource management and labor relations. Fostering the creation of a healthy work environment was a major focus of my efforts. My mentor selected me as one of six organizational leaders to represent our facility at the regional reading of the final union bargaining agreement.

In this position, I worked across services with various leaders. My chief nurse executive and mentor appointed me to represent the facility as a member in the regional network selection of a clinical information system. This exposure to regional network operations, national contracting and procurement processes, and collaborating across services was again foundational in my executive development.

This mentor shared her knowledge of the local market and the executive nursing community. We talked often about my executive career path and shared thoughts and ideas. The wisdom, guidance, and caring that I experienced with my executive mentor has developed into a 5-year friendship that continues to this day.

Both of these experiences with executive mentors have shaped my executive trajectory and were significant in positioning me for application, selection, and appointment in a national-level directorship in the enterprise and my success in the role.

Case Study Questions

1. As the author describes her experience, identify the major milestones, skills that were developed, educational opportunities that were sought, and synchronicity along the way. How did intentional planning contribute to positive outcomes? How did being in the right place at the right time play into success?

2. Identify specific messages from the author's experience that you will take with you on your personal journey. Outline how you will move forward using an action plan to integrate the lessons.

REFERENCES

Abraham, P. J. (2011). Developing nurse leaders: A program enhancing staff nurse leadership skills and professionalism. *Nursing Administration Quarterly, 35*(4), 306–312. doi:10.1097/NAQ.0b013e31822ecc6e

Allen, J., & Dennis, M. (2010). Leadership and accountability. *Nursing Management, 17*(7), 28–29.

American Association of Colleges of Nursing. (2004). *AACN position statement on practice doctorate in nursing.* Retrieved from http://www.aacn.nche.edu/publications/position/DNPpositionstatement.pdf

American Association of Colleges of Nursing. (2007). White paper on the role of the clinical nurse leader. Retrieved from http://www.aacn.nche.edu/aacn-publications/white-papers/cnl-white-paper

American Association of Colleges of Nursing. (2014). Competencies and curricular expectations for clinical nurse leader education and practice. Retrieved from http://www.aacn.nche.edu/aacn-publications/white-papers/cnl-white-paper

American Nurses Association. (2001). *Code of ethics for nurses with interpretive statements.* Retrieved from http://www.nursingworld.org/MainMenuCategories/EthicsStandards/CodeofEthicsforNurses/Code-of-Ethics-For-Nurses.html

American Nurses Credentialing Center. (2014). *2014 Magnet application manual.* Silver Spring, MD: Author.

American Organization of Nurse Executives. (2014). Nurse executive competencies. Retrieved from http://www.aone.org/resources/leadership%20tools/nursecomp.shtml

Bamford, M., Wong, C. A., & Laschinger, H. (2013). The influence of authentic leadership and areas of worklife on work engagement of registered nurses. *Journal of Nursing Management, 21*(3), 529–540. doi:10.1111/j.1365-2834.2012.01399.x

Bargininere, C., Franco, S., & Wallace, L. (2013). Succession planning in an academic medical center nursing service. *Nursing Administration Quarterly, 37*(1), 67–71. doi:10.1097/NAQ.0b013e31827857a7

Bleich, M. R. (2011). Measuring the value of projects within organizations. In J. L. Harris, L. Roussell, S. E. Walters, & C. Dearman (Eds.), *Project planning and management: A guide for CNLs, DNPs, and nurse executives* (pp. 147–160). Sudbury, MA: Jones & Bartlett Learning.

Block, L., Claffey, C., Korow, M., & McCaffrey, R. (2005). The value of mentorship within nursing organizations. *Nursing Forum, 40*(4), 134–140.

Blouin, A. S., & McDonagh, K. J. (2011). Framework for patient safety, part 1: Culture as an imperative. *Journal of Nursing Administration, 41*(10), 397–400. doi:10.1097/NNA.0b013e31822edb4d

Carriere, B. K., Muise, M., Cummings, G., & Newburn-Cook, C. (2009). Healthcare succession planning: An integrative review. *Journal of Nursing Administration, 39*(12), 548–555. doi:10.1097/NNA.0b013e3181c18010

Centers for Medicare and Medicaid Services. (2010). *Affordable care act update: Implementing Medicare cost savings.* Retrieved from http://www.cms.gov/apps/docs/aca-update-implementing-medicare-costs-savings.pdf

Centers for Medicare and Medicaid Services. (2013a). Fact sheets: CMS finalizes FY 2014 policy and payment changes for inpatient stays in acute-care and long-term care hospitals. Retrieved from https://www.cms.gov/Newsroom/MediaReleaseDatabase/Fact-sheets/2013-Fact-sheets-items/2013-08-02-2.html

Centers for Medicare and Medicaid Services. (2013b). Fact sheets: CMS to improve quality care during hospital inpatient stays. Retrieved from http://www.cms.gov/Newsroom/MediaReleaseDatabase/Fact-sheets/2014-Fact-sheets-items/2014-08-04-2.html

Chorpita, B. F., Bernstein, A., & Daleiden, E. L. (2008). Driving with roadmaps and dashboards: Using information resources to structure the decision models in service organizations. *Administration and Policy in Mental Health*, *35*(1–2), 114–123. doi:10.1007/s10488-

Chung, S. M., & Fitzsimons, V. (2013). Knowing generation Y: A new generation of nurses in practice. *British Journal of Nursing*, *22*(20), 1173–1179.

Davis, M. V., Mahanna, E., Joly, B., Zelek, M., Riley, W., Verma, P., & Solomon Fisher, J. (2014). Creating quality improvement culture in public health agencies. *American Journal of Public Health*, *104*(1), e98–e104. doi:10.2105/ajph.2013.301413

Dixon-Woods, M., Baker, R., Charles, K., Dawson, J., Jerzembek, G., Martin, G., & West, M. (2014). Culture and behaviour in the English National Health Service: Overview of lessons from a large multimethod study. *BMJ Quality and Safety*, *23*(2), 106–115. doi:10.1136/bmjqs-2013-001947

Elder, P. (2014). Take the high road in conflicts. *ASRT Scanner*, *46*(3), 18.

Garrett, B. M., MacPhee, M., & Jackson, C. (2013). Evaluation of an e-portfolio for the assessment of clinical competence in a baccalaureate nursing program. *Nurse Education Today*, *33*(10), 1207–1213. doi:10.1016/j.nedt.2012.06.015

Gordon, D. (2014). CMS to increase quality measures for MSSP ACOs: 4 things to know. Retrieved from http://www.beckershospitalreview.com/accountable-care-organizations/cms-to-increase-quality-measures-for-mssp-acos-4-things-to-know.html?tmpl=component&print=1&layout=default&page=

Graham, I. W. (2010). The search for the discipline of nursing. *Journal of Nursing Management*, *18*(4), 355–362. doi:10.1111/j.1365-2834.2010.01104.x

Greene, M. T., & Puetzer, M. (2002). The value of mentoring: A strategic approach to retention and recruitment. *Journal of Nursing Care Quality*, *17*(1), 63–70.

Griffith, M. B. (2012). Effective succession planning in nursing: A review of the literature. *Journal of Nursing Management*, *20*(7), 900–911. doi:10.1111/j.1365-2834.2012.01418.x

Hamstra, M. R. W., Orehek, E., & Holleman, M. (2014). Subordinate regulatory mode and leader power: Interpersonal regulatory complementarity predicts task performance. *European Journal of Social Psychology*, *44*(1), 1–6. doi:10.1002/ejsp.1992

Harrison, L. (2012). Using agency-wide dashboards for data monitoring and data mining: The Solano County Health and Social Services Department. *Journal of Evidence Based Social Work*, *9*(1–2), 160–173. doi:10.1080/15433714.2012.636322

Havaei, F., Dahinten, V. S., & MacPhee, M. (2014). Psychological competence: The key to leader empowering behaviors. *Journal of Nursing Administration*, *44*(5), 276–283.

Hayes, E. F. (2005). Approaches to mentoring: How to mentor and be mentored. *Journal of the American Academy of Nurse Practitioners, 17*(11), 442–445. doi:10.1111/j.1745-7599.2005.00068.x

Heathfield, S. (2001, April 25). *360 degree feedback: The good, the bad and the ugly defines and examines multirater feedback.* Retrieved from http://human resources.about.com/library/weekly/aa042501b.htm

Heenan, M., DiEmanuele, M., Hayward-Murray, K., & Dadgar, L. (2012). Hospital on a page: Standardizing data presentation to drive quality improvement. *Healthcare Quality, 15*(1), 41–45.

Institute of Medicine. (1999). *To err is human: Building a safer health system.* Washington, DC: National Academies Press.

Institute of Medicine. (2001). *Crossing the quality chasm: A new health system for the 21st century.* Washington, DC: National Academies Press.

Institute of Medicine. (2004). *Keeping patients safe: Transforming the work environment of nurses.* Washington, DC: National Academies Press.

Institute of Medicine. (2011). *The future of nursing: Leading change, advancing health.* Washington, DC: National Academies Press.

Jackson, D., Hutchinson, M., Peters, K., Luck, L., & Saltman, D. (2013). Understanding avoidant leadership in health care: Findings from a secondary analysis of two qualitative studies. *Journal of Nursing Management, 21*(3), 572–580. doi:10.1111/j.1365-2834.2012.01395.x

Jenkins, P., & Welton, J. (2014). Measuring direct nursing cost per patient in the acute care setting. *Journal of Nursing Administration, 44*(5), 257–262.

Jobe, L. L. (2014). Generational differences in work ethic among 3 generations of registered nurses. *Journal of Nursing Administration, 44*(5), 303–308.

Johansson, B., Fogelberg-Dahm, M., & Wadensten, B. (2010). Evidence-based practice: The importance of education and leadership. *Journal of Nursing Management, 18*(1), 70–77. doi:10.1111/j.1365-2834.2009.01060.x

Jones, J. (2004). Career mentor. *Emergency Nursing, 12*(2), 34–35.

Kanaskie, M. L. (2006). Mentoring—a staff retention tool. *Critical Care Nursing Quality, 29*(3), 248–252.

Karsten, M. A. (2010). Coaching: An effective leadership intervention. *Nursing Clinics of North America, 45*(1), 39–48. doi:10.1016/j.cnur.2009.11.001

Kerfoot, K. M. (2009). What you permit, you promote. *Nursing Economics, 27*(4), 245–246, 250.

Kerfoot, K. M. (2010). Leaders, self-confidence, and hubris: What's the difference? *Nursing Economics, 28*(5), 349–351.

Leggat, S. G. (2013). Achieving organisational competence for clinical leadership: The role of high performance work systems. *Journal of Health Organization and Management, 27*(3), 312–329.

Leigh, J. (2014). Modelling suggests authentic leadership from managers influences structural empowerment, job satisfaction and self-rated performance among nurses. *Evidence Based Nursing, 17*(2), 55–56. doi:10.1136/eb-2013-101424

Letcher, D. C., & Nelson, M. L. (2014). Creating a culture of caring: A partnership bundle. *Journal of Nursing Administration, 44*(3), 175–186. doi:10.1097/nna.0000000000000047

Lewis, L. C. (2014). Charting a new course: Advancing the next generation of nursing-sensitive indicators. *Journal of Nursing Administration, 44*(5), 247–249.

Lievens, I., & Vlerick, P. (2014). Transformational leadership and safety performance among nurses: The mediating role of knowledge-related job characteristics. *Journal of Advanced Nursing, 70*(3), 651–661. doi:10.1111/jan.12229

Lynas, K. (2012). Leadership scheme to develop the careers of talented candidates. *Nursing Management, 18*(9), 34–36. doi:10.7748/nm2012.02.18.9.34.c8893

Major, K., Abderrahman, E. A., & Sweeney, J. I. (2013). "Crucial conversations" in the workplace: Offering nurses a framework for discussing—and resolving—incidents of lateral violence. *American Journal of Nursing, 113*(4), 66–70. doi:10.1097/01.NAJ.0000428750.94169.f3

Malloch, K. (2010). Innovation leadership: New perspectives for new work. *Nursing Clinics of North America, 45*(1), 1–9. doi:10.1016/j.cnur.2009.10.001

McKinley, M. G. (2004). Mentoring matters: Creating, connecting, empowering. *AACN Clinical Issues, 15*(2), 205–214.

McMillan, L. R., Parker, F., & Sport, A. (2014). Decisions, decisions! E-portfolio as an effective hiring assessment tool. *Nursing Management, 45*(4), 52–54. doi:10.1097/01.NUMA.0000444882.93063.a7

McSherry, R., Pearce, P., Grimwood, K., & McSherry, W. (2012). The pivotal role of nurse managers, leaders and educators in enabling excellence in nursing care. *Journal of Nursing Management, 20*(1), 7–19. doi:10.1111/j.1365-2834.2011.01349.x

Murphy, L. G. (2012). Authentic leadership: Becoming and remaining an authentic nurse leader. *Journal of Nursing Administration, 42*(11), 507–512. doi:10.1097/NNA.0b013e3182714460

Owens, K., & Patton, J. (2003). Take a chance on nursing mentorships: Enhance leadership with this win–win strategy. *Nursing Education Perspectives, 24*(4), 198–204.

Patrick, A., Laschinger, H. K., Wong, C., & Finegan, J. (2011). Developing and testing a new measure of staff nurse clinical leadership: The clinical leadership survey. *Journal of Nursing Management, 19*(4), 449–460. doi:10.1111/j.1365-2834.2011.01238.x

Patton, D., Fealy, G., McNamara, M., Casey, M., Connor, T. O., Doyle, L., & Quinlan, C. (2013). Individual-level outcomes from a national clinical leadership development programme. *Contemporary Nurse: A Journal for the Australian Nursing Profession, 45*(1), 56–63. doi:10.5172/conu.2013.45.1.56

Pines, E. W., Rauschhuber, M. L., Cook, J. D., Norgan, G. H., Canchosa, L., Richardson, C., & Jones, M. E. (2014). Enhancing resilience, empowerment, and conflict management among baccalaureate students: Outcomes of a pilot study. *Nurse Educator, 39*(2), 85–90. doi:10.1097/nne.0000000000000023

Polito, J. M. (2013). Effective communication during difficult conversations. *Neurodiagnostic Journal, 53*(2), 142–152.

Riley, W. (2009). High reliability and implications for nursing leaders. *Journal of Nursing Management, 17*(2), 238–246. doi:10.1111/j.1365-2834.2009.00971.x

Ronsten, B., Anderson, E., & Gustafsson, B. (2005). Confirming mentorship. *Journal of Nursing Management, 13*(4), 312–321.

Sommet, N., Darnon, C., Mugny, G., Quiamzade, A., Pulfrey, C., Dompnier, B., & Butera, F. (2014). Performance goals in conflictual social interactions: Towards the distinction between two modes of relational conflict regulation. *British Journal of Social Psychology, 53*(1), 134–153. doi:10.1111/bjso.12015

Stewart, D. W. (2006). Generational mentoring. *Journal of Continuing Education in Nursing, 37*(3), 113–120.

Swanson, M. L., & Stanton, M. P. (2013). Chief nursing officers' perceptions of the doctorate of nursing practice degree. *Nursing Forum*, *48*(1), 35–44. doi:10.1111/nuf.12003

Taylor, B., Parekh, V., Estrada, C., Schleyer, A., & Sharpe, B. (2014). Documenting quality improvement and patient safety efforts: The quality portfolio. A statement from the Academic Hospitalist Taskforce. *Journal of General Internal Medicine*, *29*(1), 214–218. doi:10.1007/s11606-013-2532-z

Thompson, R., Wolf, D. M., & Sabatine, J. M. (2012). Mentoring and coaching: A model guiding professional nurses to executive success. *Journal of Nursing Administration*, *42*(11), 536–541. doi:10.1097/NNA.0b013e31827144ea

Titzer, J. L., Shirey, M. R., & Hauck, S. (2014). A nurse manager succession planning model with associated empirical outcomes. *Journal of Nursing Administration*, *44*(1), 37–46. doi:10.1097/nna.0000000000000019

Tofade, T., Abate, M., & Fu, Y. (2014). Perceptions of a continuing professional development portfolio model to enhance the scholarship of teaching and learning. *Journal of Pharmacy Practice*, *27*(2), 131–137. doi:10.1177/0897190013505869

Weberg, D. (2012). Complexity leadership: A healthcare imperative. *Nursing Forum*, *47*(4), 268–277. doi:10.1111/j.1744-6198.2012.00276.x

Welton, J. M. (2014). Business intelligence and nursing administration. *Journal of Nursing Administration*, *44*(5), 245–246.

Wocial, L. D., Sego, K., Rager, C., Laubersheimer, S., & Everett, L. Q. (2014). Image is more than a uniform: The promise of assurance. *Journal of Nursing Administration*, *44*(5), 298–302.

Wolf, G., Finlayson, S., Hayden, M., Hoolahan, S., & Mazzoccoli, A. (2014). The developmental levels in achieving Magnet designation, part 1. *Journal of Nursing Administration*, *44*(3), 136–141. doi:10.1097/nna.0000000000000041

Wong, C. A., Spence Laschinger, H. K., & Cummings, G. G. (2010). Authentic leadership and nurses' voice behaviour and perceptions of care quality. *Journal of Nursing Management*, *18*(8), 889–900. doi:10.1111/j.1365-2834.2010.01113.x

Young, M. (2014). Constructive feedback and disciplinary action. Retrieved from http://www.americannursetoday.com/constructive-feedback-and-disciplinary-action/

CHAPTER 11

Information Management and Knowledge Development as Actions for Leaders

Donna Faye McHaney and Miriam Halimi

LEARNING OBJECTIVES

1. Identify strategies nurse leaders can use to create environments that promote data mining, data use, and data enrichment.
2. Match skills and knowledge that are requisite to data analytics.
3. Explore the integration and connectivity of data systems to transform quality, safe transitions of care at all points of service.

AONE KEY COMPETENCIES

I. Communication and relationship building
II. Knowledge of the healthcare environment
III. Leadership
IV. Professionalism
V. Business skills

AONE KEY COMPETENCIES DISCUSSED IN THIS CHAPTER

II. Knowledge of the healthcare environment
III. Leadership
IV. Professionalism
V. Business skills

II. Knowledge of the healthcare environment
  - Clinical practice knowledge
  - Patient care delivery models and work design knowledge
  - Healthcare economics knowledge
  - Healthcare policy knowledge
  - Understanding of governance
  - Understanding of evidence-based practice
  - Outcomes measurement
  - Knowledge of, and dedication to, patient safety
  - Understanding of utilization and case management

- Knowledge of quality improvement and metrics
- Knowledge of risk management

III. Leadership
- Foundational thinking skills
- Personal journey disciplines
- Ability to use systems thinking
- Succession planning
- Change management

IV. Professionalism
- Personal and professional accountability
- Career planning
- Ethics
- Evidence-based clinical and management practices
- Advocacy for the clinical enterprise and for nursing practice
- Active membership in professional organizations

V. Business skills
- Understanding of healthcare financing
- Human resource management and development
- Strategic management
- Marketing
- Information management and technology

FUTURE OF NURSING: FOUR KEY MESSAGES

1. Nurses should practice to the full extent of their education and training.
2. Nurses should achieve higher levels of education and training through an improved education system that promotes seamless academic progression.
3. Nurses should be full partners with physicians and other health professionals in redesigning health care in the United States.
4. Effective workforce planning and policy making require better data collection and information infrastructure.

Introduction

Leading and managing are essential expectations of all professional nurse leaders, and they are more important than ever in today's fast-evolving technological healthcare environment. Understanding new ways of thinking and looking for opportunities to integrate technology to enhance and improve patient outcomes is important for not only nurse leaders but also nurses in general. Nurse leaders need to be role models in the utilization of technology and engage their staff in making decisions about technology design and work flow.

Nurse leaders need to be intimately familiar with the impact of technology on clinicians, patients, and clinical outcomes. Nurse leaders should be connected with clinical informatics departments and leverage their skills and knowledge to promote the adoption of technology in their units and organizations. Leaders need to be champions and adopters of technology, be knowledgeable about the tools their personnel are expected to use, and have enough of an understanding of technology and associated processes to hold their staff and leadership teams accountable for using the technology as expected. One of the primary motivators for the adoption and appropriate use of healthcare information technology is to improve the quality of care, improve healthcare team communication by providing real-time access to patient information, and develop safeguards that decrease errors. This will be achieved only by making it easy to do the right thing within technology, limiting work-arounds, focusing on iterative optimization processes, and holding clinicians accountable for utilizing technology as intended. Although electronic health records (EHRs) need to be implemented to improve safety, provide a better operating platform for the future, and create a digital culture for healthcare organizations, it is important to understand that it is not the full solution to address health care's wide and pervasive issues (Morrison, 2011).

Information technology, such as EHRs, clinical decision support systems, e-prescribing, computerized physician order entry, picture archiving and communication systems, bar coding, patient interactive education systems, automated dispensing cabinets, radio frequency identification, patient portals, biomedical device integration, smart IV pump integration, and application interoperability, are becoming frequently used technologies on clinical units (MedPAC, 2004). **Table 11-1** defines each of these technologies and terms. Nurse leaders need to be familiar with them and work with informatics leaders to identify information technology (IT) priorities for the organization. Implementing an IT solution should be based on an organizational need and should address a current problem. It is important to keep in mind that technology alone does not solve a problem. Processes, people, and cultures must all be assessed and addressed simultaneously.

The following scenario illustrates why nurse leaders need to be knowledgeable about technology tools that their staff is expected to use:

> A new admission form is rolled out to a medical–surgical unit. The form is designed with hard stops next to the fields to ensure that all mandatory admission information is completed when a patient is admitted. You are notified that you have patients for which the required documentation was not completed on admission. You notice that there is no specific pattern when this is occurring, and the gaps in documentation are occurring across all shifts. Because you know the electronic admission form has the required stops, you can audit the electronic record by looking for the time the patient was admitted then checking to see if the form was completed. You notice that the form is in a saved status, not a signed status, so the documentation is not committed to the record. As a result, you follow up with the nurses who are selecting the wrong button, give them new instructions, and hold them accountable if the issue persists.

INFORMATICS

Informatics is the science and art of turning data into information (Hebda & Czar, 2013). It is focused on bridging the realms of clinical practice and information technology (Hunt, Sproat, & Kitzmiller, 2004). Healthcare organizations often employ individuals who are specialty trained in informatics, either through

TABLE 11-1	Examples and Definitions of Technologies Found in Clinical Environments
Type of Technology	**Definition**
Electronic health record (EHR)	An EHR is part of an automated order entry and patient tracking system that provides real-time access to patient data and creates a lifetime record or a continuous longitudinal record of a patient's care. EHR functionality varies based on vendor development.
Clinical decision support system	This type of system provides support to clinicians in real time with recommendations for treatments. Clinical decision support systems cover a variety of technologies, including alerts, drug interaction and drug allergy checking, and full clinical pathways and protocols. Clinical decision support systems can be part of order entry and documentation.
Computerized physician order entry	This system is an electronic template in which orders can be entered for patient care; medications; laboratory tests; procedures; consultations or referrals; admissions, discharges, or transfers; and diagnostic tests.
Picture archiving and communication system	This technology captures and integrates diagnostic and radiological images from various devices, including X-ray, MRI, and CT. Picture archiving and communication systems store images that can be viewed from within an EHR, clinical data repository, or other tools.
Bar coding	Bar code scanning can be used for many different purposes in health care. It is frequently used to match patients to their medication orders. It can also be used for breastmilk scanning (matching patients to the correct expressed milk), blood administration, and lab draws.
Patient interactive education system	This technology places emphasis on providing entertainment and education resources to the patient bedside via a TV, keyboard, and bed speaker. Interactive patient education systems are often integrated with EHRs. Future designs will expand these systems to work outside hospital environments and will be accessible from within patients' homes.
Automated dispensing cabinet	This technology is used to distribute medication doses. Some automated dispensing cabinets are more sophisticated than others. More complex systems are interfaced with patient medication lists and will not dispense medications that are not on a patient's list.
IV pump integration	This technology allows for integration between IV pumps and EHRs, thereby allowing for a more enhanced work flow in which clinicians can continue to focus on improving patient safety during the medication administration process.
Application interoperability	Application interoperability allows electronic communication among IT systems. Areas of focus for interoperability include standardization of content and messaging and development of security and privacy guardrails.

informatics certification or advanced degrees. Some have clinical backgrounds and others have nonclinical backgrounds. As mentioned earlier, nurse leaders should familiarize themselves with these individuals and roles within the organization.

Informatics department sizes vary based on the size of the organization and the amount of technology deployed throughout the organization. Leaders need to know when to leverage the knowledge and skills of members in the informatics department. Consider inviting them to a staff meeting, or meet with them one on one when your staff is not utilizing the technology as expected to gain an understanding of where breaks in clinical processes and technologies may intersect.

The term *informatics* has been applied to various disciplines (Hebda & Czar, 2013). Healthcare informatics is a broad multidisciplinary field with many different subspecialties, such as nursing informatics, clinical informatics, and medical informatics (Sewell & Thede, 2013). The definitions for each subspecialty vary slightly, but the overarching goal of healthcare informatics is for interdisciplinary data management that drives real-time data availability, creates and allows for utilization of lifetime patient records, and embeds evidence into electronic tools. These terms are now frequently used in health care because they are reflective of the multidisciplinary demand of managing information and implementing technology within healthcare environments (Hunt et al., 2004).

The American Medical Information Association (AMIA, 2015) defines clinical informatics as "the application of informatics and information technology to deliver healthcare services. It may also be referred to as applied clinical informatics and operational informatics" (para. 1). When informatics is used for healthcare delivery, the AMIA considers it to be essentially the same regardless of the professional group involved (dentist, pharmacist, physician, nurse, or other healthcare professional). Clinical informatics is concerned with information used in health care by clinicians (AMIA, 2015). Clinical informatics includes a wide range of topics ranging from clinical decision support to images (e.g., radiological, pathological, dermatological, ophthalmological, and other images); clinical documentation to provider order entry systems; and system design to system implementation and adoption issues (AMIA, 2015).

Nursing informatics is one example of a discipline-specific informatics practice within a broader category of health or clinical informatics. Nursing informatics has become well established since its recognition as a specialty for registered nurses (RNs) by the American Nurses Association (ANA, 2008) in 1992. The ANA (2008) definition of nursing informatics is a specialty that integrates nursing science, computer science, and information science to manage and communicate data, information, knowledge, and wisdom in nursing practice. Nursing informatics supports consumers, patients, nurses, and other providers in their decision making in all roles and settings (ANA, 2008). Nursing informatics has its own scope and standards of practice for informatics nurse specialists (who have a graduate degree in informatics or a related field) and informatics nurses (who have experience but are not educated at the graduate level) (ANA, 2008). An organization's informatics department may include both types of clinicians.

Clinical and Nursing Informatics Departments

Clinical or nursing informatics departments are hospital-based departments focused on supporting clinician adoption of information technology to improve patient outcomes and bridge the gap between clinical practice and the use of information technology. Generally, informatics departments are responsible for more than just the implementation and maintenance of electronic health records. Informatics departments focus on work flow and implementation of other technologies, such as IV pumps, cardiac monitors, vital signs devices, and medication dispensing devices.

There is no standard reporting structure for informatics departments. They may report to IT departments or nursing or quality divisions. It varies based on the size and complexity of an organization. Regardless, having a working relationship with this department is essential to support clinicians at the bedside and leverage the investment in the technologies deployed on their units. Nurse leaders are positioned to provide the bridge to patient-centered care, information, and technology.

Many types of individuals and positions exist in an informatics department. Names of specific positions may vary at each organization, but personnel should fulfill one of these roles:

- Chief medical informatics officer (CMIO): This healthcare executive is responsible for bridging the gap between the medical staff and IT departments and works to make sure the design and content of systems are aligned with clinical evidence. CMIOs are generally physicians with a background or interest in information technology.
- Chief nursing informatics officer (CNIO): This is a fairly new role that bridges nursing-specific needs with IT and focuses on both the tactical and strategic needs of an organization. The CNIO works closely with the chief nursing officer to align IT strategies with the overall nursing strategy.

The CMIO and CNIO are an influential team when they are aligned appropriately and partnered effectively. CMIOs often are very familiar with community practice and physician needs and have a strong comprehension of work flows and processes from outpatient to inpatient. CNIOs are more focused on clinician work flow and understand the operational needs of an organization. CNIOs have a unique understanding of IT needs from a different angle than physician colleagues and are focused on implementing and optimizing healthcare information technology. Not every organization has a CNIO. Organizations may instead use the title director of clinical or nursing informatics.

- Informatics nurse specialist: This individual has an advanced graduate education in nursing informatics or a related field and may hold an American Nurses Credentialing Center certification (Weaver, Lindsay, & Gitelman, 2012). This person is an advocate between nursing and IT, represents nursing in IT meetings, and translates clinical practice into functional IT designs.
- Clinical liaison or informatics nurse: This person is an RN that works in informatics. He or she has experience or interest in the area but no formal educational preparation (Hebda & Czar, 2013).
- Pharmacy informatics leader: This individual focuses on the subspecialty of informatics when it is applied directly to pharmaceutical care and is knowledgeable about both pharmacy practices and informatics. This person is concerned with pharmacy needs, medication requirements (ordering, administration, and pharmacy management), and IT.
- Application specialist: This nonclinician has a strong knowledge of technology and is an expert in computer programs and data interfaces. This individual may focus on working with clinicians on purely technical issues or addressing desktop and network issues.
- Physician (adoption) coach: This person can be either a clinical or nonclinical individual who has both clinical and technical knowledge that is

necessary to guide and support physicians through the implementation process and works toward full adoption and technology optimization.

- Training coordinator: This person is responsible for conducting training and development sessions for clinical and nonclinical staff on technology. The training approaches encompass classroom learning, computer-based training, job aids, and personal instruction that can be delivered on the unit, depending on what is appropriate for the technology being deployed.
- Process liaison: This person may or may not be in the informatics department but has the responsibility to align the work flow and practices with IT by developing future state processes, identifying gaps in the current state, and working with clinicians and informatics personnel to resolve any barriers to moving toward a future state.
- Project manager: This person is responsible for the planning and execution of an IT project, including developing project plans and facilitating project meetings.

TECHNOLOGY PORTFOLIO

Technology has become pervasive in all matters within the healthcare milieu. What was once a stand-alone technology, such as an IV pump or vital signs machine, is now viewed as a part of the technology portfolio and can be integrated directly within the EHR, eliminating the burden of manual entry while also improving real-time documentation. The explosion of technology and technology integration has fundamentally changed the job descriptions of unit personnel, such as unit secretaries, who used to transcribe orders from paper and enter them in electronic systems. Technology should not be perceived as a strategy to decrease nursing time per patient day; rather, it should be viewed as a way to support clinicians and their practice and improve the patient experience. As a nurse leader, you should be familiar with the documentation requirements of your clinical staff so you can monitor it appropriately and be informed when chart reviews need to be performed if there are concerns about a nurse's performance. Knowing how technology works is also necessary to monitor performance and hold nurses accountable for their actions.

Nurse leaders need to be familiar with both daily reports and reports that can be run on demand, such as daily census reports or ad hoc reports pertaining to a unit's medication scanning rate. Nurse leaders need to be aware of which reports they need to access, how to access them, and the report formats so they can manage and lead their units and ensure that quality measures are being met.

Nurse leaders cannot shy away from technology. In today's environment, understanding technology and how it works is a requirement for successful nurse leaders. Technology is not used only for clinical purposes; it is used to complete scheduling, payroll, annual capital requests, human resources functions, and mandatory education initiatives.

Nurse leaders need to be involved in the review of new IT functionality and have an awareness of the shift new technology can bring to current job roles. Problem solving clinical challenges and work flow needs should be unbundled and thought of in a new context of how information technology can support clinical practice and elevate the patients' and clinicians' experiences. The patient experience is also being impacted by technology. Patients are being prompted to use clinical portals and interactive patient education systems and are encouraged to communicate with providers via message centers and other electronic tools.

Importance of Systems Thinking and Healthcare Information Technology for Nurse Leaders

In healthcare organizations, nurse leaders need to look beyond their own unit, division, or department and evaluate the best approach to achieve outcomes. Inter-departmental and multidisciplinary considerations should also be evaluated. There is also the risk that if there is one change (big or small) in one area, there may be an unintended or unanticipated event in other parts of the system. In healthcare IT, the roles of clinicians are so integrated that what a nurse does in the EHR can directly impact a physician, and vice versa. Acknowledging this dynamic is a critical consideration for IT planning and design. Additionally, when devices are integrated with EHRs, there must be an understanding of how all the technologies work together to prevent unknown consequences. Systems thinking is an overall holistic approach to looking at how parts are interrelated and how systems work over time and within the context of larger systems. The big picture must be understood before individual parts are addressed.

Viewing the relationships among parts, rather than individual parts alone, drives us to think differently about issues. A perspective about the larger system is essential to make decisions that progress toward optimal outcomes (Sherman, 2014). One way to visualize this is to think of a tree. Only a small part of the whole tree is visible above ground. We cannot see the roots of a tree because they are buried underground, yet they exist and are an essential part of the tree. The same is true of organizations; much of what goes on in our world is hidden from view until we seek a deeper level of understanding about what is buried beneath the surface (Sherman, 2014).

Incorporating Systems Thinking into Your Practice

A strong nurse leader needs to see the whole picture and make connections between individual events and processes, even if they seem counterintuitive (Sherman, 2014). We can all become better systems thinkers by being inquisitive, becoming knowledgeable beyond our own discipline, and asking questions about the relationships among events (Sherman, 2014). Here are some examples of systems thinking in action:

> Example 1: Sally Smith is a surgical department nurse manager. In 2014, as an outcome of Meaningful Use, it was determined that the nurses on her unit would need to start enrolling patients in the clinical patient portal. She began to realize that nursing and physician documentation was not as accurate as it should be, and the downstream impact to secure the patients' trust and their ability to engage in their own care and continuity of care could be significant. Sally called a meeting with the informatics department and physician cochairs to plan a strategy to improve clinical documentation and brainstorm about improving processes.

> Example 2: Jessica Jones is the nurse leader for a critical care division. She has noticed an increase in mortality due to late diagnosis of sepsis. In reviewing the data, she sees that the correct tests and sepsis screenings are not being completed

on admission. She knows that early identification of sepsis is crucial to surviving sepsis. She contacts the CMIO and CNIO to investigate hard wiring these practices into the EHR and looks at the work flow from beginning to end.

Example 3: A hospital was looking to change the way nurses enter medical histories so they can be integrated directly with patients' problem lists. No longer would medical histories be stand-alone data elements; rather, nursing would enter patient histories as patients stated their problems. After the system was activated, it was discovered that the change impacted physician billing because the medical history collected by nursing was used by billers to generate additional charges. There was a direct impact on revenue capture that was not considered prior to the change.

Nursing Informatics and Shared Governance

Success in any organization requires active involvement from all parties. Shared governance is one strategy that has been proven effective in actively engaging staff. Nursing informatics can be represented in a multitude of ways within a shared governance structure. It can be included in practice or education councils, or it can be its own council. Appendix A in this chapter contains a sample charter for a hospital-based nursing informatics council. There is no single way to go about creating a shared approach to informatics, but it is important to ensure that clinical nurses at the bedside have an opportunity to engage in decisions related to technology and their practice.

Shared governance structures may vary across organizations, but the outcomes of all shared governance models are similarly focused on a collaboration between direct-care nurses and leadership, who both have a voice in the process and are included in decisions that directly impact clinicians whenever possible.

By leveraging shared governance structures, nurse leaders develop and build new nurse leaders. As this process unfolds, potential nurse leaders may be considered for emerging roles within the organization (Lorenzi & Riley, 2003).

Data Analytics to Support Change

The use of data analytics can support nurse leaders through change processes. Data analytics is the science of examining raw data to draw new conclusions about information that can be used to drive change. Clinical analytics software can be used to help aggregate real-time data from physicians and nurses and produce quality metric reports that drive practice changes. By refining clinical quality data analysis and providing healthcare providers with real-time data access, reimbursement can be improved by identifying and closing gaps in care.

ETHICAL, LEGAL, AND SECURITY ISSUES

As the healthcare information highway has expanded, ethical, legal, and security issues are of paramount concern. Ethical considerations encompass establishing acceptable parameters that maintain patient confidentiality within legal and regulatory strictures. Factors related to privacy, security, and confidentiality in managing patient data, information, and knowledge must be understood and upheld at all levels of clinical practice (ANA, 2008). This includes nurses' engagement in resolving ethical issues surrounding patients, colleagues, or systems, as evidenced in such activities as participating on ethics committees and understanding the use of internal review boards. Nurse leaders' involvement in resolving ethical, legal, and security issues requires participation on interdisciplinary teams.

Ethical, legal, and security issues go hand in hand with technology. These concepts have been top issues for IT departments and healthcare organizations for many years. Ethics is defined as a system of conduct or behavior (Security, 2004). Ethics means conforming to professional standards that are defined by an organization or group of individuals, such as in nursing. Security can be defined as being safe and free from danger. Terms related to security are privacy and confidentiality. Privacy is described as being that of control. Individuals should be able to determine how much personal information to share, and how much to allow others to access. The benefit of controlling information is to provide freedom from intrusion and protect the possible misuse of shared information (Romano, 1987). Confidentiality means being entrusted with information that is held secret or secure (Saxton, 2012). These concepts share a common relationship when discussing patient information.

Many legal issues can arise from using technology and should be addressed by organizations. The Health Insurance Portability and Accountability Act (HIPAA) of 1996 was originally designed to protect workers from losing their right to insurance coverage when they leave a job (portability) and to protect integrity, confidentiality, and availability of electronic health information (accountability). HIPAA has placed attention on the implications of computerized electronic records as they relate to patients' rights (Carns, 2002). The HIPAA privacy component gives patients access to and control over their medical data. Health plans, healthcare clearinghouses, and healthcare providers must obtain prospective approval from a patient before sharing protected health information.

As a result of the privacy act, security issues concerning electronic health information arose. Security provisions must be made that cover policies, procedures, physical safeguards, and technical aspects of the management of protected health information. Security rules ensure the confidentiality, integrity, and availability of electronically protected health information. Nursing management must be aware of the legal issues surrounding patient information and employees. The current version of HIPAA legislation represents a relatively flexible set of rules that anticipates future changes in technology that can be achieved by healthcare organizations (Carns, 2002).

EVIDENCE-BASED CLINICAL AND MANAGEMENT PRACTICE

Evidence-based practice tools provide a convenient way to present vast, complex data about outcomes, efficiency, effectiveness, patient preferences, policies, and sometimes cost (Saba & McCormick, 2011). Examples of evidence-based practice tools include physician order sets and nursing care plans that are developed based on evidence-based practice content. Informatics nurses and informatics nurse specialists support evidence-based practice and clinical practice in the following ways:

- Using the appropriate evidence-based assessment techniques and instruments in collecting pertinent data to define the issue or problem (ANA, 2008)
- Synthesizing data, information, theoretical frameworks, and evidence when providing a consultation (ANA, 2008)

- Synthesizing empirical evidence on risk behaviors, theories, and frameworks when designing health information and patient education materials (ANA, 2008)
- Utilizing specific evidence-based actions and steps that are specific to the problem or issues to achieve defined outcomes (ANA, 2008)
- Evaluating the current practice environment and comparing it to existing evidence in identifying opportunities for the generation and use of data for research or to modify current practice to align with evidence (ANA, 2008)
- Identifying expected outcomes that include scientific evidence and are achievable through the implementation of evidence-based practices (ANA, 2008)
- Developing clinical practice guidelines and integrating them into practice, information technology, informatics solutions, and clinical nurses' knowledge bases (ANA, 2008)

Evidence should drive the need to use data (both external and internal) to inform decision making. Then, using the data to develop new knowledge, a culture should be created to mobilize information, knowledge, and wisdom, thereby fostering an environment in which nurses understand data and how to use the data to enhance patient care and inform their own practice.

Clinical information systems, such as an EHR, support evidence-based practice by providing the technology platform on which to integrate knowledge and garner data from data warehouses to create new evidence-based practice. The interdependence of technology and evidence-based practice is blatantly evident today in many EHRs (Ball et al., 2011). Examples of evidence-based practice in technology include the use of clinical decision support embedded in care plans and the development of clinical practice guidelines in technology, clinical documentation, and order sets. Evidence integration in EHRs makes it easy for clinicians to be guided by the evidence to support their practice and be most effective in supporting advancement in both technology and evidence-based practice adoption.

ADVOCACY FOR THE CLINICAL ENTERPRISE AND FOR NURSING PRACTICE

Nurses are one of the largest groups of clinicians that use information technology, and they have the greatest need for high-value technology to support clinical work flow. Nurses often say they spend too much time with technology or the computer and not enough time with their patients. As nurse leaders, it is essential to plan ahead to ensure that the deployed technologies are supporting the nursing work flow and nursing practice and are also adding value to the nurse–patient experience. Technology considerations and planning should be integrated into the nursing strategic plan.

Nurse leaders should explore device integration and connectivity of data systems to transform quality, safe transitions of care at all points of service and be active participants in these initiatives. Technology should support new models of care that allow nurses to practice to the fullest extent of their education and training. Transitioning nursing practice to the future requires data, data analytics, mobilizing data to support nursing research, and embedding evidence-based practice within technologies to make it easy for clinicians to access and follow it.

ACTIVE MEMBERSHIP IN PROFESSIONAL ORGANIZATIONS

It is important to stay connected to what is taking place in healthcare information technology. The field is changing rapidly, with new technologies emerging and current technologies evolving. With technology becoming an integral component of how nurses work, how patients engage in their own care, and how outcomes are measured, nurse leaders need to be knowledgeable of what is taking place. Examples of informatics-related organizations include the following:

- Healthcare Information and Management Systems Society (HIMSS): www .himss.org
- American Nursing Informatics Association (ANIA): www.ania.org
- Alliance for Nursing Informatics (ANI): www.allianceni.org

INFORMATION MANAGEMENT AND TECHNOLOGY

Healthcare informatics involves the application of computer and information science in all basic and biomedical sciences in broad terms. Medical informatics refers to the application of informatics to all healthcare disciplines and to the practice of medicine (Hebda & Czar, 2013). Nursing informatics is the use of information and computer technology to support all aspects of nursing practice. This may include direct delivery of care, education, research, and management. Nursing informatics facilitates the integration of data, information, and knowledge to support patients, nurses, and other providers involved in the decision-making process (Hebda & Czar, 2013).

Managers need to collaborate with the information systems (IS) department in the design, development, and implementation of management and clinical applications. Nurses in informatics roles act as liaisons among management, staff, and the IS department. Although nurse informatics personnel may be removed from bedside care, they remain focused on patient care while working toward improved clinical outcomes and quality care. These nurses can communicate how tasks are completed each day, providing an understanding of the work flow for IS staff. Often nurse leaders fill this role and work on projects within the organization. Nurse leaders may also become involved in many aspects of project management when an organization is considering the development and implementation of clinical systems. The informatics nurse may fill a variety of roles.

Data Management in Nursing

One of the core tenets of nursing informatics involves the concepts and relationships of data, information, knowledge, and wisdom. In the mid-1980s, Blum (1986) introduced the first three of these as a framework for understanding clinical information systems and their impact on health care (McGonigle & Mastrian, 2012). In 1989, Graves and Corcoran built on this work and defined the following concepts:

- Data: Discrete entities described objectively without interpretation (McGonigle & Mastrian, 2012)
- Information: Data that are interpreted, organized, and structured (McGonigle & Mastrian, 2012)

- Knowledge: Information that is synthesized so that relationships are identified and formalized (McGonigle & Mastrian, 2012)

In 2002, Nelson elaborated on these concepts and added a fourth concept, wisdom, as the appropriate application of knowledge to the management and solution of the human problem (McGonigle & Mastrian, 2012). Wisdom focuses on knowing when and how to apply knowledge to deal with a complex problem or specific human need (McGonigle & Mastrian, 2012).

Nurses and nursing management handle large amounts of data and information during any given day. Nurses are knowledge workers; they deal with information and generate information and knowledge as a product. Data are a collection of numbers, characters, or facts. These are usually gathered because they are needed for analysis or some other action at a later time. Information is a set of data that has been interpreted over a specific period of time, such as over the course of a day.

Knowledge can be defined as applying facts or ideas acquired by study, investigation, observation, or experience (Knowledge, n.d.). It is the synthesis of information that may have been derived from several sources, producing a concept or idea. Nurses acquire knowledge over time and use it extensively in their daily task of direct patient care. Data collection, with the aid of computer and information technology, helps to provide evidence of best practices supported by research. This collection of evidence-based information provides a substantial database of knowledge that can be applied to everyday practice situations.

How do these concepts relate to clinical practice? Consider this example:

> Henry F. is an RN who works on a busy surgical unit. He just admitted a 50-year-old from the operating room postappendectomy surgery. Upon admission, Henry completes a head-to-toe assessment, including an assessment of the surgical site. He discovers that the patient has an elevated temperature, elevated pain score, decreased pulse oximetry reading, and increased drainage from the surgical site. Henry places the patient on oxygen, delivers a dose of pain medication, and notifies the physician of potential risk for infection.

Henry used immediate data and information gathered during his assessment and provided the appropriate care to the patient. Henry also used technology to assist with care. He had knowledge of the signs and symptoms of infection, and he acted with transparent wisdom to provide care to his patient.

Data Integrity

It is not enough to collect data, interpret data, and build a database of knowledge. Data that make up the database must be maintained with optimal assurance that good-quality data exist. Data integrity is critical in the clinical environment because data serve as a driving force in treatment decision making (Hebda & Czar, 2013). Data integrity is the wholeness and accuracy of data when information is collected, stored, and retrieved by an authorized user (Hebda & Czar, 2013). If the quality of data is flawed or incorrect, the treatment outcomes will be flawed, thereby creating the potential for error and patient harm.

Data integrity errors can be introduced to EHRs in several ways: (1) collecting information but not documenting all the information (a nurse collects all medications from a patient but does not enter all of them); (2) entering incorrect information (selects the wrong dose of a home medication); (3) entering the correct information into the wrong data field (enters a weight in pounds instead of kilograms in a kilogram field); or (4) entering data in the correct field but transposing data into an incorrect field (enters systolic and diastolic information correctly, but it is transposed on the summary pages in the EHR).

Nurse leaders need to ensure that both clinical and nonclinical personnel on their units are trained accurately and are proficient at entering information into the EHR correctly. Clinical informatics departments can be leveraged to support this type of training. All staff should attend classes that emphasize appropriate system access, the use of input devices, potential harmful effects associated with incorrect data, data verification techniques, and error correction (Hebda & Czar, 2013).

Data Mining

Technology has enabled rapid advances in data capture and storage, resulting in large collections of data. These data are stored internally in relational databases, which consist of rows and columns of data. Relational databases provide an easy method for data storage, retrieval, and analysis.

The traditional method of analyzing data manually is no longer feasible. Extracting data from databases is known as data mining. Data mining is the process of using software to sort through data to discover patterns and determine or establish relationships (McGonigle & Mastrian, 2012). This process may help to discover previously unidentified relationships among data in a database, with a focus on applications (McGonigle & Mastrian, 2012). Data mining is a knowledge management function that engages software to uncover interrelationships within large data sets (Hebda & Czar, 2013). It uses multiple tools (artificial intelligence, statistical computation, and computerization) to drill down through large data sets to identify potential interrelationships (Hebda & Czar, 2013). In health care, data mining is used to do research, identify causal relationships among treatments and outcomes, track performance, chart quality improvement, and determine clinical system usage. Data mining provides trended patterns that can then be transformed into useful data (Hebda & Czar, 2013). It is used often in the healthcare environment because clinical databases hold huge amounts of information about patients and their medical conditions.

The process of data mining has become known as knowledge discovery and data mining (KDD) or data to knowledge (Hunt et al., 2004). Data to knowledge usually begins by answering questions that are being asked. Assessing the question gives managers and others an advantage toward filtering through numerous large databases. Without a clear objective of what is being asked or needed, data overload may occur instead of gaining knowledge. After the data are gathered, they must be prepared for mining by selecting and formatting the data for use. Clinical data must be defined appropriately to identify like items. For example, "CABG" and "coronary artery bypass graft" must be identified as the same thing.

KDD can be defined as the development of skills, understandings, and integrative abilities derived from data (Hebda & Czar, 2013). Knowledge discovery is pivotal in looking at data from different perspectives and shedding new light on the data set. Data mining is a powerful tool in the knowledge discovery process that can be done with a number of software packages (Saba & McCormick, 2011). Essentially, data mining is the process of finding new correlations or patterns among data (McGonigle & Mastrian, 2012).

Data mining processes may begin after the formatting has been completed by evaluating and analyzing trends and predictive attributes. Identified trends can then be interpreted and used within nursing environments. For data mining to be successful, nurse leaders and staff nurses must be proficient at understanding current issues in managing data. Nurse leaders, especially, should be aware of techniques, like data mining, that allow them to extract, predict, evaluate, and apply knowledge to daily tasks. Data mining should be used to improve efficiency and quality to improve care delivery practices and patient outcomes. Through data mining and knowledge discovery, new healthcare policies and care practices can be developed, and syndrome surveillance and detection of disease outbreaks can occur. Nurse leaders should identify what data they need to advance their organization and support future nursing research studies.

Data Cleansing and Enrichment

Data cleansing is used to clean up erroneous data that have been captured and stored in databases. Data cleansing software flags the erroneous data and generates a report. After the report is reviewed, the files or records that have been flagged may be deleted or corrected. This process should be conducted on a routine basis to keep electronic records free from errors.

Data enrichment is the process of enriching data to refine and enhance information. It is intended to make sure the data contains necessary information to get more out of it, do more with it, easily access it, and be more proactive. It ensures that the correct individuals are using valid assessment methodologies to cover the essential areas of integrity, accuracy, consistency, and completeness of data sets for clinical documentation.

Meaningful Uses for Data

An abundant amount of information is collected in health care. Administrative data, medical data, and patient information, both personal and care related, are collected. Administrative data may concern employee benefits, staffing schedules, and anything related to the overall business aspects of health care. Medical information may include information related to pharmacy inventory, supply inventory, encounters in the hospital, medical information, medications given, treatment ordered, results of tests, and other information related to clinical care. Patient information includes not only personal information but also information related to each hospital encounter that individuals may have during their life span at the facility. Nurse leaders may handle a variety of data that fall into each of these categories.

When large amounts of data are collected and handled, meaningful uses for the data must be found that will enhance the quality of care for individuals currently and in the future. Using the data efficiently is a challenge for the healthcare industry, and recognizing meaningful uses may be difficult. This may be due to limitations that facilities impose on nurse leaders or the organization's lack of awareness about products that can be used to manipulate data. Meaningful uses of data may include evaluating trends for specific patient treatment options and outcomes, tracking encounters for an individual, monitoring medication errors, identifying trends in patient lengths of stays, and much more.

Training administrators to recognize meaningful uses for data should begin early in their educational careers. It is important for nurses to understand that data are a vital part of research that provide a resource for evidence-based practice in health care today. Nurse leaders should recognize that they can play a vital role in promoting practice changes that will create dynamic environments that integrate evidence-based information to promote optimal outcomes.

Nurse leaders need to remain vigilant about how nurses document and enter information into EHRs. Data are becoming transparent to all disciplines, with the ability to access technology remotely and through patient portals. Nurse leaders must ensure that the correct information is being entered in a timely manner. Data that is entered discretely can be mined for reports and monitoring. Nurse leaders should leverage data to monitor improvements in core measures and organizational initiatives and for use during daily patient care. Data sets can be trended, such as blood pressure and blood sugar, to look at care over time. Nurses use information technology to enter data, generate information, and create knowledge and wisdom that supports their nursing practice.

Computer Networking

Networks are the infrastructure of today's electronic world and are used to transfer information from one location to another. Networks can be made up of any computer devices that are attached, providing a conduit for information to be passed. There are two main types of computer networks: local-area networks (LANs) and wide-area networks (WANs). All computers on a LAN are local, meaning they all exist in a common geographical location and have a common owner. A WAN is two or more computers that are remote, meaning they are located over a large geographical distance and are connected by leased telecommunications equipment. LANs and WANs have largely given way to intranets and extranets, discussed in the next section.

Designing networks is a crucial part of the design, development, and implementation of any healthcare information system. The organization's size and willingness to spend money must be considered. Unfortunately, many organizations spend less money and end up with less than desirable systems.

Networks require management from the time the process starts to the planning and design phase, and network management is an ongoing process. Information systems department staff may be involved in the management process, especially when troubleshooting network problems. Routine monitoring to evaluate capacity and performance should be done. A network administrator manages the server and users. Server administration includes the maintenance of daily backups and any shared resources. The management of users includes maintenance of user identification and passwords and security-related issues among users.

When considering networks and the design of systems, organizations should take into account budget and spending expenses, growth of the company and future needs, the healthcare information systems to be implemented, the number of employees using the system, and the amount of data to be stored, retrieved, and transferred, among other things. One of the most important things is to plan for the future. Nursing administrators and managers should become involved in planning, designing, developing, implementing, and evaluating networks that will be used by nurses.

Intranets, Extranets, and Virtual Private Networks

Examples of networks include intranets, extranets, and virtual private networks (VPNs). Each of these types of networks is widely used today by many organizations. These networks use Internet and World Wide Web technologies for information transfer and distribution.

Intranets are used by organizations for internal use and employ a variety of communication technologies. Intranets usually are not geographically limited but do have a common owner. Employees generally have access to intranets for organizational information and applications that are easily accessible with web browsers. Portals into the site are developed and maintained, providing centralized access to employees. Because information can be kept more current and accurate, organizations use this type of network to aid in reducing errors and improving the quality of health care.

Extranets extend beyond intranets and an organization's information by providing access to anywhere in the world. They generally use multiple types of communication technologies and are not geographically limited. Extranets are used to connect parties that have common interests. With extranets, the staff has access to information from almost anywhere, including patients' homes or their own homes, and while they are at conferences or even on vacation. Nurse leaders can access information for evaluating staffing conditions and monitoring staff ratios and patient care. Those outside the organization may also have access through some portal or gateway that allows them to provide or obtain information.

VPNs are private networks that provide stronger security with flexible remote access. Well-designed VPNs are secure, reliable, and easy to administer. Organizations may need to purchase and install software so users can connect to the organization's intranet. This software interacts with software on the organization's intranet to manage authentication and encryption (Parsons & Oja, 2014).

Wireless Networking

Wireless networking has rapidly become the norm for most computer users. Wireless access points are available in many academic areas, shopping malls, coffee shops, and neighborhoods. In some locations, entire cities are connected with a network.

Wireless technology is suited for healthcare environments in which providers are mobile and depend on current data that are generated and captured continuously during daily tasks and activities. Many of today's technologies are wireless. Handheld wireless devices continuously download data, including laboratory, pharmacy, and radiographic data, saving many hours of searching time. Bedside infusion pumps, blood glucose machines, blood pressure machines, ultrasound machines, EEG and ECG machines, and other equipment can store and download information into electronic records, saving valuable time in patient care.

Technology is rapidly changing, as are other technologies, such as radio frequency identification tags, monitoring devices to locate staff, and voice-over technology. As wireless capabilities increase, technology will continue to enhance the way nurses perform tasks and provide high-quality care at the bedside.

Internet

The largest wide-area global network is the Internet. It offers the ability to connect and communicate with any computer. When connected, the user can function on the Internet with simple point-and-click techniques, creating an interactive environment. The Internet has allowed the healthcare industry to reinvent the way medicine and health care are delivered. This transformation has great potential to provide healthcare access to many individuals who once had none.

Patients have access to vast amounts of information that provides education related to their diagnosis and care. However, patients should be warned to be cautious of information found on the Internet. Systematic evaluations of medical content on the Web have found it to be inconsistent or at a reading level too high for average consumers. There are several key points to remember when searching for information on the Internet:

- The reading level of material found on the Internet may be too high for average consumers to understand.
- Medical information may be inaccurate or inconsistent.
- Medical information can come from reputable practitioners, other providers, drug companies, practitioners who want to sell products, or other groups.
- It is crucial to evaluate the credentials of the content providers to determine their qualifications and whether the information on the site might be biased (Hanson, 2006).

More and more physicians' offices, hospitals, clinics, and other healthcare provider organizations are creating websites that patients can access for information about various diseases and treatment options that is current and accurate. Many nurses have begun to work in areas such as creating and maintaining websites, consulting over the Internet, and reviewing cases, and some nurse practitioners are even providing care across the Internet via telemedicine.

As healthcare organizations continue to transition into the electronic world, many changes are occurring. The American Recovery and Reinvestment Act mandated electronic medical records for all patients by 2014. However, many organizations continue working toward this goal. Data can be captured and stored, providing access to information that is readily available. As this movement continues, patients will be able to access their electronic records, complete medical forms before admissions or appointments, list their medications and allergies themselves, fill out their medical history, and provide insurance information and select payment options. Self-scheduling is beginning to be used, and patients will soon have the opportunity to schedule appointments as needed over the Internet.

Patients are already being assessed, diagnosed, and treated via the Internet, and as telemedicine continues to grow this effort will continue to expand. Opportunities for consultations, primary visits, and research are growing as the expansion of health care to the Internet grows. Capturing data in real-time or point-of-care environments creates large databases of information for research, providing evidence-based data that can be translated into practice fairly quickly. Video conferencing is being used to consult with colleagues concerning diagnoses and treatments. Available resources are being used to improve the clinical decision-making process.

The Internet has changed the way education is provided to nurses, patients, and students and has become the ideal vehicle for multimedia instruction and education on demand. Continuing education and higher education for nurses are available online, providing convenient times for learning. Continuing education programs are available over the Internet, and many organizations use the Internet for yearly education requirements and updating skills information. Even policies and procedures are found on organizations' intranets today. Higher-education programs can be found online, and many institutions are using technology to enhance traditional classrooms. There are many programs that are offered completely online. These programs provide classroom environments on demand and offer convenient education for individuals who need flexibility.

The Internet has changed the way healthcare organizations are doing business. Many aspects of business involve electronic transfer of information between parties. Healthcare organizations market their products, services, and facilities and recruit employees and patients via the Internet. Current employees can access their personnel records and communicate with others through email over the Internet.

Privacy and security are concerns when using the Internet. As Internet and technology use increase and change, privacy and security issues will continue to be a concern. HIPAA addressed many issues related to privacy and security. However, the ever-increasing demand for technology implementation in health care will create new issues.

Healthcare Information Systems

There are several types of healthcare information systems. Some of these systems help to manage the daily operations of general healthcare organizations, and others are classified as hospital information systems. For the purposes of this text, hospital information systems are discussed.

Hospital information systems consist of two types: administrative information systems and clinical information systems. Each of these systems plays a major role in the operations of organizations that provide health care to consumers, such as hospitals. As the demand for automation and data management increases in nursing, nurses will become more involved with evaluating, selecting, designing, and implementing information systems. They are becoming the norm for clinical areas and have been used in administrative activities for years.

Hospital Information Systems

Hospital information systems are large, complex computer systems designed to help manage the information needs of a hospital. Hospital information systems are tools that can be used interdepartmentally or intradepartmentally. These large systems are composed of smaller systems that are used for the daily operations of a hospital.

Implementing Hospital Information Systems

Nurse leaders have become more and more involved in implementing hospital information systems, both in administrative and clinical areas. Implementing information systems requires more than just installing and using the systems. A project management plan should be devised by the nurse leader, along with a project team that incorporates input for the selection, design and development, implementation, and evaluation of the information system being considered.

Nurse leaders should work closely with the IS department or the nursing informatics nurse to obtain an optimal system that will enhance the delivery of health care.

Systems

Several processes must be completed when an organization has committed to implementing technologies. Nurse leaders and other appointed or volunteer staff nurses, along with multidisciplinary team members, should determine the needs of the unit, department, or division within the organization. First, a thorough assessment should be conducted that involves looking at the current system for capturing and analyzing data for care delivery. Determining the weaknesses and strengths of the current system provides insight into what works and does not work for daily operations. The needs of the organization are determined during the assessment phase. Nurse leaders should evaluate what is currently needed and what will be needed in the future.

Second, nurse leaders, along with IS staff and administrative personnel, should evaluate and select a hospital information system that meets the needs. Several information systems should be evaluated for the closest fit to the organization's budgetary guidelines, goals, and needs.

Third, the implementation phase begins after the selection has been made. This phase involves intensive training of employees, both administrative and clinical, over some period of time. Timelines need to be developed for completing training, installing equipment and software, and testing the new system. After training and installation have been completed, the systems are brought online for use. Multiple support personnel should be available the day the system is started to help with problems that may arise or to guide employees through the process of computerized daily tasks.

Finally, the systems should be evaluated. Mechanisms should be developed during the planning phases that provide methods for support and evaluation of the system. These methods may include, but are not limited to, a call-in help desk, support technicians who are available on demand as questions and problems arise, request for help forms that can be submitted online, and suggestion boxes.

Administrative Information Systems

Administrative information systems include a wide variety of systems that work to maintain information used in the daily operations of an organization. These include financial systems, human resource systems, nonclinical patient systems such as registration and scheduling systems, and even nursing administrative systems that nurse leaders use.

Information systems that are classified as administrative systems involve any operation that is not directly linked to hands-on patient care. Operations may include nonclinical patient activities, medical records activities, business and accounting activities, and some nursing management tasks. Nonclinical patient activities may involve such tasks as patient scheduling, admissions, discharges, transfers, census functions, bed assignments, and other nonclinical activities associated with the patient. Medical records procedures include master patient index functions, abstracting (diagnosis–procedure and coding), transcription, and correspondence. Business and accounting functions may include patient insurance verification, billing, accounts payable, accounts receivable, cash processing, maintenance activities, and other business operations. Nursing management tasks may involve budget projections, employee records (annual skills and educational updates, evaluations, staffing), and other management activities required for daily operations by nurse leaders.

Clinical Information Systems

Clinical information systems involve any system that is used in patient care. However, these systems are generally associated with the nursing information system in hospitals, such as a laboratory or medication administration system. Each of the systems provides support to the care of patients. They may be general support systems or designated for a specific nursing area. Many nursing areas benefit from unique information systems. Some of these areas include surgery, infection control, labor and delivery, enterostomal therapy, oncology, mental health, orthopedics, neonatology, and intensive care. Clinical information systems can be used to improve the quality of care while enhancing the environment and reducing cost in the long term.

Many clinical information systems are designed in modular form, providing flexibility to the organization. General nursing information systems have multiple programs comprising a module that is used to perform various clinical tasks, education, and management functions. The modules may vary among vendors and software developers, but they may include medical history, patient assessment documentation, nursing care plans, medication administration, dietary information, patient education, ongoing daily care, vital signs and graphic sheet information, reports, nursing progress notes, discharge planning, and other tasks that nurses perform on a daily basis.

Clinical nurses can use clinical information systems to provide high-quality patient care. These systems provide a mechanism for capturing data that can be used to formulate treatment plans and evaluate trends. Technology, along with clinical information systems, continues to change the work environment and improve the quality of work environments for nurses.

General Applications Software for Nurse Leaders

General applications software includes communications, database management, word processing and desktop publishing, spreadsheets, personal information managers, graphics programs, and other software programs nurse leaders may need on a daily basis. Nurses use computers to perform many aspects of their daily jobs in areas such as budgeting, documentation, policy and procedures, research, inventory, scheduling, patient and staff education, maintaining personnel records, and other tasks. Because of this, nurse leaders should be prepared to encourage and support the increased use of technology in clinical and nonclinical areas of nursing. Fundamental concepts related to computers and the use of applications software are important to nurse managers and other nurses. Computer literacy is critical and will be required more and more as computers continue to be a tool of the profession.

Communications Software

Communications software provides a link for access between computers. Links may be dedicated or not dedicated. Dedicated links remain open even when not in use. Nondedicated links are open only when they are being used. Organizations tend to use dedicated links to have direct access to the organization's information resources typically through a LAN connection. Small business or home environments tend to use nondedicated links and access information only when needed. However, dedicated links have become the norm with integrated services digital network and digital subscriber lines.

Nurse leaders are not normally involved in communications software selection and installation, but they may be involved in policy development for the use of electronic communication software. Communications software to support LANs is generally taken for granted and is provided as part of the operating system that comes installed on the equipment. At work, most employees have a dedicated connection, and at home, they can dial in or connect through a portal to the remote access server and perform as if they are at work.

Database Management

Computer databases are much like filing cabinets, but they are electronic, and they include files and contents. Databases are used to store data and can be manipulated to view information based on query options. Database management systems virtually take the place of a filing cabinet to handle many informational and record-keeping needs.

Typically, relational tables are used in databases. These tables contain rows and columns in which data can be stored that relate to each other. A table is a collection of records in which one row is a record. The rows and columns consist of cells, and the cells are given data field names. Data fields are defined with the length and type of data that will be placed in the field. The fields are defined in a table definition. A database may consist of several relational tables from which data can be pulled to form reports. Reports may be printed or displayed on a computer screen for review. This process of storing and retrieving data provides ease of information management, the timely retrieval of information, and concurrent access to information by individuals at different locations.

Word Processing and Desktop Publishing

Word processing software is used to produce documents such as memos, letters, signs, books, and résumés. Desktop publishing software generally incorporates graphics into the text and is used for newsletters, posters and signs, books, and other documents that require graphics. Today, both types of software have incorporated aspects of each other, enabling a variety of documents to be produced from either type.

Spreadsheets

Spreadsheets are computer software applications that can be used to manipulate data. They contain multiple cells and rows that make up a grid. The cells may contain alphanumeric text, numeric values, or formulas that define the contents of the cell. Calculations can be performed, graphs can be produced, and statistical abilities are built in to most spreadsheets. An entire spreadsheet can automatically be recalculated after a single cell is changed. Spreadsheets can contain large numbers of rows and columns, which eases the process of organizing data. Spreadsheets are often used for creating budgets and handling large amounts of data.

Nurse leaders can use spreadsheets for developing budgets, maintaining staff records, calculating and tracking, and creating graphs pertaining to staffing and patient data. Items can be imported from and exported to other software applications.

Nursing Management Applications

Nursing management must be prepared for technology that is being implemented in administrative and clinical areas. Many applications are available for nursing management that can aid in daily tasks. Computer applications for nursing administration may include patient classification systems, acuity systems, staffing and scheduling systems, unit activity reports, utilization review, census, error reports, drug and allergy reactions, incident reports, shift summary reports, budgeting and payroll, and other systems. Nurse executives may also use application software for forecasting and planning, hospital expansion, regulatory reporting, risk pooling, surveys, preventive maintenance, and financial planning.

Today's nurse leaders have moved into the role of executive officer with obligations to report to the institution, to society, and to national accrediting agencies. **Box 11-1** details best ways to address the nurse managers' application of best informatics practices. These responsibilities and others come with the professional practice of nursing. Nurse leaders need more than a basic understanding of email and word processing; they need to have sufficient knowledge about computer technology to help improve health care and lower costs by better managing nursing information (McGonigle & Mastrian, 2012).

The applications for nursing management include a variety of options, such as calendar of events, general application software (discussed earlier in this chapter), and human resource information systems that support nursing management tasks. Calendars are useful for scheduling meetings, conferences, and educational events. Many nurse leaders use an Internet browser-based application that is available

---

BOX 11-1   Seven Tips for Managing Information and Technology

1. Create a vision for the future that fits within the organizational mission and strategic plan.
2. Learn whatever is needed so you can fulfill the vision.
3. Join initiatives that are advancing in the direction of your vision.
4. Embrace new technology; be prepared to initiate, implement, and support the technology.
5. Use automated dispensing and bar coding systems or technologies.
6. Get exposure to biometric technology.
7. Never stop educating yourself.

on the organization's intranet. The advantage to using an Internet browser-based application is that employees and managers can schedule appointments and events, such as educational opportunities, to add their names to the class role, and automatic notifications can be sent to nursing management.

Although most human resources applications support activities required for human resources departments, nurse leaders find themselves in situations when these data are most helpful. The management of human resources is a huge task for most organizations, requiring significant time and personnel. These applications can be very informative and supportive to nurse managers. Reports can be obtained that supply information such as the number of individuals who apply for available positions, the number of employees broken down by rank, what educational programs have been completed, retention and turnover rates, staff credentials and special skills, time and attendance, and much more.

With appropriate integration of the overall hospital information systems, these data can be exported and imported into other hospital information systems, nursing information systems, and other general application software.

SECURING HEALTHCARE INFORMATION

The level of an organization's commitment to security is largely driven by the sensitivity of information and repercussions for data compromise. Data security cannot be overemphasized. With the complexity of health care today, it is imperative to understand that data security management in a hospital environment is complex for many reasons, some of which are as follows:

- Need to categorize data for administrative or clinical purposes
- Diverse users, including doctors, nurses, technicians, administrators, and so forth
- Various user skill levels with regard to computer use
- Inherent complexity of communication and interaction among departments
- Stringent privacy regulations in the healthcare industry
- Rapidly changing technology

The meaningful planning, implementation, and management of data security require that key players clearly understand fundamental concepts in information systems security and their roles in helping protect critical data and information. Nurse leaders play a significant role at various levels within the hospital organization and should be involved in actively seeking ways to secure data and information. Such involvement is effective only if leaders are well informed in several aspects of information security. When nursing leaders understand the rudiments of information security, they are less likely to become intimidated and will therefore embrace their roles in effectively planning, implementing, and managing security.

Serious security concerns face organizations that use information, including hospitals and other healthcare agencies. Data that are in storage, being processed, or in transmission can be severely compromised, and organizations should take steps to ensure information security.

Ensuring that operations and processes are in place to protect and defend information and information systems by ensuring their availability, integrity, authentication, confidentiality, and nonrepudiation is vital to maintaining intact data handling. Operational processes include data restoration by incorporating protection, detection, and reaction capabilities.

Security Breaches and Attacks

Security breaches are many and varied. Whenever the issue of information breaches comes up, it is not unusual for an organization's insiders to be looking outside to catch a glimpse of the adversary. Fingers are quickly pointed at hackers, but in a significant number of security breaches, the perpetrators are insiders. A perpetrator may well be a coworker sitting next to you. Consider a disgruntled nurse who has been working in the intensive care unit for several years. This individual, who has access to sensitive patient information and life-supporting computer devices, is terminated for poor performance. Such individuals can wreak havoc if they choose to avenge any perceived inequities. Other insiders also have direct access to information systems. News reports are full of stories about personal information theft. It is believed that more thefts are not reported for fear of losing customer confidence.

There are numerous ways that security can be breached, including social engineering, shoulder browsing, salami attacks, denial of service attacks, website defacement, data diddling, and password sniffing, not to mention viruses, worms, and other malicious software such as Trojans and rootkits, to name a few (McGonigle & Mastrian, 2012). See Appendix C in this chapter for information about these types of security breaches.

Consider this example:

> You are working on the computer and see a very interesting screen saver advertisement on the Internet. The advertisement invites you to visit a website to download the screen saver. As you download and install the software, you may be unknowingly installing a Trojan. After it is installed, the attacker could do several things in your computer without your knowledge, such as collecting your personal and banking information and sending it to the attacker's computer in a remote location. In many cases, some of the most powerful antimalware software fails to detect the malicious software.

Information can be stolen from computers without touching them. This is accomplished by stealing a defining characteristic of the computer device called the Internet protocol (IP) address. Hackers simply use the IP address of someone else's computer, often referred to as IP spoofing. Even worse, an attacker can remotely take control of the victim's computer and use it to attack another computer. A single attacker can take control of several computers at a time and use them for exploits (McGonigle & Mastrian, 2012).

The use of wireless technologies is pervasive in most hospitals. Although this affords convenience, wireless networks could be among the most vulnerable networks. Today, there is a plethora of free sniffing software that can be downloaded over the Internet. These programs have the capability not only to capture login information but also to collect enormous amounts of patient and other critical information. Some of the free downloadable software, when used with other software, could even map out the specific locations of wireless devices in a facility. Such attacks require no special training. These breaches and attacks are only a few examples of vulnerabilities in an organization.

Why Do Breaches Occur?

There are potential vulnerabilities in most information systems. These vulnerabilities are weaknesses at the hardware or software level. Weaknesses in hardware include lack of adequate physical protection, which makes hardware highly vulnerable. Software vulnerabilities range from operating system weaknesses to software configuration issues. When operating systems are developed, their flexibility and user friendliness often supersede security. Vulnerabilities differ among versions of one operating system. These differences can be subtle or substantial.

Software that is installed on operating systems introduces another level of complexity to information system security. Some poorly developed applications have little chance of being secure when an attack is launched. Like the operating system platforms on which they are ported, resilience varies. The security holes in an operating system, combined with security holes in applications installed on it, could be a recipe for disaster with devastating consequences for an organization.

User behavior, if not monitored and controlled, could open doors for information systems security breaches. In most organizations, different levels of information access are assigned to users. These users are typically grouped and given rights to perform certain actions on a computer or network. For example, nurse leaders have higher access than nurses, nurses have higher access than nurse technicians, nurse technicians have higher access than patient transporters, and so on. A group is simply a collection of users with similar rights. Whether an individual is on a computer or network, he or she has certain rights. Although some rights limit what a user or group can do, others are very pervasive and allow limitless access. It is not difficult to understand what happens when such a powerful user right is compromised. The sad reality is that some users may have this potent right and not even know it. User behaviors like indiscriminate downloading and installing software from unknown websites could put malicious, clandestine codes on a computer. When this happens, the computer or an entire network could be at the mercy of a hacker.

Protecting the Organization's Information

There are several ways to protect a healthcare organization's information. The approach will depend on the importance an organization places on its information and the impact of security breaches on its operations. The core of information security is the protection of data and information confidentiality, integrity, and availability. Information protection can be elaborate and proactive or sporadic and reactive. Reactive approaches respond to incidents by providing bandage solutions in which there are no thought-out plans or systematic ways to deal with security issues. On the other hand, proactive approaches look ahead and anticipate possible adverse events. These approaches often have well-planned programs to deal with security issues. The level of attention to detail could determine the effectiveness of security measures. Most organizations use a layered defense approach, which is popular today.

The local computing environment is the total physical and organizational environment, including all data, applications, people, and facilities under the control of a single authority. The protection of a computing environment means safeguarding computers, communication devices, and operating systems and integrating software applications without reducing security. In some cases, the building itself may have to be secured with cameras. Effective security begins with a security policy that will guide the actions of the organization. Specific security measures include cryptography, incident detection, reporting, and responses.

Implications of Information Security for Nursing Leaders

Nurses collect, store, and transmit large amounts of data and information, with various sensitivities, from patients. The output of data from one unit may be the input data for another unit. The accuracy and precision of information must be maintained at all times. Patient privacy concerns are also paramount. HIPAA provides a number of administrative, physical, and technical safeguards for covered entities to ensure confidentiality, integrity, and availability of electronic health information. It has stringent stipulations with legal liability implications and penalties (U.S. Department of Health and Human Services, 2012). The Health Information Technology for Economic and Clinical Health (HITECH) Act has further tightened privacy rules. These rules and regulations mean that the security and privacy of patient information cannot be ignored and should be addressed at all levels of nursing administration.

Nurses, doctors, and other entities that nurses work with need to be actively involved in the management of patient information. Nursing leaders cannot play a passive role when it comes to securing patient information. They should engage in active defense processes right from the outset. This means that senior leadership, including nurse leaders, must commit to information assurance and set the tone for a culture and values that promote and respect patient information security. It is important for senior management to realize that the framework for a security policy extends beyond the principles of computer security. Security policies should address the basic goals of reducing risk and complying with applicable laws and regulations. Policies should also look at ensuring operational confidentiality, integrity, and availability, as has been highlighted throughout this section. Roles and responsibilities, as well as accountability, should be established and clearly understood by all.

To protect the hospital's information, nurses at all levels must recognize the need to protect information resources. Information security awareness and education campaigns may be necessary to ensure that nurses understand their role in protecting information that is entrusted to them.

Information security training for nurses should be ongoing. To sustain the survivability of training initiatives and information security assurance in hospitals, training should be a mission in which every function in the hospital has a stake. When senior leaders seek training in regulatory compliance, high-level management of information security, and other skills related to security, they are indicating their commitment to security. Training not only should be tailored to specific nursing roles but should ensure that senior leaders, program managers, the chief information officer, the information systems security officer, the systems administrator, and all employees understand not only their roles but also how they interface with one another. Information users should understand and know who to tell in case of an information breach. They also need to be able to identify when an incident has occurred. Top management needs training in information security policy formulation strategies, whereas middle management learns how to develop and implement best practices. Nursing leaders may need outside help during training.

Information security management in a hospital is challenging. There are several components to security initiatives. Nursing leaders who are seeking to initiate or augment existing programs should be involved in information security initiatives, maintain a checklist for effective security implementation, and be mindful of possible security breaches such as hacking. See Appendix B in this chapter for information on each of these items.

IMPACT OF TECHNOLOGY ON COMMUNICATION IN NURSING

Even though the basic concepts of effective communication are the same, technology has changed the way nurses communicate today. With cell phones, tablets, laptops, and other mobile devices, electronic communication has become a mainstay. Social media has also gained popularity and is a valuable communication tool for both personal and business use.

As of September 2013, 73% of online adults used social networking sites, 71% of online adults used Facebook, 17% used Instagram, 21% used Pinterest, and 22% used LinkedIn. As of January 2014, 19% of online adults used Twitter (PEW Research Center, 2015). As stated in the PEW report (2015), methods of communication are continuing to change. Email used to be the sole form of electronic communication. Although it is still the main electronic communication method, shorter messaging methods and social media continue to become more prevalent. Adults are more comfortable with technology today than ever before; as a result, medical applications and other software are used with increasing frequency to access healthcare information. The growing number of technically trained nurses will emerge as nurse leaders in today's evolving healthcare system. They will be prepared to take advantage of information technologies that are related to patient care and support.

The American Recovery and Reinvestment Act provided incentives for hospitals to adopt healthcare information technology (U.S. Department of Health and Human Services, 2012). Even with these incentives and research supporting the efficacy of electronic communication with patients, many clinicians are not using electronic technology in delivering patient-centered care. However, nurse leaders and nurses are positioned to change that by using electronic communication technology to create and help sustain patient–provider communications that improve healthcare outcomes (Weaver et al., 2012).

Nursing's Role in Influencing Behaviors by Using Technology

Serious chronic diseases and conditions, such as heart disease, cancer, diabetes, and obesity, are common, costly, and on the rise. These diseases account for many deaths in the United States and need to be addressed. Although there is no simple solution, electronic communication must be included as part of the overall plan. Effective electronic communication can be used to engage patients to participate in their overall care. Educating, reminding, and encouraging patients to monitor their behaviors, as well as providing feedback, are some of the basic tasks that nurses can do through electronic communication. By enabling patients to become more competent participants in their care through electronic communication, time, effort, and dollars can be saved while healthcare outcomes are improved (Weaver et al., 2012). Tools for communicating with patients are evolving rapidly, and nurses will play a role in new approaches to communication related to patient care. It is already known that many patients self-diagnose by seeking information about symptoms on the Internet. Making effective use of electronic technologies allows nurses and other providers to direct patients to the most reliable and relevant resources and information on the Internet.

Email

Communicating with patients via email can be very effective. Some benefits associated with email include increased efficiency, stronger patient–provider communication, easy access to education and information, and more informed decision making. These benefits affect patient behavior and ultimately health outcomes.

Social Media

Social media is well established and is here to stay. Along with email, social media represents a unique opportunity for electronic communication in health care. It can be a powerful adjunct to other communication strategies when used appropriately. Some examples are as follows:

Example 1: Nurses can connect with other nurses worldwide to share information. Nurses should present themselves as professionals and be mindful of HIPAA regulations when participating.

Example 2: Nurses can follow professional organizations through social media for an excellent source of continuing education that provides nurses with current and relevant information pertaining to the profession.

Example 3: Twitter can be a great source of healthcare information by following hashtags such as #BreastCancer. The Healthcare Hashtag Project (Symplur, 2015) maintains a catalog of hashtags to help healthcare professionals use Twitter more effectively.

Text Messaging

Text messaging is a short message delivery system using technology that enables exchanges to an individual or to a large audience. When used in health care, the benefits include convenience, ubiquity, immediacy, communication, monitoring, measurability, dissemination, and multimedia capabilities (Terry, 2008). **Box 11-2** provides advantages to using this method of information delivery.

Regardless of the communication method, implemented programs must be monitored and measured for ongoing efficacy and to determine whether the program is meeting goals that are outlined in the strategic plan. Nursing leaders need to maximize the benefits of electronic tools and programs by ensuring that they and their staff are well educated on technologies that are available to them. Nursing leaders, particularly those with expertise in healthcare informatics, must be proactive and need to understand the potential uses, challenges, and benefits of evolving technologies.

BOX 11-2   Benefits of Text Messaging

- Convenience: Many people carry cell phones and have them turned on.
- Ubiquity: Most people have a mobile device with text capability.
- Immediacy: Recipients are likely to read a text message as soon as they receive it.
- Communication: Two-way communication capability provides opportunities for direct engagement.
- Monitoring: Text messaging can be used to monitor or report symptoms.
- Measurability: Results can be tabulated and measured.
- Dissemination: Text messages can be used for emergency alerts and announcements.
- Multimedia: Texts can include links to audio, video, or websites.

SUMMARY

In the rapidly evolving technological and complex healthcare system, nurse leaders need to be proactive and armed with skills that will allow forward thinking. Processes to enhance nursing tasks and the overall functions of the healthcare system are essential. Nurse leaders will need to have the ability to manage highly skilled nurses as technology continues to advance. Knowing how to prepare themselves and those they manage is imperative and can be demanding if they lack a new way of thinking. The four basic skills of leadership, professionalism, business, and communication have evolved to a new level, and organizations need to focus on developing employees who can meet and manage the goals of the strategic plan. Nurse leaders have a critical role in the adoption of technology by being change agents and empowering their staff to be partners through a shared governance structure. Nurses use technology more than any other discipline, and their knowledge, experience, and input can and should be considered when making IT-related decisions. For IT adoption to occur and have the intended positive consequence, nurse leaders must hold nurses accountable for using technology correctly.

REFLECTIVE QUESTIONS

1. Consider ways a nurse leader can promote education in this advancing technological healthcare environment that are not already in place. What do you see for the future?
2. What evidence do we have of the effectiveness of e-communication for health?
3. To what extent will nurses play a role in deciding which technologies will be used? Do you think nurses and nurse leaders have a significant say in how technologies are used? Why or why not?

4. Consider your clinical environment and the technology that is being used. How have you contributed as a leader? What opportunities exist now or in the future that will allow you to be proactive as a leader?

5. How can shared governance be used to promote the adoption of technology? What are some of the objectives of a nursing informatics council?

6. What are some technologies that are found on a unit? How many technologies do you use in your clinical environment? Based on some of your current challenges, do you anticipate implementing any technologies in the next few years to address those issues? What outcomes do you expect?

7. What roles or individuals would you find in an informatics department? How can an informatics department support you and your staff?

8. What do perceive your role to be when implementing new technology?

9. Systems thinking requires a broad view of an entire system, not just your own division or unit. Provide several examples in which systems thinking was necessary to reach the intended outcome.

10. What are some evaluation tools that can be used to focus on evaluating errors through the perspective of systems thinking?

11. As a nurse leader, what skills are essential to be a change agent and to support staff through times of significant IT transformation?

CASE STUDY 11-1   Using Information Technology to Improve Work Flow

Wade Forehand

Jill is the director of a 40-bed medical–surgical wing that has recently gone live with a new test version of a preoperative nursing documentation flow sheet for surgical patients. Jill has been invited to attend the monthly board meeting for the hospital. In preparation for the meeting, Jill's chief nursing officer (CNO) has asked her to do some homework to present to the board. The CNO informs Jill that the board is composed of professional members of the community, many of whom are not familiar with the countless changes that are being seen in healthcare technology. Jill's CNO recommends that she prepare some notes to speak about healthcare information technology, EHRs, and their meaningful use. The CNO also requests that Jill explain the new process that her floor is actively testing in relation to the preoperative nursing documentation flow sheet. The board is particularly interested to explore how the training, transition, and compliance rates for documentation have occurred. They are also eager to hear how the staff nurses on the unit are responding to the new work flow. If Jill's unit trial is successful with the test version of the preoperative nursing documentation flow sheet, the process will be rolled out to other units in the hospital.

Case Study Questions

1. How could Jill improve her understanding to enhance the work flow? Consider online sources such as HealthIT.gov (http://www.healthit.gov/), HIMSS (http://www.himss.org/Index.aspx), and Centers for Medicare and Medicaid Services (CMS) (http://www.cms.gov/).

2. As the nursing leader, how could Jill begin to formulate an appropriate definition for healthcare information technology, EHRs, and meaningful use for the board members? Remember that the audience is composed of professionals who may have very little knowledge of health care and technology.

(continues)

CASE STUDY 11-1 Using Information Technology to Improve Work Flow (Continued)

3. Create a diagram that represents the new work flow for nursing staff since the test version of the preoperative nursing documentation flow sheet went live. Create a clear and logical process that the board members will be able to follow.
4. Create a chart using a word processing program, such as Microsoft Word, to demonstrate both positive and negative views of how nurses are responding to the new work flow process on the unit. An example is as follows:

	Positive Nursing Views	Negative Nursing Views
1. Go Live Training and Education		
2. Transition and Support		
3. Nursing Views and Opinions		
4. Compliance with New Process		

CASE STUDY 11-2 Disciplinary Action and Managing Patient Information Breaches

Wade Forehand

Sam is a nurse manager on a busy neurosurgical intensive care unit (NICU). Sam is logged in to one of the computer workstations in the hallway of the unit and is working on weekly audits. He soon notices that a commotion is occurring at the end of the hallway. The patient in this room is decompensating and is about to go into cardiac arrest. Sam rushes to the room to assist his staff with the critical patient. Because he is in a hurry, Sam forgets to exit the computer workstation and leaves the documentation system open. Sally, a volunteer in the hospital, is walking by the computer station and realizes that the system has not been shut down. She approaches the workstation to close it. Upon reaching the computer, she notices that the screen is displaying the name of her friend within her senior community center. Before she closes the computer, Sally hovers over the patient's name to discover why he is in the hospital. After reading the information, Sally closes the computer and returns to her volunteer post. Later that evening, Sally called her friends from the senior center to talk about the information she learned.

Several days after the information was shared, the hospitalized patient discovers that Sally was involved. He decided to report this incident to hospital administrators. An investigation by the HIPAA compliance officer is initiated.

Case Study Questions

1. Begin by exploring what ethical principles have been compromised by both Sam and Sally.
2. What role, if any, did technology play in this situation?
3. From the perspective of a nursing leader, how should this investigation be handled?
4. Should disciplinary action be pursued for either Sam or Sally? Explain your answer for both individuals.

CASE STUDY 11-3   Maximizing Communication through Technology

Wade Forehand

As a nursing leader, you may often find that you have to deal with difficult circumstances and individuals who may be challenging. Being an effective leader requires you to have the skills and competencies that are necessary to communicate in these situations.

As the shift supervisor in a busy hospital, you receive an email from one of the unit directors. The email comes across to you as abrasive and insulting. You feel that the unit director is questioning your ability to make staffing decisions for the hospital. Your role requires you to look at each unit's staffing, staffing requests, patient census, and patient acuity to make judgments about where to send the additional floating staff members. There are many factors involved in your staffing decisions. You feel that the unit director does not understand that you have to consider each care area, not just her specific unit.

Case Study Questions

1. From your personal experience, consider how each individual may feel and why.
2. From the perspective of the shift supervisor, compose an email in response to the unit director who you feel is questioning your professional ability. Suppose that just before you send your reply, the unit director calls to speak with you. She apologizes because she feels her email may have been harsh and possibly misunderstood. She attempts to explain her situation and her unit's needs. After the discussion, you have a mutual understanding, and no hard feelings persist. In considering your potential email reply to the unit director, was it a positive form of communication or a negative form?
3. What are the potential effects of sending either a positive email or a negative email as a form of communication?
4. Consider some communication strategies you might be able to incorporate into your email reply to ensure that you are communicating in a positive and constructive manner.

REFERENCES

American Medical Informatics Association. (2015). Informatics areas: Clinical informatics. Retrieved from http://www.amia.org/applications-informatics/clinical-informatics

American Nurses Association. (2008). *Nursing informatics scope and standards of practice.* Silver Spring, MD: Nursesbooks.org.

Ball, M. J., Douglas, J. V., Dulong, D., Newbold, S. K., Sensmeier, J. E., Skiba, D. J., & Kiel, J. M. (2011). *Nursing informatics: Where technology and caring meet* (4th ed.). New York, NY: Springer.

Blum, B. I. (1986). Clinical information systems—a review. *Western Journal of Medicine, 145*(6), 791–797.

Carns, A. (2002, November 11). The checkup is in the e-mail: A new service lets patients have online consultation with doctors. So why aren't many people using it? *Wall Street Journal,* p. R9.

Corcorna, S. (1989). The study of nursing informatics. *Image: The Journal of Nursing Scholarship, 21*(4), 227–231.

Hanson, C. W. (2006). *Healthcare informatics.* New York, NY: McGraw-Hill.

Hebda, T., & Czar, P. (2013). *Handbook of informatics for nurses and healthcare professionals* (5th ed.). Upper Saddle River, NJ: Pearson Prentice Hall.

Hunt, E. C., Sproat, S. B., & Kitzmiller, R. R. (2004). *The nursing informatics implementation guide.* New York, NY: Springer.

Knowledge. (n.d.). In *Merriam-Webster dictionary.* Retrieved from http://www.merriam-webster.com/dictionary/knowledge

Lorenzi, N. M., & Riley, R. T. (2003). *Managing technological change.* New York, NY: Springer Science + Business Media.

McGonigle, D., & Mastrian, K. G. (2012). *Nursing informatics and the foundation of nursing* (2nd ed.). Burlington, MA: Jones & Bartlett Learning.

MedPAC. (2004). *Information technology in healthcare.* Retrieved from http://www.medpac.gov/documents/reports/chapter-7-information-technology-in-health-care-(june-2004-report).pdf

Morrison, I. (2011). *Leading change in health care.* Chicago, IL: AHA Press.

Nelson, L. (2002). Protecting the common good: Technology, objectivity, and privacy. *Public Administration Review, 62,* 69–73.

Parsons, J. J., & Oja, D. (2014). *New perspectives on computer concepts 2014.* Boston, MA: Cengage Learning.

PEW Research Center. (2015). Social networking fact sheet. Retrieved from http://www.pewinternet.org/fact-sheets/social-networking-fact-sheet/

Romano, C. A. (1987). Privacy, confidentiality, and security of computerized systems. *Computers in Nursing, 2,* 99–104.

Saba, V. K., & McCormick, K. A. (2011). *Essentials of nursing informatics* (5th ed.). New York, NY: McGraw-Hill.

Saxton, R. (2012). Communication skills training to address disruptive physician behavior. *AORN Journal, 95*(5), 602–611. doi:10.1016/j.aorn.2011.06.011

Security. (2004). In *Webster's collegiate dictionary and thesaurus.* New Lanark, Scotland: Geddes and Grossett.

Sewell, J., & Thede, L. Q. (2013). *Informatics and nursing: Opportunities and challenges* (4th ed.). Philadelphia, PA: Lippincott Williams & Wilkins.

Sherman, R. O. (2014). Becoming a systems thinker. Retrieved from http://www.emergingrnleader.com/systemsthinkinginnursing/

Symplur. (2015). Why the healthcare hashtag project? Retrieved from http://www.symplur.com/healthcare-hashtags/

Terry, M. (2008). Text messaging in healthcare: The elephant knocking at the door. *Telemedicine Journal and E-Health, 14,* 520–524. doi:10.1089/tmj.2008.8495

U.S. Department of Health and Human Services. (2012). *Justification of estimates for appropriations committees.* Retrieved from http://www.cms.gov/About-CMS/Agency-Information/PerformanceBudget/Downloads/CMSFY12CJ.pdf

Weaver, B., Lindsay, B., & Gitelman, B. (2012). Communication technology and social media: Opportunities and implications for healthcare systems. *Online Journal of Issues in Nursing, 17*(3), 3.

Appendix A

NURSING INFORMATICS COUNCIL CHARTER AND BYLAWS

The following Nursing Informatics Council Charter and Bylaws was developed by, and is in use at, Holy Cross Hospital in Silver Spring, Maryland. Permission has been granted by Holy Cross Hospital to use this as an example for this text. (It has been edited for publication.) Miriam Halimi developed this information during her employment at Holy Cross Hospital. It is still in use today.

Nursing Informatics Council
Charter and Bylaws
I. Role

The Nursing Informatics Council is an interdepartmental venue that [aims] to advance the use of health IT to improve patient safety and patient outcomes. This Council [considers] the organizational imperatives and initiatives and identifies areas of primary improvement. This Council is responsible for the knowledge expansion of nursing informatics within the nursing community at the organization.

II. Purpose

- To promote the advancement and expansion of knowledge for the practice of informatics
- To raise awareness of the importance of the nursing role in the use of clinical information systems
- To promote improvements in the delivery of patient care through the use of technology
- To provide a venue for staff to offer feedback regarding the technology incorporated into the clinical environment
- To share the vision of the organizations' long-term plans for the IT initiatives and its future technology implementations
- To develop a team [comprising] leaders in the informatics and technology revolution to improve quality and patient outcomes
- To provide a communication mechanism for the dissemination of information regarding system changes at the unit level
- To implement new strategies to enable staff to perform "real-time" documentation on both paper and electronic systems
- To develop core informatics competencies for nursing
- To act as clinical superusers for your division
- To provide a forum for the sharing of educational best practices
- To develop innovative training methods for new functionality
- To identify collaborative methods to work with other disciplines for improving the use of the electronic medical record

III. Membership

General Membership

The general membership of this committee will consist of individuals who are active Clinical IT Trainers or individuals identified by the Nursing Leaders (should have two representatives per nursing division), members of the Department of Clinical Informatics, including:

Training Coordinator
Clinical Liaison/Informatics Nurse
Director, Clinical Informatics
Informatics Nursing Specialist
One member of the nursing leadership team
Two Clinical Educators

Officers and Officer Responsibilities

1. Chairperson
   a. Prepares with co-chair the council meeting agenda
   b. Coordinates teleconference
   c. Delegates council assignments
   d. Facilitates council meetings
   e. Prepares and distributes meeting agenda and accompanying documents for review prior to the next meeting
   f. Serves as mentor for the co-chair
2. Co-chair
   a. Assists with duties and responsibilities of the chair as stated above and facilitates meetings in the absence of the chair
   b. Acts as timekeeper for the meeting
3. Secretary
   a. Records attendance and meeting minutes
   b. Submits attendance and meeting minutes to the chairperson at the end of each meeting
   c. Maintains all council communication and correspondence
   d. Places meeting minutes on organizational intranet
   e. Maintains current membership list

Membership Responsibilities

1. Attends all meetings (either in person or via teleconference), or at least one person from each [department attends]
2. Represents the interests of their unit/department in all transactions [with] the council
3. Reviews any material submitted as agenda items in advance of meetings
4. Actively participates in discussions of agenda items
5. Acts as a resource for information regarding council activities
6. Facilitates communication [among] the Council and unit/department-specific councils

Term of Office

1. Members shall serve as long as they remain involved [with] the Genesis training team.
2. Members not on the training team will [serve] a 2-year term.

Process for Resignation

1. The process for resignation requires a written letter to the chair of the council. If a midyear vacancy occurs within the council, a replacement member will be sought by those who work within the same service line as the departing member.

IV. Meetings

1. The Council shall meet monthly for approximately two hours.
2. Agendas shall be set and distributed prior to the meetings. Once on the agenda, items shall remain active until action by the Council renders them closed or resolved.
3. Special ad hoc meetings may occur as a result of [system-wide] initiatives.
4. Minutes of each meeting shall be reported by the Secretary and approved by the Council. Copies of these minutes shall be posted on the organization's intranet.

V. Responsibilities:

1. An annual evaluation of the process of communication, operations, and outcomes of the Council will occur annually in July.
2. Based on the results of the annual evaluation, review of the bylaws will be conducted.

VI. Reporting Relationship

1. An annual report with submission of council goals will be presented to the Coordinating Council.
2. Each year, the Council will evaluate its structure and process to ensure it is supporting the PPM and strategic goals.

VII. Decision-making Authority

1. A quorum greater than 50% of the membership must be present to conduct business.
2. All decisions are reached using a consensus model that invites each nurse to have a voice in the decisions being made by the Council.
3. All professional nurses are invited to observe open council meetings.

VIII. Council Year
The Council will begin on the first of July and end on the 30th of June.

Appendix B

CHECKLISTS FOR EFFECTIVE SECURITY IMPLEMENTATION

Things to consider when undertaking information security initiatives:

1. Embarking on information security initiatives is a step in the right direction. Protecting patient information is a regulatory compliance issue that must be taken seriously.
2. The technical and administrative complexity in managing such programs could be overwhelming. Significant time needs to be put in to the entire project, particularly during the planning stage.
3. It is critical to get buy-in from top management before starting a project on information systems security.
4. Ensure that you clearly understand all parties involved, including their roles and accountability.

5. It is important to have some technical understanding of information systems.
6. Have a grasp of information flow within the hospital and the interfaces involved.
7. Determine the human and financial resources needed to achieve established goals.
8. Spend time familiarizing yourself with laws and regulations governing patient information privacy.
9. Establish rapport with the information technology department and work closely with them.
10. There will be obstacles along the way. Learn to be persistent.
11. Ensure that your organization has an information security policy.

Administrative and technical checklist for effective security implementation:

1. Adopt a security approach that is layered.
2. Divide users into groups based on their information needs and assign only those rights needed to do their work.
3. Make sure that information system devices are placed in secure locations and are physically locked to prevent unauthorized access.
4. Password protect the computer boot process.
5. Use operating systems, such as Windows New Technology-based systems, that allow you to lock down files and folders.
6. Have a strong password policy.
7. Depending on the sensitivity of information, audit computer use.
8. Implement software and hardware firewalls as appropriate.
9. Have a written acceptable computer use policy.
10. Implement intrusion detection systems at the boundaries of your internal network.
11. Make sure computer devices are protected from electrical spikes, surges, and brownouts.
12. Ensure that critical servers are housed in controlled environments with air conditioning, fire prevention, and protection.
13. Ensure that critical information is backed up frequently.

Recommendations made by Foundstone to remove hacking:

1. Isolate or remove compromised hosts from the organization's network.
2. Do not plug USB storage devices into potentially compromised machines and then plug them into other systems—this may expand an incident.
3. Secure or disable all wireless access points and dial-in modems.
4. Suspend all outbound Internet traffic if you suspect a hacker may be sending sensitive information to remote hosts.
5. Ensure that all sensitive communication is encrypted during containment and remediation.
6. Monitor network traffic.
7. Patch and harden all Internet-facing applications and operating systems.
8. Review all critical code to ensure it has not been modified.
9. Monitor all email for phishing.

10. Ensure up-to-date antivirus software is running on all desktops and servers.
11. Activate your response team.
12. Do not change anything unless instructed or approved by management and the legal team.
13. Notify management as soon as possible.
14. Document everything you know, retain evidence, and maintain a chain of custody.

Appendix C

SECURITY BREACHES

Data diddling: Data diddling refers to the alteration of existing data. This modification often happens before data are entered into an application or as soon as data are processed and output from an application. Unauthorized data modification could render the integrity of critical information worthless and in some cases could mean the difference between life and death in a hospital environment (McGonigle & Mastrian, 2012).

Denial of service attack: A denial of service attack renders workstation computers or servers inaccessible by legitimate users. These attacks are often launched against critical servers that host email, web, and database services. The attack not only can be costly to an organization financially but also could result in loss of life in a hospital.

Malicious software: Malicious software, such as Trojans and rootkits, is extremely dangerous software that, after installation, can remain in the system for a long time without being detected. This software is often stealthily installed by unsuspecting computer users. Free downloads are common ways of inviting such trouble.

Password sniffing: Password sniffing and cracking are attacks that are easy to do. During password sniffing, the attacker uses tools to gain awareness of network traffic and capture passwords being sent between computers. Many tools used for such attacks are free downloads from the Internet. These tools are also incredibly easy to install and use. Gaining unauthorized access to another person's password could be devastating for individuals and a hospital as a whole. Sometimes this can go undetected for long periods of time.

Salami attack: A salami attack occurs when the attacker pilfers small amounts of information from several places and goes unnoticed. This attack may initially start at a single location and soon be extended to steal from similar servers located in different geographic regions. All the attacker needs to do is elevate the access rights on the network.

Shoulder browsing or surfing: Shoulder browsing or surfing is a subtle but serious concern. This occurs when a person sits or stands by another who is busy working on a computer. This person appears to be making conversation or saying something of importance to the busy individual. The person doing the browsing looks on the monitor and makes mental notes of information. It might seem on the surface that not much information can be stolen this way. Over time, several pieces of information can be gathered and put together to constitute significant intelligence (McGonigle & Mastrian, 2012).

Social engineering: Social engineering occurs when a person tricks another person into sharing confidential information, such as by posing as someone authorized to have access to that information. This type of security breach is quite common and fairly easy to stage. In a hospital, patient privacy is protected by laws and regulations that, if not followed, could result in lawsuits and other serious consequences. If an imposter dedicates some time to learning the language of nurses, buys a decent pair of scrubs, and gathers some amount of boldness, he or she could slip through the cracks and steal critical patient information. This could be detrimental to the hospital's operations.

Viruses: Viruses are often small software programs that attach to legitimate software installed on a computer and are designed to carry out specific actions, and they have the capability to spread. These actions could range from simply drawing annoying pictures on a computer screen to erasing all data from a hard drive.

Website defacement: Website defacement is another invasive attack in which the attacker alters website content. It is often used for purposes of espionage.

Worms: Worms do not need to attach to other software. They are often self-replicating and self-propagating. Worms are notorious for taking up useful network bandwidth and bringing the network to a crawl or completely stalling it. They could also replicate erratically and fill up hard drive space.

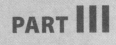

Leading to Improve the Future Quality and Safety of Healthcare Delivery

CHAPTER 12

Laws, Regulations, and Healthcare Policy Shaping Administrative Practice

Carolyn Dolan and James L. Harris

LEARNING OBJECTIVES

1. Discuss how laws and regulations shape healthcare policy and administrative practice.
2. Identify foundations of health law and policy and their interrelatedness to administrative leadership.
3. Distinguish differences and complementary elements of delivery systems and payment structures underpinned by laws and regulations.

AONE KEY COMPETENCIES

I. Communication and relationship building
II. Knowledge of the healthcare environment
III. Leadership
IV. Professionalism
V. Business skills

AONE KEY COMPETENCIES DISCUSSED IN THIS CHAPTER

II. Knowledge of the healthcare environment
III. Leadership
IV. Professionalism

II. Knowledge of the healthcare environment
- Clinical practice knowledge
- Patient care delivery models and work design knowledge
- Healthcare economics knowledge
- Healthcare policy knowledge
- Understanding of governance
- Understanding of evidence-based practice
- Outcomes measurement
- Knowledge of, and dedication to, patient safety
- Understanding of utilization and case management
- Knowledge of quality improvement and metrics
- Knowledge of risk management

III. Leadership
- Foundational thinking skills
- Personal journey disciplines
- Ability to use systems thinking
- Succession planning
- Change management

IV. Professionalism
- Personal and professional accountability
- Career planning
- Ethics
- Evidence-based clinical and management practices
- Advocacy for the clinical enterprise and for nursing practice
- Active membership in professional organizations

FUTURE OF NURSING: FOUR KEY MESSAGES

1. Nurses should practice to the full extent of their education and training.
2. Nurses should achieve higher levels of education and training through an improved education system that promotes seamless academic progression.
3. Nurses should be full partners with physicians and other health professionals in redesigning health care in the United States.
4. Effective workforce planning and policy making require better data collection and information infrastructure.

Introduction

Healthcare costs continue to escalate while the quality of care is often inconsistent and fragmented. In comparison to other wealthy countries, the United States is high in cost and low in quality. Fifty percent more is spent in the United States on health care per capita than any other country. Fifteen percent of the gross domestic product is spent nationally on health care, and it is projected to increase by 20% before 2050 (Congressional Budget Office, 2009). The ongoing debate about healthcare reform and financing escalating costs will impact new and existing laws, regulations, and healthcare policy in the immediate future and beyond. This complexity requires all administrators to become full partners with stakeholders from various spheres while being knowledgeable of how laws, regulations, and healthcare policy shape administrative practice.

Health care will continuously be defined and controlled by those whose political power and influence is the greatest. If nurse administrators fail to engage themselves, partner with stakeholders in the formation of healthcare policy, and exert pressure on lawmakers and regulatory agencies, the future of administrative practice could be jeopardized and regulated by a few brokers. This could readily yield deleterious consequences further restricting practice, healthcare management, and education of future providers and administrators.

To provide context for this chapter, a historical overview of the law, sources of law and examples, and how a bill becomes a law will be presented, including legal precedents. A discussion of laws and regulations that affect health care will be provided. Three foundational components of healthcare policy (public, organizational, and professional) will also be discussed in terms of how they shape administrative practice. Examples of laws that impact how care delivery systems and initiatives respond to mandatory requirements and impact administrative practice and health care will be presented from a legal and policy perspective using legal cases.

HISTORICAL CONTEXT OF LAW

Black's Law Dictionary defines law as "the regime that orders human activities and relations through systematic application of the force of a politically organized society, or through social pressure, backed by force, in such a society, the legal system" (Law, 1999, p. 889). The explanation continues as Posner (1993) posits that the word *law* comes with at least three distinctions: (1) primitive law is a social institution; (2) law is a set of propositions; and (3) the law is composed of a set of rights, duties, and powers.

Historical man recognized the potential gains to be realized by a society governed by law. Endeavoring to attain such a system necessitated the establishment of a set of governing principles, rules, and regulations. American civil order can be traced to the voyage of the *Mayflower* and a famous document, the Mayflower Compact, drawn up by the would-be separatists (the pilgrims) between themselves and their king. From a practical standpoint, the pilgrims sought an agreement to keep the peace since the ship had missed its mark (Virginia) and did not land where planned. There was concern that some would not be bound by any law in the new world. They proceeded to establish the Massachusetts Bay Company, electing first John Carver and then William Bradford as governors. The Massachusetts Bay Company quickly realized that its inhabitants were now "freemen" and would be able to vote in the colony's newly established system of representative government. Thus, what had begun as an idea was transformed into an experiment—men ruling themselves without a king (Blum et al., 1977).

Civil law (codified law) and English common law (precedents and judicial law) were the predominate types of established law in the civilized world. Although the supreme law of the United States is the Constitution and the Bill of Rights, the Constitution was preceded by two other important documents: the Declaration of Independence and the Articles of Confederation (Library of Congress, 2014).

American law, which is influenced by many sources, is the behavior, proposition, penalty, regulation, or rule that is mandated by the legislature and the courts. Influences that ultimately shape laws that are applied in the United States can be divided into two basic categories: common law (how the courts have ruled in the past based on legal precedents derived from an adversarial system of trial by jury or judge, known as case law or uncodified law) or civil law (codified law based on a compilation of regularly updated rules and regulations that are primarily enacted by the legislature). Both the courts and the legislatures have strong religious underpinnings as evidenced by links to the Roman Catholic Church and the Anglican Church in common law and the civil code. Models of right and wrong, shaped by Judeo-Christian tradition, are interlaced with Western historical practices, mores, and traditions. For example, in the days of early American settlers, community rules or rights (customary) in agrarian areas were passed down as codes of belief and were often biblically based (Exodus 20:15, "Thou shalt not steal"). Books were scarce in the New World, and codes of behavior were taught by the family, community, tribe, or colony and evidenced over time until eventually inscribed as law (Cooper, 2004).

SOURCES OF LAW

Multiple examples are prevalent in the sources of law that guide many decisions today. The U.S. Constitution has been called a living document that established not only the federal government but also our system of laws (U.S. History, 2014). The writers were learned men who had studied the great lawmakers, such as Polybius, Cicero, Locke, Montesquieu, and Blackstone, among others. At the time of its signing in 1787 by delegates to the Constitutional Convention in Philadelphia, the U.S. Constitution represented the greatest synopsis of law ever written. To ensure that America remained governed by the governed and was never subjected to an autocracy, the delegates devised the three-branch system of separation of powers. This is the governmental structure upon which the American legal system rests today. It determines many actions that govern the management of health care (Our Government/The White House, 2014).

U.S. law is a meshed form of common law that was divided into federal and state components at the nation's inception, not as one body but as one union of 13 colonies. In 1776 and again in 1789, first at the signing of the Declaration of Independence and then at the activation of law via the U.S. Constitution, our nation, which was represented by 13 united but separate colonies that all claimed independence, separated itself from England and established a new republic, the United States of America.

The federal government has four sources of authority at law: constitutional, statutory, administrative, and common. Common law relies on legal precedents or stare decisis as authority in rulings. Case outcome after case outcome is passed down as the legal issue becomes settled. Legal precedent informs future court decisions and becomes strongly persuasive, if not virtually binding. Over time, common law may evolve significantly from its original version through emerging judicial interpretations and subsequent revisions to law. Within the sources of the authority of law there are four keystones: substantive, procedural, criminal, and civil. If federal and state laws conflict, the federal law takes precedence.

The architecture of the American legal system includes five main pillars:

- Constitutional law (judicial decisions)
- Statutory law (U.S. Congress statutes and codes)
- Administrative law (executive regulations)
- Common law (precedent, case law)
- State law (generally applies principles of federal law) (Our Government/The White House, 2014)

For example, administrative law (whether federal or state) is a source of law that is responsive to matters of executive agencies (Administrative Law, 2014). The judges, administrative directors, and other appointees are selected through the presidential tier of government. State governments are structured similarly. This is important in understanding how state boards of nursing derive their powers of licensure, regulation, and discipline of the nursing profession. **Tables 12-1** and **12-2** display the three-branch system of governmental power according to federal and state government structures.

TABLE 12-1   Three-Branch System of Governmental Power

U.S. Constitution		
Legislative	Executive	Judiciary
Senate-House	President	SCOTUS
Speaker of the House	Vice president	Court of appeals
Senate pro tempore		District courts

Generally, individual states' governments follow the federal government structure. In order of individual succession to power, the vice president is followed by the speaker of the House of Representatives, and then the Senate pro tempore, as depicted in Table 12-2.

Under the separation of powers intent of the U.S. Constitution, the executive branch vests several duties and privileges in the president. The president has war power as the commander in chief, treaty making in international affairs, veto power over legislative bills, an unlimited power to pardon, and the privilege of appointing executives to head offices. Exclusive of the office of the vice president, the president enjoys nine cabinets and appoints the heads of 15 departments under the authority vested by the executive branch. The departments under the executive branch are the offices of the Vice President, Management and Budget, Policy Development, White House Office, Council of Economic Advisers, Office of Science and Technology Policy, Council of Environmental Quality, National Security Council, and Administration. The departments include Agriculture, Defense, Energy, Homeland Security, Interior, Labor, Transportation, Commerce, Education, Health and Human Services, Housing and Urban Development, Justice, State, Veteran's Affairs, and Treasury (Executive Branch, 2014).

The U.S. Supreme Court is the highest federal court and is composed of nine Supreme Court justices who are appointed for life through the executive branch. The court is located in Washington, D.C., and hears cases by certiorari (the process of an issuance of a writ to a lower court directing it to send the court record to the higher court for review).

The court of appeals is composed of 13 circuits (including the Washington, D.C., court) throughout 94 judicial districts in the 50 states and U.S. territories. Judges are appointed and are known as Article III judges; they are appointed for life (Judiciary Branch, 2014). **Table 12-3** displays sources of law and examples that are relevant to contemporary health care.

TABLE 12-2   State Governmental Power

State Constitution		
Legislative	Executive	Judiciary
Senate-House	Governor	State supreme court
	Lieutenant governor	Court of appeals
	Executive departments	Circuit or district courts
		Lower courts

TABLE 12-3   Sources of Law and Examples

Source of and Role of Law	Federal Examples	State Examples
U.S. Constitution (supreme law) Role: Interprets the law, no higher court, no higher challenge Lower courts: Appeal matters of law to the highest court if the issue has *standing*, presents a new issue that is not *moot*, and is *ripe*	1. SCOTUS: *Roe v. Wade*, 410 U.S. 113 (1973) 2. The Affordable Care Act (ACA) was enacted by Congress. However, a question was presented to SCOTUS after its passage. In *National Federation of Independent Business v. Sebelius* No. 11-393 by certiorari, the Supreme Court decided that the ACA penalty for not buying healthcare insurance is a tax (2014). 3. 10th Amendment	1. Abortion: Regulation by state. After consideration of "undue burden," state requiring "parental notification" (e.g., MN Stat. §§ 144.343(2)–(7) (1988)) was not found to create an undue burden. 2. ACA: Issue clarified 3. 10th Amendment: Power not given to the federal government or prohibited to the states by the U.S. Code (USC) is reserved to the states.
Congress-statutory: To establish (make) law through codes and statutes States: To make lake through legislature (codified law by codes and statutes)	1. HR4449, Patient Self-Determination Act: Amendment to Social Security Administration (SSA), which required Medicare and Medicaid providers to implement access and opportunity about advance directive program. Also see *Washington v. Glucksberg*, 521 US 702 (leading right to die case, eventually went to the Supreme Court of the U.S.). 2. Affordable Care Act 42 USC § 111-152	1. Natural death acts: Examples include VT. Stat. Ann. Tit. 18 §§5252-5262 (Supp, 1985), Alabama State Code §§ 22-8A-1-10 (2014) 2. ACA: State funding of Medicaid (e.g., MyMaineConnection; Maine Children's Insurance (Chips) Program, 2014) 3. Colorado regulatory Dept. of PH FCCR 1006-2 (2014): Recreational use of marijuana Washington RCW 46.61.503 (2014): Recreational use of marijuana for persons over age 21.
Executive (nationally, president; state, governor) Administrative: States under police power; establish nurse practice acts Role: To establish laws through regulations and rules	1. U.S. Department of Health and Human Services, child abuse laws, elder abuse, Environmental Protection Agency (EPA) (see executive agencies for more examples) 2. Title VII of CRA-Anti-Discrimination Act of 1964	1. DEA 21 CFR §1304. 03 (6) (Drug Enforcement Agency, Code of Federal Regulations) Other: State departments of health, environmental protection departments 2. State regulations specific to nursing practice: State Nurse Practice Act (NPA), such as FL Chap XXXII 464.001-.027 (NPA) (2014) and TX Peer Review: Texas Code (NPR) §303.001(5)] (2014)

(continues)

TABLE 12-3 Sources of Law and Examples (Continued)		
Source of and Role of Law	**Federal Examples**	**State Examples**
Common law (case law) Role: To establish substantive law based on stare decisis	1. 29 USCA §2000e-2(a) (termination of employee)	1. *Stark v. Circle K Corp.* (Montana, 1988) (breach of contract) 2. *Big Town Nursing Home, Inc. v. Newman CCA TX*, 1970, 461 zd.ze.2d 195 (1994) (false imprisonment for failure to discharge)

Each of the branches of government is entrusted with a different role in the development and oversight of American law. The legislature (U.S. Congress) is entrusted with many powers, including the power to declare war, control immigration, conduct investigations, compel disclosures pertaining to its legislative function, and determine when and if new law is needed or if current law should be changed (repealed, amended, or revised). Under the necessary and proper clause of the Constitution, the role of lawmaking is a somber one and should be treated with diligence and careful adherence to procedure and process. Congress is to enact law to protect the public welfare, morals, and safety (Roles of Congress, 2014).

A bill must have bicameral (Senate and House) support to be passed. After the bill is passed, it is presented to the executive branch, the president, who is slated with implementing or executing new law via the power of the pen by signing or vetoing (Roles of the President, 2014). Finally, the judiciary branch is entrusted to oversee the U.S. Constitution and to interpret federal and state laws within light of the Constitution and to decide whether law upholds it. The balance of powers at work in the development and interpretation of law is the legal process that distinguishes our system of government from any other in the world.

HOW A BILL BECOMES A LAW

A bill can enter the house by a number of means. One example is when a lobbyist introduces it for a special interest group. For example, advanced practice nurses (APNs) in Alabama, via the Nurse Practitioner Alliance of Alabama, have pressed for prescriptive authority of controlled substances for many years. Association members paid for professional lobby representation at the state level to press for their bill to reach the house. Finally, in 2013 negotiations with the Medical Association of the State of Alabama's lobbyists led to the passage of Code of Alabama §§ 41-22-6 and 22-2-250, allowing a partial victory for APNs to prescribe controlled substances III–V via the Alabama Qualified Controlled Substance Certificate Program as administered by the Board of Medicine (State of Alabama, 2014). Though it was not the legislative victory in autonomy that was hoped for, the expansion of the law demonstrates how APNs were able to expand the law and provide greater access to care for Alabama patients (Alabama State Nurses' Association, 2014).

Constituents may write to their representative, or a group of interested citizens may express their dislike about a matter and request action. The steps of a bill being introduced are as follows:

1. The bill is introduced as a House bill (HB) or Senate bill (SB), assigned a number, and sent to committee.
2. It may be killed (squashed) in committee, revised, or sent to the floor.
3. The bill will be heard.
4. The bill is approved or rejected and becomes enrolled and engrossed.
5. The engrossed version is sent to the White House for the president to review.
6. The president can sign the bill into law or veto it.
7. A veto can be overturned by a two-thirds majority of Congress (357 members of the 535, 435 representatives and 100 senators must approve the bill).
8. If two-thirds of the Congress approves, a bill becomes law (U.S. Constitution).

HOW A BILL IS CHALLENGED

When a new law is needed or when an old law must be changed, certain factors must be considered. Article III of the Constitution gives guidance to the judiciary on when to hear a case or controversy (The Judiciary, 2014). This remains constant in health care even today. Three key factors are essential requirements before the court may hear a case. First, the facts of the case must show that the plaintiff has sustained an injury. This is known as standing. In *Linda R.S. v. Richard D.* (1973), the court agreed with the Texas District Court that ruled on the matter of the Texas penal code regarding a mother of an illegitimate child who sued for child support under Texas statutory law. The law did not apply to deadbeat dads of illegitimate children; therefore, the mother of the child was the not the proper plaintiff and lacked standing.

Second, a court must determine that the issue is not moot. Mootness distinguishes cases and controversies from issues that are nonjusticiable (no longer affecting the rights of the litigants), such as when a defendant has died. However, the Supreme Court makes exceptions to the rule of mootness, as in *Roe v. Wade*, since Jane Roe's pregnancy had long ended after the court heard the case (*Roe v. Wade*, 410 U.S. 113, 1973). The court may reason that when an important right has been denied, and without judicial review that right is likely to continue to be denied, the court will hear the case despite mootness.

The third essential requirement of justiciability is ripeness. This requirement insists that the controversy has matured or is adverse to the point of immediacy and that all available remedies have been sought and are ineffective. A legal matter that is not moot, that is ripe, and that is brought by a party with standing has relevance to society now. Therefore, standing, mootness, and ripeness are the three specific doctrines that determine judicial review under the case and controversy requirement. Upon appeal and by grant of certiorari, the Supreme Court may hear a case when there is an important federal question of law (Barron & Dienes, 1983).

Ongoing modern controversies among the states include the recreational use of marijuana, assisted suicide at the end of life, stem cell research, the definition of marriage, and the right to late-term abortion, to name a few. In addition, the advent of electronic health records and rapid advances in technology, such as robotics and telemedicine, have created new controversies and cases that promise to explore issues of law never before addressed.

Although an act may become legalized in a state, it may remain federally illegal. For example, the use of marijuana for recreation remains federally illegal and is illegal in all states except Colorado and Washington. Federal law maintains marijuana as a Schedule I substance that is controlled under the Controlled Substance Act of 1970, despite a growing societal acceptance of its use. This hot-button issue reached a new level when, on August 28, 2013, Eric Holder, in a joint meeting with the governors of both states, outlined the parameters for federal oversight but stated that his office would implement a trust but verify policy. The attorney general, in an acknowledgment of the states' violation of federal law, stated that no preemptive action would be taken against the states by the Department of Justice presently. He further provided specific expectations for developing regimens of enforcement that would be required of the states. The passage of the marijuana for recreational use by Colorado and Washington demonstrates how the public may dispute a federal law until the state is pressed to act by its sovereign authority to change the law. A Pew survey in March 2013 illustrated society's changing opinion of marijuana legalization for all purposes. The research found that 72% of Americans believe that governmental efforts enforcing marijuana laws are not cost efficient, and 60% did not favor federal enforcement (intrusion) on states in which marijuana has been legalized (Public Opinion, 2014).

Constitutionally, although states may impose stricter laws than federal laws, states may not pass laws that weaken or negate federal law. Under the supremacy clause, if federal and state law conflict, federal law preempts state law (Department of Justice, 2014). Because the Supreme Court typically does not take on political cases, the use of marijuana for recreation may not be addressed; however, the actions by the states may create a climate for other constitutional issues to emerge that will capture the court's attention and demand its scrutiny.

Legal theories and bases impacting U.S. Supreme Court rulings imposed by a constitutional case are initiated with a challenge. Society or an individual may decry a long-held legal practice and press the political process toward change. For example, the rights of the dying collectively initiated changes in the common law by bringing conflicting cases regarding surrogacy before the court. When the legal question arises, the Supreme Court, following its Article III interpretive role, is pressed to hear the case and possibly define or interpret the law. After the court decides the constitutional question (there is no higher court on which to appeal), new laws, rules, and regulations or amendments may follow from the legislative and rule-making bodies.

By the time a case enters the Supreme Court docket, lower courts have decided laws, and lawmakers have enacted laws along the way. The right to die and assisted suicide questions are among the most anguishing for both those affected and lawmakers. The matter remains unsettled, but clearly society is speaking on the subject, and history (and law) is being made. Evidence is replete with research concerning the value of advance directives and an individual's right to make choices concerning one's death. Further, medically futile situations are forcing families to face the difficult and complex task of deciding what to do about end-of-life treatments, or their termination, when there is no advance directive to guide them (Painter, 2009).

Author Raymond Whiting attributes choice in death as fundamental to constitutional guarantees of individual rights and is no different than free speech or the free exercise of religion. He theorizes that one's right to die is a right of self-determination and privacy, and the state should not interfere as long as the individual is no threat to others (Whiting, 2002). Certainly, the debate has been ongoing for at least 100 years in this country.

In 1997, the Supreme Court was asked to consider whether the due process clause of the 14th Amendment ensures a person's right to assisted suicide in *Washington v. Glucksberg*. The court said no because of the state's interest and the common law precedents against assisted suicide. The Washington Death with Dignity Act, RCW 70.245, passed on November 4, 2008, allowing terminally ill residents of the state to seek assistance in lethal doses of medication if they choose to end their life (*Washington v. Glucksberg*, 2014).

To illustrate regional differences more vividly, in 2012 the Georgia state senate passed a bill making assisted suicide a felony, and the following year Vermont's state legislature became the first in the nation to pass a physician-assisted suicide law by statute. Prior to the Vermont act, Oregon and Washington (supra) had passed laws based on citizens' referendums, and Montana had passed an assisted suicide law through the courts in the civil case *Baxter v. Montana* (2009).

There were other right-to-die cases and controversies in the courts long before these highly visible cases. The outcomes of two famous cases, *In re Quinlan* (1977) and *Cruzan v. Director* (2014), led to Montana Senator Danforth's success in proposing the 1990 Self-Determination Act, requiring hospitals that receive federal funds to provide access and explain to patients the right of refusal of treatment. *Quinlan* was one of the first right-to-die cases. It involved a New Jersey court decision that allowed the father of a young woman who was determined to be in a vegetative state to have mechanical ventilation removed to not prolong her life artificially. The *Cruzan* case was a 5 to 4 decision by the Supreme Court that refused to allow artificial means of support (a feeding tube) to be removed when there was no advance directive, on the basis of the state's interest. However, it upheld the legal standard that competent persons are able to exercise the right to refuse medical treatment under the due process clause on the basis of an individual's right to privacy. In *Cruzan*, because there was no "clear and convincing evidence" of what Nancy Cruzan wanted, the court upheld the state's policy.

Although the debate over assisted suicide had been ongoing since the turn of the century, the *Cruzan* case was a great victory in the minds of many people. Finally, an individual could control the questions of how, when, where, and who would be present, to some extent. Although the federal Self-Determination Act (and the Natural Death Act), in addition to multiple states' acts that preceded and followed the federal act, attempted to address the legal issues surrounding end-of-life matters, questions have continued to the present day (The 1990 Self-Determination Act, 2014).

In 2005, the *Schiavo* case in Florida presented the question of what is a persistent vegetative state. The case provided a highly emotional, political, and religious backdrop when the case of the deeply comatose individual, who had not left an advance directive, became public. For many, the outcome of the case (that remained in the state appellate court system) was predictable. The clear and convincing evidence issue surrounding *Schiavo* was addressed previously in the case of *Cruzan v. Director* (2014) when the court held that Cruzan could not be disconnected from her feeding tube because her wishes were not known (in accordance with state law). In *Cruzan*, the court tied their logic to the 14th Amendment's due process clause, emboldening the right-to-die movement.

Therefore, the courts have supported a constitutional basis for the right to die, but not the right to assisted suicide. Because a right to privacy was explicit in the Florida Constitution (Article I, §23), the *Schiavo* case was determined at the state level. However, society's outpouring of anguish over the decision was extreme as Mrs. Schiavo languished and her parents pleaded. For several days there was constant media attention. The case went before trial and appellate courts at the state level before going to the U.S. district court. It was denied certiorari by the U.S. Supreme Court and remanded to the Florida Supreme Court, where the decision of the appellate court was upheld based on strong medical testimony that Terri Schiavo, having suffered massive and irreversible brain damage and having not left expressed end-of-life directives, had given testimony to her next of kin, her husband, Michael Schiavo, who testified that she would have chosen to die rather than to go on living in a chronic vegetative state with no hope of recovery.

The *Schiavo* case was interesting in many respects. Due to the outpouring of sympathy for the parents, the Florida legislature took an extraordinary measure in passing a law to allow the governor to issue a one-time stay on the court's order. Governor Jeb Bush, in his authority as governor, ordered the reinsertion of the nasogastric tube as the case remained in the appellate court system until its final ruling (Dorf, 2003).

States continue to debate the assisted suicide question, and several have passed death with dignity acts in an attempt to avert such a legal controversy. Many aspects of the issue remain unsettled, and individual rights for the terminally ill, which include assisted suicide, vary from state to state. Such questions are often central political issues concerning the sovereignty of state's rights, separation of church and state, a basic fundamental right of privacy, or another issue of freedom granted under the prevailing law of the U.S. Constitution. Such questions make social issues some of the most difficult and interesting cases.

In December 2013, Jahi McMath sustained irreversible brain death after cardiac arrest and was pronounced dead in a California hospital. After 2 weeks, the family refused to allow the child to be removed from artificial means of support. The hospital sued to have the body disconnected from the ventilator and won. Charitable agencies, in support of the mother, donated funding to have the body transported to an undisclosed location in New York, where the child remains on a ventilator to this day (O'Connor, 2014). The McMath case may teach new lessons regarding communication; ethics; relationships among family, providers, and hospitals; and the rights of parents when medical care is deemed hopeless.

In 2014, private and government-sponsored health care may not reimburse care that is considered medically futile. In McMath's case, the hospital ethics committee supported the decision to terminate artificial support. Such dilemmas have importance for nursing. Nurses must continue to remain beneficent and cognizant of laws while respectful of the patient and patient's family. In the article "Ethical Aspects of Withdrawing and Withholding Treatment," Wainwright (2007) encourages nurses to be proactive and lead the way in end-of-life and medical futility controversies. Nurses, to be proficient for the task, must embrace their own values and beliefs and be able to distinguish treatment from care to remain inviolate in their duty of care.

Definitions of death and life continue to be legal areas in which issues are most misunderstood, challenged, and argued. The impact of local culture, political and societal influences on human behavior, and law is evident as rules of society evolve and are revised. It is a dynamic state in which the application of the law changes from generation to generation. Some legal scholars argue that the constitutional guarantees of life, liberty, and the pursuit of happiness never change under the law, only their application.

The law not only guides human conduct but also may determine, distinguish, and establish it for the aggregate. Law, then, is the expression of the legislative will of the people or an act by the judiciary. It literally gives and takes away rights and privileges, passes judgment, and determines penalties and punishments (Law, 1999).

LAWS THAT AFFECT HEALTH CARE

Laws affect any practice. Healthcare agencies are not exempt from complying with multiple laws and regulations, whether federal, state, or territory. Public law consists of three types of law (constitutional, criminal, and administrative) and defines the citizens' relationship with the government, whereas laws that affect relationships between individuals are civil. Multiple categories of public law affect nursing practice whereby nurses must accommodate a patient's wishes. For example, if a patient's religious beliefs forbid the receipt of blood or blood products, nurses and other healthcare providers must accommodate such wishes. While these beliefs are controversial to many, nurses cannot interfere with one's right to have a procedure, such as an abortion (*Roe v. Wade*, 1973).

CONSTITUTIONAL LAW

Constitutional law pertains to any of the individual states' or the federal government's constitution. More broadly defined, constitutional law is

> the body of the judicial precedent that has gradually developed through a process in which courts interpret, apply and explain the meaning of particular constitutional provisions and principles during a legal proceeding. Executive, legislative, and judicial actions that conform with the norms prescribed by a constitutional provision. The text of the U.S. Constitution is marked by four characteristics; a delegation of power, in which the duties and prerogatives of the executive, legislative, and judicial branches are delineated by express constitutional provisions; a Separation of Powers, in which the responsibilities of government are divided and shared among the coordinate branches; a reservation of power, in which the sovereignty of the federal government is qualified by the sovereignty reserved to the state governments; and a limitation of power, in which the prerogatives of the three branches of government are restricted by constitutionally enumerated individual rights, Unenumerated Rights derived from sources outside the text of the Constitution, and other constraints inherent in a democratic system where the ultimate source of authority for government action is the consent of the people. (U.S. Constitution, 2014)

Since the basis of all law is measured against the standard of the U.S. Constitution, most of this chapter has been devoted to a discussion of the history and principles that infused its writing. A thorough understanding of the core of law should provide the reader with the basis for the interpretation of all other sources and types of laws and their applications and uses. Law may be further classified by its substance or its procedure in that substantive law focuses on the actual source (type) of law, while procedure looks at the process by which it is regulated, in terms of violation, prosecution, and civil practice. For example, in torts, after the statute of limitations has been reached, a claim becomes stale and cannot be brought against a defendant (Aiken, 2004).

CRIMINAL LAW

Criminal law is made up of statutes, rules, and regulations for conduct as provided by the government or a governing body (e.g., city, state, federal). Criminal law includes misdemeanors and felonies, definitions of crime, penalties, punishments, and terms of prosecution. Because crimes are against the public, penalties may include service, fees, and imprisonment or, in extreme cases, death. Criminal procedure refers to the area of law that specializes in the prosecution of crimes fairly, properly, and in accordance with constitutional protections (Criminal Procedure, 2014).

Criminalization of Nursing Mistakes

In 2004, Julie Thao, an experienced obstetrics registered nurse from Wisconsin, was sued for malpractice and wrongful death (torts) related to a terrible medication error resulting in the death of a 16-year-old. Thao was also charged with felony criminal neglect by the state district attorney (Felony Charges against Julie Thao, 2014). A criminal neglect charge is similar to manslaughter, which carries a prison sentence of up to 6 years and a penalty of $25,000. In Thao's case, the board of nursing, under the auspices of its administrative role, heard the case, suspended her license, and imposed specific practice restrictions. Thao's attorney, Stephen Hurley, was quoted as saying, "What we're telling nurses and all medical professionals is that we demand perfection" (Shalo, 2007, pp. 20–21).

The just culture paradigm identifies three behaviors that lead to errors: human, at risk, and reckless. Some people are of the opinion that Mrs. Thao demonstrated all these behaviors in the commission of the mistake that led to the taking of an innocent life. Since Thao had worked a double shift and had failed to adhere to the system's bar coding safety mechanism and inadvertently hung the wrong medication, many viewed her behavior as more than human error (a lapse, a slipup). But virtually all healthcare professionals agreed that she was not blameworthy to the extent of being charged with criminal conduct.

The case of Julie Thao garnered national attention as nursing and other healthcare organizations came out in public support of Thao. The Pennsylvania Institute for Safe Medication Practices (ISMP), the Wisconsin Board of Nursing, the Hospital Association, and the American Nurses Association all supported Thao.

The criminalization of nursing errors is a disturbing trend today as civil (common law) disputes in tort are also prosecuted in criminal court. When a nurse who has committed an unintentional nursing error resulting in injury to a patient is prosecuted for a crime, it has far-reaching implications for all licensed healthcare professionals. Society has repeatedly placed its trust in nursing. When news of bad acts, bad outcomes, or bad actors become public, damage to the profession's image and integrity occurs.

In the article "The Criminalization of Mistakes in Nursing," nurse attorney Nayna Philipsen (2011) contrasts a nursing mistake with a crime. For example, the Jasmine Gant (discussed later) and Julie Thao stories can cause grievous harm and even loss of life. In that nurses typically do not seek to injure patients under their care (albeit the potential for negligence is ever present), an act or failure to act—such as in neglecting to report abnormal vital signs or a laboratory critical value, or a change in a patient's mental status—may ultimately harm the patient. Such harm is on account of an unintentional act.

A nurse's omission in any of the preceding examples, and many more that could be hypothesized on a busy unit by a stressed nurse, would meet the requirement of one of the elements of negligence: breach of the standard of care. It would not demonstrate that the nurse intended to harm the patient or that the nurse intended to breach the duty of care, but a claim may follow in a civil suit and the nurse could be found liable for the failure to act. Conversely, crimes are intentional acts of omission or failures to comply with a requirement set by law. The state or federal government brings the action, and the case is prosecuted through the courts with punishments that may include fines, penalties, or imprisonment. In addition to civil and criminal proceedings, disciplinary actions on nurses' licenses may occur at the board of nursing level, such as what happened in the case of Julie Thao, who incurred a cause of action in civil court. The family sued St. Mary's Hospital on behalf of the infant son, and the case settled for $1.9 million, an indictment by the district attorney, and disciplinary action by the Wisconsin Board of Nursing (Wisconsin Department of Regulation and Licensing, 2014).

Paradoxically, at a time when The Joint Commission was setting new standards for anonymous reporting of occurrences and health care was moving away from blaming individuals to a systems-based root cause analysis approach to problem solving in a just culture environment, several high-profile cases, such as the Jasmine Gant death, raised the public conscience. Despite the controversy and media attention, the commission maintains the principled view that for health care to become safer, it must become systems based and stop looking toward perfecting individuals. The need to provide patient safety in the complex healthcare environment will continue to remain a dynamic medical, legal, and ethical challenge for professionals.

Federal and state governments have administrative laws that affect nursing practice and licensing requirements within each state and territory. Administrative law, commonly called regulatory law, has two major functions: rulemaking and enforcement (adjudication). For example, the U.S. Public Health Service, the Occupational Safety and Health Administration (OSHA), and the Centers for Disease Control and Prevention are all under the executive branch and are governed by administrative or regulatory law. The heads of these departments are generally an agency body, board, or the president, depending on the structure of power (legislative, independent) within the government. All governmental agencies are listed, described, and available for public review through the *United States Government Manual* or the *Federal Regulatory Directory*, which are available at the Library of Congress Reference Desk. The chief duties of the executive agencies are outlined under the Administrative Procedure Act (5 U.S.C. 551, et seq.). The primary sources for administrative rulemaking are the *Federal Register (FR)* and the *Code of Federal Regulations (CFR)*. The *FR*, *CFR*, and *United States Government Manual* are available electronically from the U.S. Government Printing Office (2015).

Another commonly recognized federal administrative law is the Health Insurance Portability and Accountability Act (HIPAA) of 1996, also known as the Privacy Rule (45 CFR Parts 160 and 164). The Privacy Rule makes up a large component of HIPAA and is a subpart of the regulations found in the Standards for Privacy of Individually Identifiable Health Information, the national standards for the protection of information. Administered by the Office of Civil Rights (OCR), these standards (regulations that carry the force of law) identify the legitimate use and disclosure of individuals' health information (audio or video, paper, electronic, etc.) and control of how the data may be used. The overarching goal of the standards is information protection that also allows for the flow of information so high-quality health care can be provided, health data can be shared for third-party payment, or care can be furthered, such as referrals or transfers, without compromising confidentiality. The Privacy Rule, the Security Rule, and the Enforcement Rules are the three major administrative regulatory standards that ensure the OCR successfully accomplishes its mission of protecting personal health information. The source of federal law that empowers the OCR to implement these regulations is 45 CFR Parts 160, 162, and 164 (Health Insurance Portability and Accountability Act, 2014).

Another commonly identifiable federal administrative law is the Occupational Safety and Health Administration (OSHA) Act of 1970. Under the U.S. Department of Labor, OSHA ensures that employees have safe work environments (U.S. Department of Labor, 2002). More information about OSHA is available from the U.S. Department of Labor (2015).

Although the preceding cases, laws, and codes are cornerstones that govern administrative practice and nursing legal actions, there are other areas that administrators must be cognizant of while managing healthcare situations involving legal matters. Such areas are included in the following discussion.

Workplace disruption has become more commonplace and presents a challenge. All healthcare organizations should implement a zero-tolerance policy related to disruptive behavior. The policy should include a professional code of conduct and educational and behavioral strategies to assist nurses and other healthcare professionals in addressing such activity. Some 2 million American workers are victims of workplace violence annually. It can range from threats and verbal abuse, to physical abuse, to assaults and homicide within and outside the workplace. The Joint Commission has been explicit in stating that healthcare facilities must address the problem of behaviors that threaten the performance of the healthcare team. Intimidation and disruptive behaviors can promote medical errors, contribute to poor patient and staff satisfaction, increase care costs, and cause staff to seek new positions in more professional environments. Safety and quality are directly dependent on teamwork, communication, and collaboration within the workplace (Longo, 2010; The Joint Commission, 2008).

In 2008, the *Consensus Model for APRN Regulation: Licensure, Accreditation, Certification, and Education* was created to guide states and jurisdictions in the implementation and oversight of APNs (National Council of State Boards of Nursing, 2014). Although the model is not a law, its uniform and nationally recognized title is of utmost importance for any profession that is concerned with public protection. Uniformity is essential for consumers and employers; it allows consumers of healthcare services to more fully understand the role and functions of an APN.

With the advent of competency-based education and privileging and credentialing of staff, including nurses, administrators must be aware of the legal ramifications inherent in validating competencies and credentialing nurses who initiate evidence-based practice protocols and engage in independent practice. As a healthcare agency accreditation body, The Joint Commission ensures that competencies are validated during triennial and for-cause visits.

Nurse practice acts and boards of nursing are examples of state administrative laws. Under the 10th Amendment of the U.S. Constitution and the general welfare clause, the creation of regulations involving health and welfare has traditionally been the role of state governments. The primary method of control over nursing practice is the nurse practice act (NPA). However, since this one law (or set of laws) cannot guide every aspect of the nursing profession, each state's (and territory's) NPA establishes a board of nursing tasked to administer or carry out the elements necessary to clarify or implement more specific rules and regulations needed for the nursing profession to practice safely and protect the public (Russell, 2012).

The NPA is enacted by the legislature of the state and is made available for public review prior to becoming law. The police power (legal administrative power) authorized under the 10th Amendment of the U.S. Constitution empowers states to preserve and protect the safety, health, welfare, and morals of their communities via nursing boards that have decision-making power that carries the full force of law.

Each state regulates nursing practice in three ways. First, the NPA is a statute created and approved by the state legislature to provide broad guidelines for the practice of nursing and nurse licensure requirements. Second, the board of nursing is an appointed group of individuals who represent all levels of nursing practice, other healthcare professionals, and lay citizens. This board is responsible for disciplining nurses and creating nursing rules and regulations. Third, the NPA provides nursing administrative rules and regulations that comprise the details of how the NPA will be enforced by law (National Council of State Boards of Nursing, 2011).

THE BOARD OF NURSING

State boards have been regulating nursing for more than 100 years. When there is a complaint to the board of nursing regarding a nurse's performance, statutory authority provided by the NPA vests the full investigatory, prosecutorial functions under administrative law by the board of nursing to review the facts and determine the outcome as an arm of its disciplinary function. If the board finds that the nurse violated state criminal law (e.g., drug diversion), actions against the licensee may include referral to substance treatment programs, criminal investigations, fines, and penalties. Other potential actions following a disciplinary proceeding on a nursing license, as outlined by nurse attorney Tonya Aiken, include dismissed charge, investigations agreement, letter of reprimand, probation, suspension, or revocation (Aiken, 2004).

Boards of nursing are required by their state governments (their citizens) to protect consumers (their citizens) from harm. Under their constitutional police power, boards of nursing regulate and discipline the nursing profession (their citizens). Although North Carolina became the first state to license nurses in 1903 (Johnson, 2014), all states and territories are regulated under the National Council of State Boards of Nursing. Upon license renewal, registered nurses are required to self-report legally significant data impacting their license. Although it may vary from state to state or compact, any felony or misdemeanor charges of violence or substance use must be acknowledged. Further, all states require continuing education hours for nurses as a condition for renewal of their license, as well as other practice mandates, to maintain the professional privilege of practice. For example, Florida statutory law defines an APN and outlines specific continuing education license requirements in its law (Florida Administrative Code, 2014).

Many offenses, injuries, and infectious diseases may also need to be reported. Nurse administrators must remain vigilant to ensure that nurses report any child or elder abuse and neglect, that criminal background checks are completed for prospective employees, and that any issues are reported about nurses who practice under the influence of substances. These are only a few reporting activities. Annually, state boards of nursing spend many dollars dealing with nurses who are found guilty of impaired practice due to substance abuse (C. Dearman, personal communication, June 1, 2014).

CIVIL LAW

Civil law is a body of rules that delineate private rights and remedies affecting relationships between individuals or between an individual and a state (property issue). Civil law is distinct from criminal or public law and involves contracts and torts. Defendants in civil cases are rendered in breach of contract or liable in tort, as opposed to being guilty of a crime, and are customarily court ordered to fulfill the contract terms or are assessed financially for damages (pain, suffering, economic losses) sustained by the plaintiff (Peterson & Kopishke, 2010).

CONTRACTS AND CONTRACT LAW

Most contract law is a branch of civil law. A contract occurs between individuals or business entities. Contracts are involved in many human transactions involving employment, personal relations with others, the sale of goods, property (land), and business relationships. Contracts may be verbal or written, but in most transactions there is a written, signed document establishing certain elements. Three pertinent points needed for a contract to become binding between two entities are as follows:

1. There is mutual assent; in other words, there was a process in which at some point the parties mutually agreed to be bound. This is also known as manifestation of assent to be bound. Generally, contract creation between

parties involves negotiation to the point of consensus. The clearer the proposal (or terms), the less likely a contract will be misinterpreted as merely negotiations in contemplation of a contract. Should an issue of fact arise, the more specific the proposal, the more likely the trier of fact will be able to determine the existence of a contract.

2. There is an offer and acceptance. The offerer makes the offer with the knowledge that there is a promise (a liability) to be fulfilled, and the offeree exerts the power to accept or not accept the offer.

3. The written contract contains specific terms, including the expression of the offer, identity of the offeree, subject matter, price or amount to be paid, method of delivery, and performance, quantity, and nature of work. Specific terms of performance are more likely to result in good outcomes.

The intent to enter into the contract, and the terms of the bargain or contract, should be expressly clear to both parties. The terms should be explicit since an ambiguous contract may prevent the court from enforcing its terms. Courts have said they do not write contracts between parties and will not guess as to the terms. When one party fails to perform on their responsibility to a contract, it is known as a breach of contract, and the injured party will seek a remedy by filing suit (a claim similar to filing a tort claim). Fulfilling the obligation of the contract is often the remedy ordered by the court. Contracts may also govern transactions between businesses (Rohwer & Schaber, 1997). **Box 12-1** provides an overview of terminology that is relevant to employment contracts.

Contracts may be oral or written. "If a contract is written, it will be more likely to be understood and carried out to the satisfaction of both parties than an oral agreement that's terms may be misunderstood. Contract terms may be expressly or distinctly outlined or implied (yet recognized by both parties)" (Aiken, 2004, p. 67). Nurses agree to contract with employers from pay period to pay period,

---

BOX 12-1 Employment Contract Terminology

- Legal age and mental capacity: Competent individuals or parties
- Essential terms: Agreed-upon terms of the individuals or parties stating what each must or must not do
- Mutual assent to be bound: Mutual agreement by both individuals or parties regarding the terms and obligations imposed by the contract
- Consideration: Something of value that supports one's contract and makes it enforceable; may be performance, forbearance, money, or another thing of value
- Breach: Failure to perform upon agreement
- Termination: Anything that ends the contract, such as death, insanity, destruction of an essential element, illegality, fraud, counteroffer, revocation
- Remedy: If the contract is sufficiently definite, the court may grant the relief the plaintiff seeks (performance, money, etc.)

Source: Rohwer & Schaber, 1997

without signing anything, simply by accepting a paycheck. Generally, the terms of a contract run from one pay period to the next, and an employee may terminate or be terminated with a 2-week notice (in writing) effective prior to the next term. An employee may not actually sign a contract with an employer and still be bound in a written contract with an employer. A handbook or unit policy manual can be considered a contract and carries the force of law until terminated (Aiken, 2004). Commonly in health care, actual written contracts such as those between hospitals and third parties or agencies that employ registered nurses are used. Under these circumstances, the nurse is known as an independent contractor and does not work for the hospital, but the agency or the nurse may work independently based on the terms of the employment contract.

Contract terms may be binding depending on whether the nurse agrees to certain actions, such as policy adherence, specific duties, confidentiality, and, in certain instances, tours of duty. In government and state care facilities, contracts are often explicit that the employee represents the best will of the agency. The contract may specify that the employee may not represent personal views or perspectives that are of a political nature when working. For example, government employees are prohibited from supporting and discussing political candidates who are seeking office during the course of their assigned duty at the place of employment. The employer offers a contract with a payment (or salary or fee for service), and an employee or independent contractor or offeree accepts the offer and performs the service or the work as specified in the contract. Some protections in health care are guaranteed in all work service contracts, such as federal rights under Title VI (to guard against civil rights discrimination), the Americans with Disabilities Act, wage and hour safeguards (to guarantee reasonable compensation), and OSHA, and they do not need to be specified in contractual terms.

The following example concerning a nursing work contract that was found on a recent nursing blog illustrates the importance of having explicit terms of a work contract outlined and agreed upon to protect the facility and the employee:

> Once again I am thankful I work for a unionized nursing unit. As part of our contract we are only allowed to be pulled to areas we are cross trained in or that have similar patient populations. If we are pulled to a another unit we are to task only without primary patient care responsibility. It sounds like common sense but when have hospital administrators ever been accused of having common sense when it comes to nursing assignments. Also, in the contract, they cannot bring in an agency nurse to work my unit to float me out to a unit the agency nurse won't work. No one floats if there is a per diem or agency nurse on the unit. A hospital across town is famous for this and we have inherited a number of their critical care staff who were tired of being pulled to the med/surg floor when a critical care agency nurse was called in to take their assignment in ICU. (Employment Contracts, 2014, p. 1)

In addition to work contracts, administrators enter into multiple contracts with suppliers and various business entities to render specific services. It becomes imperative for administrators to be knowledgeable of contracts and seek counsel before entering into any agreement. A flawed contract can easily result in litigation if it is not fully executed, and it can be costly to the institution in legal fees and profits. Consider the following: an administrator signs a contract that appears to be valid, only to discover that it deeply discounts reimbursements for a procedure that is frequently performed by orthopedic surgeons. This example and multiple others require the following actions:

- Assess the overall and specific impact
- Identify the long-term financial impact
- Negotiate better performing contracts through standardization of products and bulk purchasing
- Ask what the value of health is, how it is measured, and the cost of health and caring by providers

TORTS

Civil law includes torts. A tort is defined as wrongs other than a breach of contract in which one may seek redress in civil court. Torts result in injury or harm to an individual, as opposed to crimes against the state. Torts may include the denial of another their legal rights, failure to adhere to one's public duties, or breach of a duty owed someone resulting in harm to the person in whom the duty was owed. Torts may be intentional or unintentional. Intentional acts occur knowingly with intent and result in harm (damages) to another or another's person; unintentional acts are those that occur negligently without the actor's intent to cause harm. Negligent acts may also be reckless or wanton. Traditionally torts are categorized as belonging in one of three categories: intentional, negligent, and strict liability. Quasi-intentional tort is another category of intentional act in which harm to the person is presumed. In strict liability, the doctrine of res ipsa loquitur (the thing speaks for itself) applies. This tort is based on an absolute duty, not intent or negligence.

Negligence is the failure to exercise the standard of care that a reasonably prudent person would have exercised in a similar situation; any conduct that falls below the legal standard established to protect others against unreasonable risk of harm, except for conduct that is intentionally, wantonly, or willfully disregardful of other's rights.

In civil law torts, healthcare professionals are most often sued for negligence (malpractice), the breach of duty to comply with the standard of care resulting in harm to the plaintiff for which damages are sought. Occasionally, claims of other torts may apply. A claim of action in tort will be filed through the civil court system at the state level, typically in the county where the tort occurred. The case will proceed only if certain requirements (also known as elements) are met. The elements of malpractice are as follows:

1. There was a duty owed the patient for the nurse to practice the standard of care.
2. There was breach of the standard of care and the nurse's action was not reasonable given the set of facts.
3. There was harm (or damages incurred) to the patient as a direct result of the nurse's action.
4. There was a causal relationship between the breach of the standard (defendant's act) and the harm to the patient (plaintiff).

If essential elements are met, the case may go to trial or be settled. The medical record is the key source of evidence. Documentation is imperative. If one is found at fault, they are found liable or guilty of malpractice (negligence). In a civil proceeding, a preponderance of evidence is the burden of proof necessary for a finding of liability. This is a lesser burden than the prosecutorial burden of a criminal procedure. Further, all crimes are reported to the board of nursing. After a licensed professional is sued, a notation is also recorded in that person's state board file (although this is a civil proceeding) and in the National Practitioner Database, whether the provider is proven liable or not. Serious employment implications may result by having a mark on one's record.

To show malpractice, the facts must indicate by a preponderance of evidence that it was foreseeable that the harm would occur, and but for the breach it would not have occurred. The goal of torts is to make the damaged plaintiff whole by monetary means. The patient's harm (or death) is considered compensable.

A patient who has been harmed will generally file a civil suit against the nurse in the circuit court of the county in which the tort occurred, asking for a trial. This is known as a civil action in tort. Although there may potentially be various types of torts that a patient could bring, malpractice (medical negligence) is the most common. An example of a hypothetical claim of action filed in tort is provided in **Box 12-2**.

BOX 12-2   Claim of Action

IN THE SUPERIOR COURT OF KING COUNTY JANE DOE

Case No. 123456789

Plaintiff v. COMPLAINT for PERSONAL INJURY

Memorial Hospital of King County

Defendant and Defendants 1–3, inclusive.

Nan Nurse

Tom Nurse

Dee Nurse

Comes now the plaintiff in the aforementioned matter and states as follows:

FACTS

On or about July 3, 2014, Plaintiff was admitted as a patient to the ER service of Dr. A. B. Harris into Memorial Hospital of King County for fever of 102.4, chills, and right side pain. Subsequent to an examination and basic lab tests, a diagnosis was made of pyelonephritis. Shortly after arriving, she began to vomit intractably and shake violently, and these symptoms could not be controlled with usual treatment of promethazine given by mouth which she could not keep down. At about 7:15 p.m. she was admitted to the third floor urology–nephrology wing, an IV of 0.9 NS was ordered for rapid infusion of 150 ml/hour for 8 hours. Nan Nurse started the intravenous infusion at the prescribed amount but failed to recognize that the intravenous catheter had not cannulated a vein but was in the surrounding tissue of Mrs. Doe's wrist, which had previous nerve damage from a bicycle accident. Therefore, Mrs. Doe had no way of telling Ms. Nan Nurse that the catheter was not in the correct site. Ms. Nan Nurse rapidly infused the 0.9 NS along with 4 mg of IV Zofran (ondansetron) and Mrs. Doe was left for over 1 hour without observation, at which time she sustained gross swelling, extensive tissue damage, and further pain. Due to the medication she had received in the ER she was drowsy and completely unaware of the extent of the . . .

When a fact pattern meets the four elements of negligence, the case may move forward to jury trial, bench, or settlement. In most negligence cases the outcome will be to settle the dispute and avoid going to trial where a jury or judge will try the facts and decide if the tort occurred as alleged and to what extent damages are owed. In medical malpractice, the opinion of an expert may be crucial to the outcome of a case because experts testify to the standard of care, the duty that was owed, and the reasonableness of the actions of the nurse (whether prudent) (Peterson & Kopishke, 2010). Only a registered nurse can establish the standard of care for a nurse and serve as an expert witness for nursing (Aiken, 2004).

The most common causes of action for nursing malpractice reported by the National Practitioner Database are falls, medication errors, failure to monitor, failure to notify or communicate, documentation (failure to document or falsification), and equipment harms. The highest risk areas for nurses are obstetrics, anesthesia, emergency, and surgery.

In most cases of negligence, an expert witness is needed to determine whether the standard of care was met. The expert nurse will be someone who has similar education and experience and is familiar with the area of specialty. The nurse will be asked whether he or she would have acted or made the same decision if given the same facts to determine whether the standard was breached. To demonstrate a breach of duty, a reasonable and prudent person test is engaged by the courts. This asks what a reasonable and prudent nurse would do in a similar situation. Only a registered nurse can testify to the standard of care of another registered nurse. There are various ways to assist the court or trier of fact in determining the standard of care, such as nurse practice acts, job descriptions, expert witness testimonies, hospital or unit policies, certification or professional standards, manufacturer manuals, professional association standards, and regulatory standards such as those provided by The Joint Commission. **Table 12-4** lists commonly faced torts by nurses, a definition of each, and clinical examples.

Tort-Related Terms

Administrators and practicing nurses should be aware of the following tort terms:

- Breach: A fraction or violation of trust or faith at law.
- Certification: The formal recognition of the specialized knowledge, skills, and experience demonstrated by the achievement of standards identified by a nursing specialty to promote optimal health outcomes (Peterson & Kopishke, 2010).
- Competent: Duty qualified; answering all requirements; having sufficient capacity, ability, or authority; possessing the requisite physical, mental, natural, or legal qualifications; able, adequate; sufficient; capable, legally fit (Peterson & Kopishke, 2010).
- Duty of care: An expected action or observation that is owed the patient after the relationship between the professional and the patient has been established (Peterson & Kopishke, 2010).
- Expert witness: A witness who, by virtue of special knowledge, skill, training, or experience, is qualified to provide testimony to aid the fact finder in matters that exceed the common knowledge of ordinary people (Peterson & Kopishke, 2010).

TABLE 12-4   Torts

Tort	Definition	Example
Battery	An intentional act of harmful or offensive contact with another's person (apprehension is nonessential, damages are nonessential, and intent can be transferred). An object can be used to cause battery (e.g., throwing a rock). In health care, any touching of a patient without consent (implied or expressed) may meet the elements of the tort of battery (§46 Rest. Torts, 2nd).	*Kathleen K. v. Robert B.* 150 Cal. App. 3d 992, 198 Cal. Rpt. 273 (1984). Intentional transmission of sexually transmitted disease.
Assault	An intentional, unlawful, offensive act that places the other person in apprehension of an unpermitted contact (§46 Rest. Torts, 2nd).	*Vietnamese Fishermen's Ass'n v. Knight of the K.K.K.*, 518 F. Supp. 993 (S.D. Tex., 1981). Enrobed members rode around in shrimp boats with guns, frightening fishermen.
False imprisonment	The unlawful, intentional confinement of another within fixed boundaries so the confined person is conscious of being harmed by the confinement (§Rest. Torts, 2nd). Also, a crime committed by the act of restraining another person in a bounded area where there is no means of escape (locked door, car, physical restraints, chemical restraints, or barriers); includes the unauthorized or invalid use of legal authority (detainment without warrant or arrest) and threats of immediate harm (Legal Information Institute, n.d.).	*Peterson v. Sorlien*, 299 N.W. 2d 123 (Minn. 1980).
Intentional infliction of emotional distress	An intentional tort that occurs when one, without a privilege to do so, acts intentionally in such a way that is extreme and outrageous enough to cause severe emotional distress to another (§46 Rest. Torts, 2nd).	*Ford v. Revlon, Inc.* 153 Ariz. 38, 734 P.2d 580 (1987). Employer liable for coworkers' continued vulgar remarks.
Trespass to land and trespass to chattel (property)	The unlawful entry, failure to exit, or act of causing another to go onto another person's land. The wrongful taking of another's property. Trespass may be unintentional (negligent) and criminal (common-law larceny).	*Fadig v. Municipality of Anchorage*, 785 P.2d 911 (Alaska App. 1990).
Invasion of privacy	Public disclosure or invasion of a person's privacy without consent by the use or misuse of personal information, data, or photographs such that a reasonable person would object. The protection extends to medical records (U.S. Department of Health and Human Services, n.d.).	*U.S. v. Warshak et al.*, U.S. 632 f ed 266 (Sixth Cir., 2010).
Negligence	The failure to exercise the standard of care by an act of commission or omission that a reasonable, prudent person situated similarly would have done.	*Quaid v. Baxter Healthcare Corp.* No. 1-08-2727 (2009). Twin neonates received 1,000 times the amount of ordered heparin.

(continues)

TABLE 12-4 Torts (Continued)		
Tort	**Definition**	**Example**
Defamation, libel, and slander	Quasi-intentional torts, which are intentional torts that involve speech, whether oral (slander) or written (libel), that damages another person's reputation or interest in privacy. Defamation pertains to a specific act of false communication to a third party that causes harm to that person. Truth is an absolute defense to the claim of defamation. Breach of confidentiality through violation of HIPAA may create a civil claim in quasi-intentional tort, such as sharing patient information inappropriately (social media and other forms of communication).	*Poliner v. Texas Health Systems* 2006 WL 770425. Sharing peer-review information.

- Malpractice: Action that a person would not do in delivery of care.
- Negligent: Simply, the failure to exercise the standard of care.
- Res ipsa loquitur: Latin for the thing speaks for itself.
- Respondeat superior: Latin for let the master answer.
- Scope of practice: The breadth of practice by virtue of training, education, and legal privilege (licensure or certification).
- Standard of care: The degree of care that a reasonably prudent person in that profession should exercise under the same or similar circumstances (Peterson & Kopishke, 2010).
- Statute of limitations: The specified time allowed from discovery and the filing of a claim of action, typically related to malpractice or negligence (Peterson & Kopishke, 2010).

Malpractice cases continue to produce effects in the healthcare environment that result in increased costs, declining profit margins, and organizations that reorganize or merge with other institutions to remain solvent. Medical negligence is the third leading cause of death in the United States, right behind heart disease and cancer. It is estimated that medical errors kill roughly 200,000 patients annually in the United States. In 2012, more than $3 billion was awarded in malpractice claims, averaging a payout every 43 minutes. Statutes of limitations (deadlines for filing a lawsuit in order to not be permanently barred) vary from state to state, as do procedural requirements that must be met before a medical malpractice lawsuit is filed (Cheeks, 2013).

Although there are numerous examples of nursing malpractice cases, frequently cited cases cluster around four areas: treatment; communication; medication; and monitoring, observing, and supervising. Treatment cases include the following examples:

- Failure to follow approved medical staff protocols or provider orders
- Delay in initiating a provider order
- Failure to timely recognize and treat symptoms that result in emergency situations
- Early termination of a treatment

Communication cases include the following:

- Failure to report a change in condition to the provider
- Failure to obtain a provider order prior to implementing treatment
- Failure to respond to patient concerns or communicate information to treatment teams

Medication cases include the following:

- Wrong medication dose, route, or patient
- Failure to document medication
- Missed dose or treatment with provider notification

Monitoring, observing, and supervising cases include the following:

- Patient abandonment
- Failure to check status and document findings at designated times, such as when a patient is restrained, placed in seclusion, or placed on a 1:1 status
- Inadequate management of a preoperative or postoperative patient

Nurses and nursing administrators must be aware of the scope and standards of care and authoritative statements on how professional nurses should practice in the event of a malpractice claim. While scope and standards of care are not prescriptive, they provide a framework for the expectations of a professional who critically thinks and performs tasks and functions competently (Brewer, 2014).

Patient safety is a basic tenet of professional practice, and being an advocate for a safe environment is embedded in the American Nurses Association Code of Ethics (2015). As patient safety advocates, nurses are in pivotal positions to promote the adoption of psychologically safe environments that are conducive to reporting mistakes and asking for help, education, or feedback (Tocco & DeFontes, 2014). In environments absent of psychological safety, staff members are reluctant to report mistakes, and this punitive approach shuts off information that is needed to identify faulty systems and create safe ones. In a punitive system, no one learns from mistakes.

As previously identified in the Thao case, an alternative to a punitive system is application of the just culture model. The model creates an environment that encourages individuals to report mistakes so the precursors to errors can be better understood and safer procedures can be created (Agency for Healthcare Research and Quality, n.d.). The just culture concept dates to 1997 when John Reason proposed that such a culture is the middle component between patient safety and safety culture (Reason, 1997). Just culture seeks to answer two questions: (1) What is the role of punitive sanction in the safety of the healthcare system? and (2) Does the threat or application of punitive sanction as a remedy for human error hurt the system safety efforts? (Marx, 2001).

In addition, the just culture model describes three classes of human behavior that establish predictability in error occurrence. The first is human error—doing other than what should have been done. The second is at-risk behavior, which occurs when a choice is made that increases the risk that is not recognized or is mistakenly believed to be justifiable. The third is reckless behavior, in which activities or actions are taken with a conscious disregard for extensive and indefensible risk (Marx, 2001, 2008).

Although it is not stated as such in the American Nurses Credentialing Center's (2014) five model components for the Magnet Recognition Program, just culture is consistent with its components. The components include Transformational Leadership; Structural Empowerment; Exemplary Professional Practice; New Knowledge, Innovations, and Improvements; and Empiric Outcomes. As the healthcare industry continues to experience changes and redesign, today's leaders must be transformative to meet the care demands of the future. Structures and explicit processes will continuously create avenues for innovation. Opportunities to develop staff that support structures and processes are central to meeting organizational goals. Understanding the role of nurses will lead to professional practice. Leaders have a professional responsibility to redesign and refine practice environments that will advance and spread evidence. As care models are tested and created, measureable and sustainable outcomes will shape practice, and more organizations will become Magnet designated (American Nurses Credentialing Center, 2014).

For a number of years, just culture has proven to be effective in reducing errors and improving patient safety. Just culture was historically adopted by aviation and other industries, but lessons learned have proven useful in healthcare systems where errors have serious, if not catastrophic, results.

Of considerable influence on error reduction and the partnership between patients and healthcare professionals is the Patient's Bill of Rights. On June 22, 2010, President Obama announced new interim final regulations, the Patient's Bill of Rights, that included a set of protections that applied to healthcare coverage 6 months after the enactment of the ACA. These new protections created a strong foundation of patients' rights in the private health insurance market that exemplifies Americans in charge of their own health and well-being (Centers for Medicare and Medicaid Services [CMS], 2014). Nonadherence to the covenants contained in the Patient's Bill of Rights will result in litigation where federal agencies and state boards of nursing become involved with resultant actions against professionals.

HOW HEALTHCARE POLICY SHAPES ADMINISTRATIVE PRACTICE

The preceding sections have addressed laws that affect nursing practice. Participation in identifying and enacting workable solutions in healthcare settings can be enhanced when one understands health policy and the processes used to establish laws and regulations. The opportunities are limitless and include a great voice for nursing in health policy (Institute of Medicine, 2011).

Russell and Fawcett (2005) identified three types of policies that extend substantive knowledge for nursing and that are applicable to administrative practice (public, organizational, and professional):

> Public policies are those that are developed by nations, states, cities, and towns. The health policies promulgated by public entities typically have a broad impact on individuals, groups, communities, and health organizations. Health care institutions, such as hospitals, clinics, and home health agencies, to guide practice of a particular institution, develop organizational policies. Professional policies are standards or guidelines developed by discipline-specific and multidisciplinary associations to provide direction for those individuals and groups who work for or with the associations. (Russell & Fawcett, 2005, p. 320)

Whether it is a public, organizational, or professional policy, healthcare services, personnel, and expenditures are interrelated in nursing and health policy.

Russell and Fawcett's model consists of four increasingly broad and interacting levels that encompass the concepts of the nursing metaparadigm (human beings, environment, and nursing) posed by Fawcett (2005). The levels are not hierarchical but are rather increasingly broad as nursing and health policies advance to health-care systems. Level 1 emphasizes health policy by focusing on quality relative to the efficacy of nursing practice on the outcomes of individuals, families, groups, and communities. Level 2 focuses on health policy related to quality and cost associated with the effectiveness and efficiency of nursing practice and the healthcare delivery subsystems created by providers on outcomes of individuals, families, groups, and communities. Level 3 highlights health policy associated with access by focusing on societal demands for equity of costs and the distribution of care delivery burdens. Level 4 stresses health policy links to quality, cost, and access in relation to social and economic quality and cost-effective services and health-related resources.

Much dialogue has ensued as to how the model should be used for policy analysis and evaluation. The model proved useful as competency-based learning opportunities were designed. The model can also guide policy analysis and evaluation aligned with access, quality, cost, efficiency, and effectiveness. Whatever the practice environment or level of the practicing nurse, administrators can use components of the model to evaluate practice. Nurses are central to using policy to leverage widespread social change, especially public policy (Ridenour & Trautman, 2009). This supports the notion that health policy priorities shape and influence the welfare of others and the development and implementation of organizational policies.

Health administrators would be remiss not to consider each of the four levels as policies are developed, implemented, and evaluated. Quality, cost, and safe practice are expectations of the American public and are imperatives to survival in the current environment of competition.

Being knowledgeable of the laws embedded in policy, as well as those governing delivery systems and payment structures, is a basic and core competency that any healthcare administrator must possess. Otherwise, serious and long-standing issues will impact the individual professionals and organizational stability. Laws become precedents that affect healthcare systems, as discussed in the following section.

DELIVERY SYSTEMS AND PAYMENT STRUCTURES

The ACA positions consumers to be at the center of their health care. It offers all Americans the stability and flexibility necessary for informed choices about health care. Therefore, administrators are challenged to have an expanded lens when reformulating value-driven processes at all levels within healthcare systems (Porter O'Grady & Malloch, 2015). Otherwise, financial stability is jeopardized and sustainable quality outcomes diminish.

Two primary tenets underpin the ACA: insurance reform and healthcare delivery reform. There is a plethora of federal, state, and local responses to the reforms, and healthcare administrators must be aware of specific laws and regulations therein. Beyond the changes outlined in the ACA is survival during these challenging and stimulating times. An overview of various systems and payment structures is provided in the following paragraphs.

On January 31, 2013, the Centers for Medicare and Medicaid Services announced the healthcare organizations that were selected to participate in the Bundled Payments for Care Improvement initiative. Organizations will enter into payment arrangements that include financial and performance accountability for episodes of care. The initiative is inclusive of four models that lead to higher quality and more coordinated care at a lower cost to Medicare (CMS, 2014). Traditionally, Medicare made separate payments to providers for each of the individual services provided. This approach resulted in fragmented care with minimal coordination across providers and healthcare settings. Payment rewards the quantity of services rather than quality. Evidentiary reports show that bundled payments can align incentives for providers and hospitals, allowing closer alignment across specialties and settings.

The concept of value in health care is widely discussed among industry stakeholders; rarely is it defined the same way. As healthcare reform laws are fully implemented, value-based purchasing is a payment methodology that rewards quality of care through payment incentives and transparency. The key elements of value-based purchasing include the following:

- Contracts that explicitly detail the responsibilities of employers as purchasers with insurance, managed care, and hospital and physician groups as suppliers
- Information to support the management of purchasing activities
- Quality management to drive continuous improvement in the process of healthcare purchasing and in the delivery of healthcare services
- Incentives to encourage and reward consumers
- Education to assist employees become better healthcare consumers

In a system of value-based purchasing, employers and other purchasers gather and analyze information about the costs and quality of competing providers and health plans. They contract selectively with plans or provider organizations based on demonstrated performance. Quality data becomes a factor in setting plan prices. The best-performing plans and providers are rewarded with a greater volume of enrollees and patients.

Another innovation in healthcare reform is accountable care organizations (ACOs). ACOs are groups of physicians, hospitals, and other healthcare providers who voluntarily join together to provide coordinated care to Medicare patients. Coordinated care helps ensure that patients, especially those with chronic illnesses, get the right care that is timely, with a goal of avoiding unnecessary duplication of services and preventing medical errors. When an ACO succeeds, high-quality care with fewer expenditures follows, and the ACO will share the savings it achieves for the Medicare program (CMS, 2014).

Closely aligned with ACOs is the Medicare Shared Savings Program; the aim is to facilitate coordination and cooperation among providers to improve the quality of care for Medicare fee-for-service beneficiaries and to reduce costs. Eligible providers, hospitals, and suppliers may participate in the program by creating or participating in an ACO (CMS, 2013).

Although the jury is out on the effects of these delivery and payment systems, each has promise because quality, safe, and cost-effective care is the cornerstone in managing patients and remaining solvent. However, administrators must remain vigilant and informed. Care reforms will continue to be driven by cost reduction methods and coordination of services. Otherwise, systems have the potential for losses and can be subject to litigation if fraudulent practices occur. Teamwork and knowledge are powerful forces that are central to success within any organization.

SUMMARY

Laws shape health policy and are the cornerstones that govern health care in an era confronted with multiple challenges. How healthcare administrators respond to change and ensure that legal and ethical domains of care are upheld will continuously impact successes, failures, and responses to a challenging landscape. Being mindful of legal entities is not limited to administrators, but is a mandate for all practicing professionals. This chapter provided an overview of laws that impact delivery systems today and in the future as well as the impending need for administrators and providers to be advocates for policy that will shape care.

REFLECTIVE QUESTIONS

1. What is the difference between a bill and a law?
2. What steps are central for healthcare administrators to respond proactively to the numerous changes in health care today and in the future?
3. What elements constitute transparency in health care, and how can you ensure they are included within current areas of practice?
4. How does health policy govern healthcare delivery, and what impact can you have on shaping policy?

CASE STUDY 12-1   To Report or Not to Report? Joe's Dilemma

Lonnie K. Williams

Joe was recently appointed as the chief nursing officer (CNO) of a 25-bed rural community hospital that was unionized. The former CNO of 42 years had recently retired and recommended Joe for the position. This was Joe's first CNO position after graduation with a master's degree in business administration. His previous management experience was as a nurse manager of the facility for 2 years, where he was one of two BSN graduates. He has 6 years of nursing experience.

The staff at the facility have multiple years of experience, and all are residents of the community or adjoining towns. The staff is close-knit and supportive of each other and their families. Additionally, the newly appointed chief executive officer (CEO) is from an academic medical center and has managed ambulatory care services at that facility.

During Joe's first week of employment as the CNO, he was approached by the housekeeping supervisor, who requested an appointment to discuss a situation. Joe eagerly agreed and met with the supervisor. The supervisor stated that over a period of 3 years she and other housekeeping staff had observed the evening shift registered nurse (RN) injecting herself with medications in the upper thigh and often discarding the syringes in the employee lounge. When she was asked if she was okay, she always replied, "This is only for my condition." The housekeeping supervisor also said that many of the housekeeping

(continues)

CASE STUDY 12-1   To Report or Not to Report? Joe's Dilemma (Continued)

staff often said patients complained of pain, even though this RN had administered pain medication "using a needle." The supervisor stated that this had previously been discussed with the retired CNO, but no changes occurred. Joe told the supervisor he would handle the situation.

Joe was at a loss about the best course of action. Should he confront the nurse, investigate further, make a note of this meeting in the RN's personnel file, make a note for his management files, or even request the supervisor to complete a memorandum stating the information? Joe decided that he would observe the RN himself and initiate a pain management performance improvement project.

During the first few weeks of the quality improvement initiative, patients repeatedly complained about increased pain. Joe observed that the RN had several syringes in her lab coat pocket as she walked toward patient rooms. When Joe confronted the nurse, she stated, "These are for patients and not for you to worry about because I am the staff RN and you are the boss. If there is a problem, just call my union representative."

Joe remained at a loss for the best course of action and decided to discuss the issue with the chief of pharmacy, who was the RN's spouse. The chief of pharmacy said not to worry because patients have complained about her for years, and they get discharged home with plenty of medications for pain. Joe elected not to discuss this with anyone else, including the CEO. He received a call later that evening from a facility that he had recently interviewed with for a service line job. He had taken the CNO position as an interim position while he waited for an offer from that facility. Joe eagerly accepted the new position with a start date later that week. Joe abruptly resigned from the CNO position without addressing the issue.

Case Study Questions

1. What is the first action that Joe neglected from a legal and ethical perspective?
2. What course of action should Joe have initiated, and what legal issues did he incur for himself and the facility?
3. Review the reporting responsibilities of any licensed RN to state licensing boards and identify actions that Joe should have initiated after the first discussion with the housekeeping supervisor. What actions would you take if you were in Joe's position?

REFERENCES

Administrative Law. (2014). Retrieved from http://hg.org/adm.html
Agency for Healthcare Research and Quality. (n.d.). Retrieved from http://www.arhr.gov/
Aiken, T. (2004). *Legal, ethical, and political issues in nursing* (2nd ed.). Philadelphia, PA: F. A. Davis.
Alabama State Code. (2014). Alabama Code §§ 22-8-A-1-10. Retrieved from http://codes./p.findlaw.com
Alabama State Nurses' Association. (2014). Prescriptive authority for CRNPs. Retrieved from http://www.npalliance.org/
American Nurses Association. (2015). *Code of ethics for nurses.* Retrieved from http://www.nursingworld.org/codeofethics
American Nurses Credentialing Center. (2014). *2014 Magnet application manual.* Silver Springs, MD: Author.

Ashley, R. C. (2003). Understanding negligence. Retrieved from http://www
.aacnjournals.org/content/23/5/72.full

Barron, J. A., & Dienes, C. T. (1983). *Constitutional law: Judicial review*. St. Paul,
MN: West.

Baxter v. Montana 2009 WL 5155363 (Montana, 2009). Retrieved from http://
www.americanbar.org/content/dam/aba/migrated/aging/PublicDocuments
/baxtr_v_mont_sum.authcheckdam.pdf

Big Town Nursing Home, Inc., v. Newman CCA TX, 1970, 461 zd.ze.2d 195. (1994).
In *Prosser, Wade, & Schwartz's, torts: Cases and materials* (9th ed.). St. Paul, MN:
Foundation Press.

Blum, J., Morgan, E. S., Rose, W. L., Schlesinger, A. M., Jr., Stampp, K. M., & Wood-
ward, C. V. (1977). *The national experience: A history of the United States* (4th
ed.). New York, NY: Harcourt.

Brewer, K. (2014). Scope and standards-of-practice documents: Guiding you to
leadership success. *American Nurse Today, 9*(1), 50–51.

Calder v. Bull, 3 U.S. 386 (1798).

Centers for Medicare and Medicaid Services. (2014). Fact sheets: CMS finalizes
FY 2014 policy and payment changes for inpatient stays in acute-care and long-
term care hospitals. Retrieved from http://www.cms.gov/Newsroom.Media
ReleaseDatabase/Fact-Sheets/2014-Facts-sheets-items.2014-01-10-2-.html

Cheeks, D. (2013). 10 things you want to know about medical malpractice.
Retrieved from http://www.forbes.com/sites/learnvest/2013/05/16/10-things
-you-want-to-know-about-medical-malpractice/

Colorado Regulatory Dept. of PH FCCR. (2014). Retrieved from http://www
/colorado.gov/pacific/cdphe/regulations

Congressional Budget Office. (2009). Health. Retrieved from http://wwwcbo.gov
/publications/collections/health.cfm

Cooper, C. O. (2004). *A history of water law, water rights and water development in
Wyoming 1868–2002*. Riverton, WY: Cooper Consulting.

Criminal Law. (2014). Retrieved from http://www.legal-dictionary.thefree
dictinonary.com/Criminal+Law

Criminal Procedure. (2014). Retrieved from http://www.law.cornell.edu/

Cruzan v. Director, Missouri Dept. of Health 497 U.S. 261. (2014). Retrieved from
http://www.casebriefs.com/.../curzan-v-missouri-dept-of-health-2/

Democratic Form of Government. (2014). Retrieved from http://www.ushistory
.org/gov/lc.asp

Department of Justice. (2014). DEA 21 CFR ξ1304. 03 (6). Retrieved from http://
www.deadiverson.usdoj.gov/21cfr/2104cfrt.htm

Dorf, M. (2003). How the Florida legislator and governor have usurped the judicial
role. Retrieved from http://writ.news.findlaw/dorf/20031029.html

Employment Contracts (2014). Retrieved from http://www.allnurses.com/general-
nursing-discussion/have-you-ever-334124.html

Encyclopaedia Britannica. (2014). Retrieved from http://www.britannica.com/

Executive Branch. (2014). Retrieved from http://www.whitehouse.gov/

Fadig v. Municipality of Anchorage, 758 P.2d 911 (Alaska App., 1990). (2014).
Retrieved from http://www.courtlistener.com/alaskactapp/6Qww/fardig-v
-municipality-of-anchorage/

Fawcett, J. (2005). *Contemporary nursing knowledge: Analysis and evaluation of nursing models and theories* (2nd ed.). Philadelphia, PA: F. A. Davis.

Felony Charges against Julie Thao. (2014). Retrieved from http://community.the-hospitalist.org/

Florida Administrative Code. (2014). FL Statute 466.003, Rule 64B9-4.010(1). Retrieved from http://flrules.org/...redaFile.asp?...6

Florida Chapter XXXII 464.001-.027 (NPA). (2014). Retrieved from http://www.strainceu.com/

Ford v. Revlon, Inc. 153 Ariz. 38, 734 P.2d 580. (1987). Retrieved from https://www.courtlistener.com/ariz/7btk/ford_v_revlon_inc/

Gladstone, W. (2014). Retrieved from http://www.archive.org.strem/s5princetonrev04newyuoft/sprinctonrev04newyuoft_djvu.txt

Health Insurance Portability and Accountability Act of 1996 (HIPAA) 45CFR, 160-164. (2014). Retrieved from http://www.hhs.gov/ocr/privacy

History.com. (2014). Slavery in America. Retrieved from http://www.history.com/topics/black-history/slavery/

Horne, C. (1915). The code of Hammurabi: Introduction. Retrieved from http://www.fordham.edu/halsall/ancient/hamcode.asp#horne

Independence Hall Association. (2014). The New England colonies. Retrieved from http://www.ushistory.org/

In re Guardianship of Schiavo, Part II of the Opinion, Judge Greer. (2014). Retrieved from http://writ.news.findlaw.com/dorf/20031029.html

In re Quinlan. 70 N.J. 10 (197) 355 A.2d 647 (1977).

Institute for Safe Medication Practices. (2014). The just culture community. Retrieved from https://wwwlsmp.org.

Institute of Medicine. (2011). *The future of nursing: Leading change, advancing health*. Washington, DC: National Academies Press.

Johnson, P. (2014). Education of health professionals: The RIBN initiative. Retrieved from http://www.ncmedicaljournal.com/archives/?75109

Johnston, A. (1887). The first century of the Constitution. *Princeton Law, 4*, 175.

The Judiciary. (2014). Role of the judiciary on when to hear a case. Retrieved from http://constitution.laws.com/article-3-of-the-constitution

Judiciary Branch. (2014). Retrieved from http://www.uscourts.gov/

Kathleen K. v. Robert B. 150 Cal. App. 3d 992, 198 Cal. Rpt273. (1984). Intentional transmission of sexually transmitted disease. Retrieved from http://www.Leagle.com/

Knox, L., & Skip, E. L. (2014). Breakin' the law. Retrieved from www.europeanhistory.boisestate.edu/

Law. (1999). *Black's law dictionary*. St. Paul, MN: Garner West Group.

Legal Information Institute. (n.d.). False imprisonment. Retrieved from https://www.law.cornell.edu/wex/false_imprisonment

Library of Congress. (2014). The Declaration of Independence, the US Constitution, and the Bill of Rights. Retrieved from http://www.archives.gov/...decl...

Linda R.S. v. Richard D., 410 U.S. 614 (1973). Retrieved from http://supreme.justia.com/cases/federal/us/410/614/case.html

Longo, J. (2010). Combating disruptive behaviors: Strategies to promote a healthy work environment. *OJIN: The Online Journal of Issues in Nursing, 15*, Manuscript 5. doi:10.3912/OJIN.Volu15No01Man05

Louisiana Civil Code. (2014). Retrieved from http://legis.la.gov/legis/LawSearch
.aspx

Marx, D. (2001). *Patient safety and the "just culture." A primer for health care executives*. New York, NY: Columbia University.

Marx, D. (2008). *The just culture algorithm*. New York, NY: Outcome Engineering, LLC.

MN Stat. §§ 144.343(2)(7) (1988). *Hodgson v. State of Minn*. 853 F.2d 1452. Retrieved from https://laws.findlaw.com/us/497/417.html

Montana. (1988). 29 USCA§2000e-2(a) *Stark v. Circle K Corp*.

Montesquieu, de B. (1748). *Spirit of laws*. JG Bell & Son. Retrieved from http://www.constitution.org/cm/sol.htm/

Moral Law. (2014). *Moral law and man's duty to society*. Retrieved from http://www.eyler.freeservers.com/JeffPers/jefpco3b.html

MyMaineConnection: Maine Children's Insurance (Chips) Program. (2014). Retrieved from http://www.mejp.org/content/need-health-Insurance

National Archives and Records Administration. (2014). Magna Carta and its American legacy. Retrieved from http://www.archives.gov/exhibits/featured_documents/magna_carta/legacy.html

National Center for Constitutional Studies. (2015). The Declaration of Independence and the Constitution of the United States. Retrieved from http://www.nccs.net/introduction-to-americas-founding-documents.php

National Council of State Boards of Nursing. (2014). *The consensus model for APRN regulation*. Retrieved from https://www.ncsb.org/421.htm

National Council of State Boards of Nursing. (2011). *What you need to know about nursing licensure and boards of nursing* [Brochure]. Chicago, IL: Author.

National Federation of Independent Business v. Sebelius No. 11-393 by certiorari. (2014). Retrieved from http://www.supremecourt.gov/search.aspx?Search=Natil.+Fed+of+Indpt.+Bus.+v+Sebelius+No.+11-393+by+certiorari&type=Site/

Natural Law. (2014). Retrieved from http://humanityawakens.wordpress.com2013/10/06/understanding-natural-law-vs

O'Connor, L. (2014). McMath case may set precedent for parental rights. Retrieved from http://www.huffingtonpost.com.2014/01/07/jahi-mcmath-precendent_n_4557342.html

Paine, T. (2014). Common sense. Retrieved from http://www.ushistory.org/paine/commonsense/

Painter, R. (2009). Developments in Texas advance directives. *Houston Lawyer*, (September–October).

Peterson, A. M., & Kopishke, L. (2010). *Legal nurse consulting principles* (3rd ed.). Boca Raton, FL: CRC Press.

Peterson v. Sorlien, 299 N.W. 2d 123 (Minn. 1980). Retrieved from http://www.law.cornell.edu/wex/false_imprisonment/

Philipsen, N. (2011). The criminalization of mistakes in nursing. *Journal of Nurse Practitioners*, *7*, 719–726.

Poliner v. Texas Health Systems (2006) WL 770425. Retrieved from https://www.jpands.org/vol13no4/poliner.pdf

Porter O'Grady, T., & Malloch, K. (2015). *Quantum leadership: Building better partnerships for sustainable health* (4th ed.). Burlington, MA: Jones & Bartlett Learning.

Posner, R. A. (1993). *The trouble with jurisprudence*. Cambridge, MA: Harvard University Press.

Powers, T. (1973). *War at home: Vietnam and the American people*. Boston, MA: GK Hall.

Public Opinion. (2014). Public opinion of legal marijuana in Colorado and Washington. Retrieved from http://www.whotv.com...public-opinion -legalization-of-marijuana-more-...

Quaid v. Baxter Healthcare Corp. No. 1-08-2727. (2009). Retrieved from http:// caselaw.com

Quill v. Vacco 521 US 793. (1997). Retrieved from http://www.nationalcenter.org /Vacco.html

Reason, J. (1997). *Managing the risks of organisational accidents*. London, UK: Ashgate.

Reston, J. (1963, August 29). "I have a dream . . .": Peroration by Dr. King sums up a day the capital will remember. *New York Times*.

Ridenour, N., & Trautman, D. (2009). A primer for nursing on advancing health reform policy. *Journal of Professional Nursing*, *25*(6), 358–362.

Roe v. Wade, 410 U.S. 113 (1973). Retrieved from http://www.lawnix.com/cases /re-wad.html

Rohwer, C. D., & Schaber, G. D. (1997). *Contracts* (4th ed.). St. Paul, MN: WestLaw.

Roles of Congress. (2014). Retrieved from http://www.house.gov/

Roles of the President. (2014). Retrieved from http://dailycaller.com/2014/01/14

Russell, G. E., & Fawcett, J. (2005). The conceptual model for nursing and health policy revisited. *Policy, Politics and Nursing Practice*, *6*(44), 319–326.

Russell, K. (2012). Nurse practice acts guide and govern nursing practice. *Journal of Nursing Regulation*, *9*(3), 36–42.

Shalo, S. (2007). To err is human, but for some nurses a crime. *American Journal of Nursing*, *3*, 20–21.

State of Alabama. (2014). *Board of medical examiners, chapter 540-X-18*. Retrieved from http://www.albme.org/Documents/Rules/Tem/540-X-18%20Final.pdf

State of Florida. (2014). Florida constitution. Retrieved from http://www.leg.state .fl.us.../Index.cfm?...Constitution...3...

Texas Code (NPR)§303.001(5). (2014). Retrieved from http://www.bon.state.tx.us /faq_peer_review.asp

The 1990 Self Determination Act. (2014). Retrieved from http://www.american .bar.org/...patient-self-determin...

The Joint Commission. (2008). Sentinel event alert. Retrieved from http://www .jointcommission.org/SentinelEvents/SentinelEventAlert/sea 40.htm?

Tiffany, J. A. (1867). *Treatise on government and constitutional law being an inquiry into the source and limitation of governmental authority according to American theory*. Albany, NY: Weed, Parsons.

Tocco, S., & DeFontes, J. (2014). Managing our fears to improve patient safety. *American Nurse Today*, *9*(5), 34–36.

U.S. Department of Health and Human Services. (n.d.). The privacy rule. Retrieved from http://www.hhs.gov/ocr/privacy/hipaa/administrative/privacyrule/index .html

U.S. Department of Labor. (2015). OSH Act of 1970. Retrieved from https://www .osha.gov/pls/oshaweb/owasrch.search_form?p_doc_type=OSHACT

U.S. Government Printing Office. (2015). Federal digital system. Retrieved from http://www.gpo.gov/fdsys/search/home.action

U.S. v. Warshak et al., US 632 f ed 266 (Sixth Cir., 2010). Retrieved from http://www.ca6.uscourts.gov/opinions.pdf/10a0377p-06.pdf

USHistory.org. (2014). 15. Drafting the constitution. Retrieved from http://www.ushistory.org/us/15.asp

Vietnamese Fishermen's Ass'n v. Knight of the K.K.K., 518 F. Supp. 993 (S.D. Tex., 1994). In Prosser, W. L., Wade, J. W., & Schwartz, V. E. (Eds.), *Torts, cases, and materials* (9th ed.). Foundation Press Eagan, MN.

VT. Stat. Ann. Tit. 18 §§5252-5262 (Sup0 1985). Retrieved from http://www.lexisnexis.com/hottopics/vtstatutesconstctrules/

Wainwright, G. (2007). Ethical aspects of withdrawing and withholding treatment. *Nursing Standard, 21*(33), 46–50.

Washington Death with Dignity Act, RCW 70.245. (2014). Retrieved from http://www.doh.wa.gov/YouandYourFamily/IllnessandDisease/DeathwithDignityAct.aspx

Washington RCW 46.61.503. (2014). Retrieved from http://app.leg.wa.gov/Rcw/default.aspx?cite=46.61.503

Washington v. Glucksberg, 521 U.S. 702, 117 S.Ct. 2258, 117 S. Ct. 2302; 138 L.Ed.772. (2014). Retrieved from http://www.casebriefs.com/blog/law/constitutional-law/constitutional-law-keyed-to-Sullivan/substantive-due-process-rise-decline-rivival/Washington-v-glucksberg-7/

What Would the Founders Think? (2011). George Mason, the framer who refused to sign the Constitution. Retrieved from http://www.whatwouldthefoundersthink.com/george-mason-the-framer-who-refused-to-sign-the-constitution

Whiting, R. (2002). *A natural right to die: Twenty-three centuries of debate.* Westport, CT: Greenwood Press.

Wisconsin Department of Regulation and Licensing. (2014). *In the matter of disciplinary proceedings re Julio Thao, LS06121NUR247.* Retrieved from https://online.drl.wi.gov/decisions/2006/ls0612145nur-00075545.pdf

Women's Suffrage Movement. (2014). Retrieved from http://womenshistory.net.com

The Work of a Nation. (2014). Retrieved from http://www.cia.gov/library/.html

CHAPTER 13

Anticipating and Managing Risk in a Culture of Quality, Safety, and Value

Shea Polancich and Marylane Wade Koch

LEARNING OBJECTIVES

1. Examine challenges to achieving high-quality health care and patient safety in the United States.
2. Identify evolving approaches that address healthcare improvement and patient safety, including use of internal data (microsystems analysis) and external data (research evidence).
3. Identify and discuss components of a quality improvement program.
4. Define tools used in the quality improvement process.
5. Discuss the importance of problem identification and resolution, monitoring and feedback, customer satisfaction, and research in providing high-quality health care and patient safety.
6. Discuss strategies to anticipate risk and avert harm.

AONE KEY COMPETENCIES

I. Communication and relationship building
II. Knowledge of the healthcare environment
III. Leadership
IV. Professionalism
V. Business skills

AONE KEY COMPETENCIES DISCUSSED IN THIS CHAPTER

II. Knowledge of the healthcare environment
III. Leadership
IV. Professionalism

II. **Knowledge of the healthcare environment**
   - Clinical practice knowledge
   - Patient care delivery models and work design knowledge
   - Healthcare economics knowledge
   - Healthcare policy knowledge
   - Understanding of governance

- Understanding of evidence-based practice
- Outcomes measurement
- Knowledge of, and dedication to, patient safety
- Understanding of utilization and case management
- Knowledge of quality improvement and metrics
- Knowledge of risk management

III. Leadership
- Foundational thinking skills
- Personal journey disciplines
- Ability to use systems thinking
- Succession planning
- Change management

IV. Professionalism
- Personal and professional accountability
- Career planning
- Ethics
- Evidence-based clinical and management practices
- Advocacy for the clinical enterprise and for nursing practice
- Active membership in professional organizations

FUTURE OF NURSING: FOUR KEY MESSAGES

1. Nurses should practice to the full extent of their education and training.
2. Nurses should achieve higher levels of education and training through an improved education system that promotes seamless academic progression.
3. Nurses should be full partners with physicians and other health professionals in redesigning health care in the United States.
4. Effective workforce planning and policy making require better data collection and information infrastructure.

Introduction

One of the most challenging aspects of health care today is to deliver safe, high-quality care within the confines of fiscal responsibility. In 2009, approximately $2.5 trillion was spent on health care in the United States, with less than optimal results. The key to challenging this less than desirable outcome of high cost and low quality may require renewed focus and adherence to the principles associated with both the improvement and safety sciences.

All individuals who work within a healthcare facility should have an understanding of the challenges associated with the delivery of high-quality, low-cost health care. Nurse leaders are particularly positioned to address these challenges and lead organizational change. Leading interdisciplinary teams is part of this mandate (Siriwardena et al., 2014). With this understanding should come a cadre of individuals who are equipped with the competencies and skills necessary to improve care delivery at the microsystem level, and as such there should also be a complement of individuals who are trained to extend any improvements made at the microsystem level up to the macrosystem level (Batalden, 2010).

Nurses at all levels, from staff nurses to executive nurses, are uniquely positioned to develop and lead improvements. Frontline nurses are at the sharpest end of health care and are, in fact, the quality and safety leaders for patients. These individuals become the last line of defense for safe, effective, quality care (Davis & Adams, 2011; Eggenberger, 2012; Marshall, 2013; Rutherford et al., 2008; Thompson, 2009). Nursing leaders and managers, particularly those trained at the graduate level, should assume leadership roles in quality and safety at the bedside and throughout the system. Effective improvement strategies developed at the bedside should have an impact both horizontally and vertically.

To achieve successes in improvement and safety at the bedside, individuals need to be educated in the theoretical underpinnings of improvement science and the practical skills for examining a microsystem and developing evidence-based interventions. However, education about theoretical content alone is insufficient to develop the required competencies to successfully develop, lead, and manage bedside improvement (Dearmon et al., 2012; Porter-O'Grady, 2011). Experiential application of improvement skills will be required. The purpose of this chapter is to describe key components necessary to foster the quality and safety competencies that are needed for developing and implementing evidence-based quality and safety projects.

The topics in this section include the following: identifying techniques for determining the internal impetus for change at the unit level by understanding and analyzing the microsystem; describing an effective strategy for developing the burning clinical question; identifying a method for determining the external support for change by describing the strategies for literature synthesis based on searching and appraisal of the literature; discussing the importance of a framework that supports the improvement, from theoretical to conceptual to methodological frameworks; describing an improvement model and the scientific underpinnings associated with the evolution of the model for improvement (MFI); and, finally, providing a discussion on analysis and measurement for improvement. As quality and safety competencies are developed, systems are poised to anticipate risk, mitigate loss, and design care models that yield sustainable value. Nurse leaders with knowledge in quality and safety will be essential to identify concerns and support the implementation of quality and safety improvements as they lead organizations.

EVOLVING PERSPECTIVES IN HEALTHCARE QUALITY MANAGEMENT

Nursing quality assurance programs began in hospitals in the 1960s with the voluntary implementation of nursing audits. These programs were designed to set standards for nursing care delivery and to establish criteria by which to evaluate these standards. However, healthcare professionals came to understand that high-quality care could not be ensured by audits. The Joint Commission determined that to ensure good quality, continuous improvement must be demonstrated. Synonyms for quality management programs have emerged, such as quality improvement, continuous quality improvement, and performance improvement. Quality control, which is part of quality management, refers to conforming to standards.

Accreditation agencies mandate that most aspects of health care must be incorporated into quality management programs. Divisional or departmental programs need to support an organization's mission. Quality management plans should incorporate customer satisfaction and patient rights and safety (The Joint Commission, 2014). Leadership must embrace quality as a continuous organizational goal.

Several groups besides The Joint Commission have stepped up to address improving the quality of health care in the United States. One of these is the Institute of Medicine (IOM), which began focusing on assessment and improvement in 1996. In the IOM's 2001 *Crossing the Quality Chasm* report (Institute of Medicine [IOM], 2001a), quality was described as evidence-based care producing desired health outcomes from services delivered. This report supported the evaluation of quality based on Donabedian's quality theory that addresses structure, process, and outcome. Implementation of the IOM guidelines included establishing the mission and vision, creating a quality management plan to provide an organizational framework that supports quality management, using evidence-based clinical practice, and providing utilization management (Donabedian, 2002). Other studies and reports from the IOM include the following:

- *To Err Is Human: Building a Safer Health System* (IOM, 1999)
- *Envisioning the National Health Care Quality Report* (IOM, 2001b)
- *Leadership by Example: Coordinating Government Roles in Improving Health Care Quality* (IOM, 2002)
- *Priority Areas for National Action: Transforming Health Care Quality* (IOM, 2003)

In 2010 the Robert Wood Johnson Foundation released a report containing testimony from The Joint Commission's Nursing Advisory Council. The recommendations address patient care quality and safety, focusing on clinical nursing practice, nursing education, and nursing research. Particular attention was paid to transforming care at the bedside, with the focus of rapid cycle change.

To read the report, go to http://www.rwjf.org/content/dam/farm/reports/issue_briefs/2014/rwjf411417.

Microsystems

To improve a system or a process, nurse leaders must begin with the end in mind. What should drive improvement at the bedside? Is it an ineffective process? For example, ask how long it takes, on average, to discharge a patient from the unit and if the process is both effective and efficient. Another goal may be to transform outcome measures that are perceived as worse than average when compared to a benchmark. For example, ask if the unit is at the top-performing decile for falls and if it has been a sustainable pattern for an extended period of time. Improvement begins on the unit and should be a by-product of an effective internal assessment and analysis of the microsystem of care at the clinical unit level. Internal data quantify the need to improve specifically for the unit and provides a baseline for comparison when interventions are developed and implemented (Batalden, 2010).

Microsystems Defined

What is a microsystem? What does this term actually mean? The majority of the work on clinical microsystem analysis and the associated terminology was developed at Dartmouth Institute under the leadership and guidance of Paul Batalden. According to the Dartmouth definition, the clinical microsystem is a combination of a small team of people who work together on a regular basis, or as needed, to provide care for a discrete subpopulation of patients. Included in the microsystem definition are the patients that receive care. In addition, the microsystem has clinical and business aims, linked processes, shared information and information technology, with measurable outcomes for the services provided. This microsystem exists within the confines of a larger macrosystem (Batalden, 2010).

The essential elements of a clinical microsystem include a core team of healthcare professionals; a defined population or populations of individuals who are cared for by the healthcare team; information and the infrastructure for information technology; the environment in which care is delivered, including equipment; and the processes associated with the care that is delivered (Batalden, 2010). A clinical microsystem is specifically focused or centered on the patient and the delivery of direct patient care. An alternate definition of a microsystem is a small work unit that supports the clinical care delivery process. In these situations, the stakeholders or those who receive the delivered product may be a group other than the patient. In these situations, a microsystem may provide support to the care delivery unit, but the impact to the patient may be indirectly provided. Administrative areas and informatics departments are examples of indirect clinical microsystems that impact the macrosystem process and provide a service that impacts patient care. Nurse leaders analyze both the direct clinical microsystem and the indirect microsystem that provides vital data necessary to improve the delivery of care to the patient in a healthcare system.

Microsystem Analysis and the Five Ps

Why would a nurse leader analyze the microsystem? Microsystem analysis is an essential component of healthcare improvement because a robust analysis provides the following outcomes: first, microsystem analysis provides supporting data or a rationale for an improvement; second, quantitative data provide a baseline for the improvement aims that can be measurably examined and are not based on speculation or result in impossible goal expectations (Batalden, 2010).

According to Batalden and colleagues (2003), a comprehensive examination of the clinical microsystem includes an analysis of the Five Ps of the microsystem. These five components include the purpose, the patients (populations), the processes, the patterns, and the providers. Systematic data collection is required for each of these five elements. Workbooks that are publicly available from the Dartmouth website provide detailed tools for examining each aspect of the microsystem (Microsystems Academy, 2015). These workbooks have been arranged to include templates for inpatient care, outpatient (ambulatory) care, and specialty care, such the emergency department.

Purpose

Beginning with the purpose, each phase of the microsystem analysis provides data that pinpoint areas for improvement. The purpose of a unit may be very specific and well defined. However, in this age of healthcare reform, healthcare organizations, in particular academic medical centers, do not have the luxury of completely specialized units (Batalden et al, 2003). For example, when an organization is at capacity on census and an open bed becomes available, there is a high probability that specialization will not be accommodated due to system demands and patients' needs for care. Healthcare organizations have entered an age in which boarding patients in the emergency department results in a lack of specialization for emergency care. It becomes a unit that must adhere to publicly reported evidence-based care that was previously the responsibility of an inpatient unit. Specialty intensive care units are now housing and providing intensive care to a varied population that could range from trauma care to cardiac intensive care. It is becoming more evident as healthcare needs grow and capacity remains constant for a unit's purpose to evolve to more global goals of the appropriate care for every patient, every time.

Patients or Populations

In alignment with the purpose, understanding the patients or populations who receive care in a microsystem provides crucial information. As with the purpose, the patient population on a unit may vary. What may have been common in past years may be fluctuating to accommodate a changing healthcare system. Therefore, understanding the most commonly treated diagnoses on the unit provides vital information to achieve the mission of evidence-based care for all patients on a unit (Nelson et al., 2003). For example, understanding a shifting pattern on a unit with primarily cardiac patients may reveal that due to capacity issues, a larger volume of pneumonia patients is being transferred to the unit. This could lead to the development of care protocols or guidelines specific to a patient population that would otherwise be treated and housed on a different unit.

Processes

Understanding the processes is another important component of microsystem analysis. Processes are the work flow of a microsystem (Nelson et al., 2003). What steps are taken to perform a task that is essential to the delivery of care? Processes are the infrastructure that supports the functioning of a unit. As such, when a process is ineffective or fails, the results can be detrimental to the health of a patient. Understanding how a process currently flows is the first step in understanding how a current process may fail. Early failure detection may enhance risk mitigation and prevent future system failures.

To examine a process, nurse leaders consult a visual organizational strategy or a flowchart. The first step in the development of a flowchart is to observe the actual steps of the process. Observation is essential because many times there are preconceived ideas about how the process should function versus how it actually functions (Nelson et al., 2003). Throughout the observation process, the nurse leader makes notes of each step in sequence and is careful to note any subprocesses. After the entire process is detailed in sequential steps, it is transferred to a visual flow diagram. Several types of tools are available for flow diagramming that range in price and complexity. However, a simple depiction of the process steps and decisions points are all that are necessary to examine the work flow and determine whether there are areas that may benefit from improvement. These improvements may range from inefficiencies associated with time management to failure points that may result in patient harm.

Patterns

The next component of the microsystem analysis is to examine the patterns. This is a comprehensive data collection and analysis process. Data related to structural, process, or outcome measures may provide insight into areas of the microsystem that may warrant improvement or assist in prioritization of areas of risk or opportunity. Structural measures are metrics that may provide detail about the functioning of the infrastructure of the unit (Nelson et al., 2003). For example, metrics such as daily census highlight the operational capacity of a unit. Process metrics are measures that may provide detail on the functioning of a process supporting clinical care. For example, the average time to discharge is a process metric that highlights the efficiency or effectiveness of the discharge process. Outcome metrics are measures that may provide detail about clinical outcomes for a patient population. For example, the unit mortality rate may provide information on treatment effectiveness. Collecting information and observing data from any of the types of metrics may show trends or patterns over time that may warrant examination and future action or improvement.

Providers

The final component of the microsystem analysis is to examine the providers working within the unit. Detailing the number of full-time equivalents assigned to a unit may provide nurse leaders with an opportunity to improve staffing or decrease inefficiencies and costs (Nelson et al., 2003). For example, if a pattern of increasing errors associated with medication reconciliation occurs in a unit, a review of the providers may uncover a lack of available clinical personnel to complete the task effectively. Perhaps support to invest in a clinical pharmacist may be gleaned from these data.

Overall, a microsystem analysis is a comprehensive analysis of the work unit. Using a standardized and data-driven approach, each of the Five Ps synergistically provides detail on the operations and outcomes of the work unit and may highlight opportunities for improvement (Nelson et al., 2003). In addition, the robust quantification of information provides a baseline assessment of metrics that may be used to set improvement targets of benchmarks associated with interventions created to improve processes or patterns. Although a clinical microsystem analysis is geared toward a clinical work unit, the rigor of the process may be expanded to other small working units. As such, even nonclinical support areas may benefit from a standardized quantification and analysis of the unit infrastructure and supporting processes and outcomes. Although nurse leaders do not perform the actual assessment, they have an important role in supporting those who do the work and articulating the discipline and systematic approach needed to see the work through the implementation, evaluation, and sustaining phases.

The analysis also provides internal data that can be used as a comparator for evidence contained in the literature. How does this microsystem compare to external data from studies outside the organization? Individuals who develop an improvement project should utilize both internal and external data.

An Example from the Field

While doing the microsystem analysis, intensive care nurses in a 15-bed medical intensive care unit (MICU) in Hospital ABC noted the following pattern. From January to December of 2012, the catheter-associated urinary tract infection (CAUTI) count had ranged from 0 to 5 per month. However, in January 2013 the count per month began to increase. From January 2013 to January 2014, the CAUTI count per month ranged from 7 to 13. This increase was identified during a microsystem analysis that specifically examined patterns. In the same microsystem analysis it was discovered that there are 10 medical staff providers who regularly see patients on this unit for a particular service. Five of the providers are nurse practitioners, and five are attending physicians. While the process was examined, it was discovered that there was variation in diagnosis and treatment patterns among the nurse practitioners and attending physicians.

The team asked the following questions: Where do I go from here? What should my next steps be? The microsystem analysis yielded a pattern for analysis and improvement (**Figure 13-1**). It was provided to the unit for review so potential strategies to decrease the CAUTI rate could be developed.

Using this internal data, the unit decided that the pattern was a risk to the welfare of the patients. Any increase in the number of infections was deemed to be enough of a risk to warrant improvement.

Developing the Burning Clinical Question

After a thorough microsystem analysis, there are often multiple areas that may be opportunities for improvement. This may result in several questions that warrant an

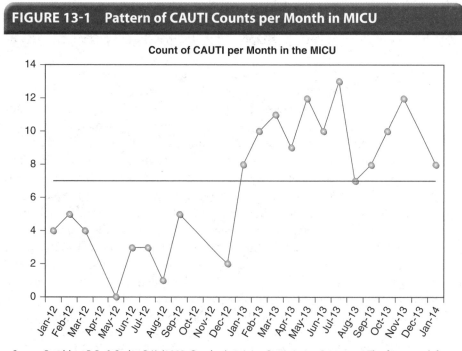

FIGURE 13-1   Pattern of CAUTI Counts per Month in MICU

Source: Batalden, P. B., & Stoltz, P. K. (1993, October). © Joint Commission Resources: The framework for continual improvement of health care. *Joint Commission Journal on Quality and Patient Safety*. Reprinted with permission.

evidence-based approach to improvement. One of the more utilized approaches to developing a clinical question for study is to develop a PICOT question: population, intervention, comparison, outcome, time frame (Melynk & Fineout-Overholt, 2015).

A PICOT question uses a structured format to define all aspects of a burning clinical question that may arise from a microsystem analysis. The P defines the population of interest. The I defines the intervention that will be applied to the population. The C is the comparison for the intervention, and in many cases it is current practice. The O is the outcome of interest that will be studied based on the intervention. Finally, the T is the time frame for studying the impact of the intervention on the proposed outcomes. Other forms and types of PICOT questions include prediction or prognosis, diagnosis or diagnostic test, etiology, and meaning. However, the PICOT question for an intervention is frequently used for improvement projects that require an intervention (Melynk & Fineout-Overholt, 2015).

Developing a PICOT Question: Application to Microsystem Pattern

The example of the microsystem analysis regarding an increase in CAUTI rates is a great starting point to develop a PICOT question for an intervention. From that example we will create a PICOT question for which we may want to implement an improvement based on the most current evidence.

A team in the MICU came together to discuss the most appropriate clinical question. This process may result in multiple questions because there are multiple provider types in the room; there are physicians and nurse practitioners, and the staff nurses are the primary care providers who manage urinary catheters. Each provider has a different scope of practice; therefore, the intervention may vary based on the perspective of the provider.

For this example we will focus on the function of the nurse practitioner. Because the nurse practitioner typically follows established protocols for diagnosis and treatment, the following PICOT question may be developed:

> In MICU adult patients (aged 18 years or older) who have a recent or indwelling urinary catheter and a laboratory-confirmed UTI (bacteria count), how does the implementation of an evidence-based algorithm for CAUTI treatment (antibiotics for symptomatic patients/antibiotics for asymptomatic patients) compare with current practice and impact the MICU CAUTI rate in the next 3 months?

This question will be used to search and synthesize the literature related to urinary tract infections, specifically in the MICU adult patient population. The nurse practitioner and the MICU team will come together to develop an evidence-based algorithm for CAUTI treatment that may be standardized to reduce variation and possibly promote an expected outcome of decreasing the number of CAUTI infections per month.

Literature Search and Synthesis

After the internal data have been established through the microsystem analysis and after the clinical question has been developed, a literature search and synthesis should be completed to gather external evidence to address the identified problem, support the intervention, and establish external benchmarks for improvement, if available.

Searching the most current literature is a key skill that must be developed when improving care at the bedside. In this age of technology, searching for information in an electronic database may be accomplished in a matter of minutes. However, this skill does require specific competencies in the electronic database search process.

Commonly Used Databases

In searching the most current evidence for clinical questions, the Cumulative Index to Nursing and Allied Health (CINAHL) and MEDLINE through PubMed are appropriate sources for nursing and medicine. MEDLINE was developed by the National Library of Medicine and contains journal citations and abstracts for biomedical information from around the world. Access to MEDLINE is publicly available through PubMed (National Center for Biotechnology Information, n.d.). Medical Subject Headings (MeSH) is the National Library of Medicine's controlled vocabulary thesaurus (U.S. National Library of Medicine, 2013). MeSH consists of sets of terms naming descriptors in a hierarchical structure that permits searching at various levels of specificity. The understanding and use of MeSH terms facilitates searching within the MEDLINE database.

EBSCO hosts the CINAHL database. It provides access to hundreds of journals for nursing and the allied health professions, with archives dating back to 1937. In addition to full-text articles, CINAHL also contains evidence-based care sheets and quick lessons, which contain information about diseases and the most effective evidence-based treatment options. CINAHL is typically accessible from biomedical libraries located on the campuses of most academic medical centers.

Searching the Literature: Application to Microsystem Patterns and Processes

The key to effectively searching the literature is identifying key terms specific to the clinical question. Based on the example clinical question identified earlier in this chapter, a need has been identified to decrease the number of CAUTIs in the MICU. In this example, the intervention is specific to evidence-based diagnosis and treatment for adult patients, with a focus on the scope of the nurse practitioner role.

To begin the search, think broadly about the background or the global topic. Using MEDLINE, the search term *urinary tract infections* will likely yield numerous results. From this search one may find terms or phrases that help limit the results more specifically to the foreground topic of *adults* with *urinary tract infections* in a *medical intensive care unit*. Even more specifically, *evidence-based practice protocols or algorithm use* may also be added to the search.

Because the search is being performed in MEDLINE, the MeSH headings may also provide additional information and strategies to narrow the search. The National Library of Medicine provides details on how to identify MeSH terms (U.S. National Library of Medicine, 2015).

After the search terms have been identified, inclusion criteria for the search must be determined. For example, many databases have functionality that allows filtering by items such as human or nonhuman, age, type of study, and level of evidence.

Although MEDLINE and CINAHL are often effective for producing results, it is wise to not limit searches to particular sources. Google Scholar and publicly available websites, such as the Agency for Healthcare Research and Quality (AHRQ) (www.ahrq.gov) and the National Guideline Clearinghouse (www.guideline.gov), provide a wealth of information that may be relevant to the topic under investigation. In fact, evidence-based clinical projects across the country have been archived on the AHRQ Innovations Exchange website. These entries provide detail, including the types and level of evidence, supporting interventions and outcomes that were tested and tried within the clinical domain.

Rating the Evidence

After a literature search has been completed, it is necessary to rate the evidence to effectively synthesize the findings. Although great detail will not be provided here about rating the evidence, selecting a rating scale is important (Melynk & Fineout-Overholt, 2015). The scale provided here is just one example of the types of ratings that may be used when evaluating each journal article. The rating scale for an evidence appraisal includes evaluating research from the highest level (Level I) to the lowest level (Level VII). For example, Level I includes evidence from a systematic review or a meta-analysis of all relevant random controlled trials (RCTs). Level III is the rating for evidence obtained from well-designed controlled trials with randomization. Level VII, as the lowest level, is evidence from the opinions of authorities or reports of expert committees (Melynk & Fineout-Overholt, 2015).

Organizing the Literature Search: Development of an Evidence Table

An evidence table is a valuable tool to organize the information obtained from a literature search. In addition, it serves as a guide or checklist for the items that are needed to compose a robust literature synthesis. After an evidence table is completed, the synthesis of the literature follows a natural progression from all the organized information. It is a matter of translating the table into words. An example of an evidence table includes components of research evidence, including the type of research design or method, the sample or setting, data sources, major variables studied and their operational definitions, data analysis, findings, level of evidence (I–VII), and appraisal worth. An assessment of the research evidence can assist with determining the highest level of evidence (rating) and if the available evidence is strong, moderately strong, or weak. This guides the author in determining the next steps toward improvement. Using an evidence table as a tool to determine the best and highest level of evidence also provides a systematic way to synthesize the literature. For example, the table provides a summary of individual studies and guidelines from which a synthesis of the research evidence can be done.

The literature search and synthesis process is a necessary skill for developing an improvement project. This process is not a limited or one-time activity. The process should be used at multiple points in the development of an improvement project, from the development of the initial clinical PICOT question to the exploration of an evidence-based intervention. Improvement that is not evidence based is likely limited or may produce less than desirable outcome, unless no evidence exists.

Theoretical, Conceptual, and Methodological Frameworks

The value of a theoretical, conceptual, or methodological framework is often overlooked when developing an improvement project. However, these frameworks provide structure or scaffolding for an improvement project (Melynk & Fineout-Overholt, 2015). Much time and energy has been invested in the development of frameworks. The use of a framework helps to bind theory and practice together. In essence, does what we expect to happen actually occur? There are many types of frameworks, including physiological, health promotion, systems change, teaching and learning, total quality management, and self-efficacy. Methodological frameworks may also include the MFI, which serves as a methodological guide for developing, implementing, and evaluating a process improvement intervention (Langley et al., 2009).

Identifying a Conceptual and Theoretical Framework: Application for Improvement

Using the CAUTI example in the MICU and a proposed intervention for an evidence-based algorithm for treatment, there are a number of frameworks that may be applicable. The use of a physiological system theory or methodological framework may be appropriate. For example, the physiological nature of the urinary tract is a valid component of the problem. However, there is also a component associated with the system for the delivery of care. Variation among providers may be enabled by the processes or the structure of the unit, resulting in less than desirable outcomes. In addition, the problem may be addressed methodologically from an improvement perspective.

For this example, the use of Donabedian's theoretical framework of structure, process, and outcome will be used. Donabedian was a pioneer in introducing quality assurance in health care and proposed that quality in health care is the product of two factors: the science and technology of health care, and the application of that science and technology. He further proposed that there is a triad approach for assessing healthcare quality. This triad is defined as structure, process, and outcomes (Donabedian, 2002).

Structure designates the conditions under which clinical care is provided, including but not limited to material resources, human resources, and organizational characteristics. The process is defined by the activities that constitute caring for a patient, which include but are not limited to care delivery processes, diagnosis, treatment, and prevention. The outcomes consist of both the desirable and the undesirable changes in the patient health or population health and include mortality, morbidity rates, and patient satisfaction.

Translating this framework to the CAUTI example, there is a defined structure in the MICU where care is delivered; it consists of human and material resources. There are processes for delivering care to patients who have urinary catheters. Finally, the resulting morbidity outcomes associated with the delivery of care to patients who have urinary catheters is less than desirable. Therefore, an assessment should be made of each component of the triad.

The Science of Improvement

The identification of a problem is not enough. Identification should lead to improvement. Using a rigorous process such as microsystem analysis should lead to quantifiable internal information that highlights a less than desirable outcome or process. Too often there is a desire to continue to assess the situation, which can lead to data paralysis and lack of action. Although there is a limit to what can be done given financial and human resource constraints, less than desirable data outcomes should be actionable (Langley et al., 2009).

When the problem has been identified and a literature search provides external support for the phenomenon, the next logical step is to intervene or improve. There is valid science behind improvement. Lloyd (2004) specifically details the scientific underpinnings for all improvement being founded in the scientific method.

Lloyd (2004) integrates the deductive (general to specific) and inductive (specific to general) phases of the scientific method. Both phases consider the information for decision making, the theoretical concepts (ideas and hypotheses), the selection and definition of indicators, and data collection (plans and methods). After the data collection step, data are analyzed and output to an interpretation of the results (asking why). Information gleaned from the process is used for decision making. Theory and prediction are central to the improvement phases.

Given the strong foundation for improvement, developing an improvement project is scientifically validated and may be standardized through a rigorous methodological approach.

The MFI and Plan-Do-Study-Act

There are many tools available for developing and implementing an improvement project. However, MFI and Plan-Do-Study-Act (PDSA) will be described as a foundational approach. The MFI–PDSA model is a valuable tool because it provides a structure for asking the appropriate questions that are foundational to an improvement project, and then it provides a method for testing an intervention through iterative small tests of change using the PDSA cycle. The model was developed by Associates in Process Improvement based on the significant work done by W. Edwards Deming (Langley et al., 2009).

Three Guiding Questions

There are three guiding questions to answer before beginning an improvement project with the MFI. The first question to ask is, What am I trying to accomplish? (Langley et al., 2009). This question will drive the entire project; it is therefore important to understand what the ultimate goal is. This may seem simple, yet there are complexities that may not be recognized on the surface. For example, think of the time-out process, which is a pause prior to a procedure to verify the correct patient, procedure, site, and side. According to The Joint Commission, this process is a National Patient Safety Goal with a required 100% compliance rate. When addressing the first question of the MFI, the most logical answer is to achieve 100% compliance with the National Patient Safety Goal for time-outs. However, is this truly the correct response? If an organization were to develop a checklist to assess the components of the time-out, what does this actually assess? In most cases, it represents the documentation of the time-out, but does this always assess the behavioral components of the time-outs? In this instance, two plausible answers to the first question of the MFI may be to be 100% compliant with documentation of time-outs and to be 100% compliant with a random sample of behavioral observation of time-outs.

The second question of the MFI is equally important: How will I know a change is an improvement? (Langley et al., 2009). This question requires that a quantifiable measure be developed to assess an improvement intervention. A microsystem assessment of the patterns or processes will provide a variety of outcome or process adherence data that may serve as the baseline for improvement. In some instances there are no data, so the baseline may be zero until iterative PDSA cycles are completed. However, measuring an improvement will provide a quantifiable outcome for an intervention that is implemented.

The third question of the MFI focuses on the intervention: What changes can I make that will result in an improvement? (Langley et al., 2009). The answer to this question will provide the details for the change to be implemented and measured.

The MFI three guiding questions are used to frame the improvement, which is then tested and evaluated in a small test of change, a rapid-cycle process called the PDSA cycle.

PDSA Cycle

The PDSA cycle evolved from the work of Walter Shewhart. He was a mathematician and engineer who discovered that the key to manufacturing a quality product relied on a standardized process of creating the specification, putting the specification into production, building, and then inspecting the outcome. This model, developed in 1939, became known as the Shewhart cycle (Moen & Norman, 2010). The Shewhart cycle involves three steps:

> Step 1: Specification
> Step 2: Production
> Step 3: Inspection (Moen & Norman, 2010, pp. 22–28)

W. Edwards Deming became a student of Shewhart, and the cycle evolved into the Deming wheel. There are several components of the Deming wheel: design the product (with appropriate tests); make it; test it in the production line and in the laboratory; sell the product; test the product in service through market research; find out what users think about it and why nonusers have not bought it.

In 1986, the model evolved again, specifically asking pointed questions to guide improvement of a process. Six steps were identified from the evolution of the Deming wheel:

1. What could be the most important accomplishments of the team? What changes might be desirable? What data are available? Are new observations needed? If yes, plan a change or a test. Decide how to use the observations.
2. Carry out the change or test, preferably on a small scale.
3. Observe the effects of the change or test.
4. Study the results. What did we learn? What can we predict?
5. Repeat step 1 with the accumulated knowledge.
6. Repeat step 2 and the subsequent steps.

Ultimately, the evolution of the cycle started by Shewhart in 1939 and modified by Deming became the PDSA cycle in 1993 (Deming, 1993). The PDSA cycle involves a circular motion and multiple iterations in a cycle. *Plan* involves planning a change or test aimed at improvement. *Do* is carrying out the change or test (preferably on a small scale). *Study* is the aspect of examining the results to determine what was learned and what went wrong. *Act* involves adopting the change, abandoning it, or running through the cycle again.

Application to Practice: MFI–PDSA Cycle

Throughout this chapter the CAUTI example has been used to demonstrate an application of the discussion. We will continue with the example in this section, beginning with the three guiding questions of the MFI. **Figure 13-2** provides the details for these questions.

An example of a PDSA cycle is as follows. The cycle flows from the three guiding questions from the MFI:

Plan:
Develop an evidence-based protocol with the outcome goal of reducing CAUTIs in adult patients in the MICU.

Do:

1. Assemble a team to meet, develop a charter, and finalize the aims and outcome metrics (using baseline information from a microsystem analysis).
2. Search the literature and develop an evidence-based protocol.
3. Implement the protocol within the defined microsystem.
4. Provide appropriate education and implementation assistance.
5. Develop a data collection tool and processes.
6. Gather data about the processes and outcomes.

Study:
Analyze the collected data and discuss what was learned with the team members.

Act:
Implement the protocol or do another PDSA cycle.

Through this example, the MFI–PDSA cycle was used to develop, implement, and study an improvement intervention that was based on an understanding of the microsystem of care. Using such a systematic approach may provide quantifiable and actionable data that may be used to successfully develop interventions that will result in improved patient and process outcomes (Langley et al., 2009).

FIGURE 13-2   Three Guiding Questions of the MFI

- Topic: Catheter-Associated Urinary Tract Infection
  - What are we trying to accomplish?
    - **To reduce the CAUTI rate** in the MICU
  - How will we know a change is an improvement?
    - To reduce the CAUTI rate in the MICU by **10% or 5 infections avoided** *(baseline was assessed, then the numbers are calculated against baseline)*
  - What changes can I implement that will result in an improvement?
    - To reduce the CAUTI rate in the MICU by 10% or 5 infections avoided by **implementing an evidence-based protocol**

Measurement for Improvement

A detailed discussion of measurement for improvement is outside the scope of this chapter. However, the importance of measurement warrants mention of the need to quantify improvement projects. Nurse leaders must have an understanding of measurement for improvement to guide staff engagement. Robust statistical processes for improvement combine descriptive, parametric, and nonparametric statistical methods with statistical process control (SPC). Understanding traditional statistical methods not only is important for the analytical processes that may be essential when evaluating or studying an improvement project but also provides the critical background for being a good consumer of research or evidence. Appraising the literature requires some knowledge of the appropriate statistical methods used to conduct the research studies that become the evidence for change (Langley et al., 2009).

Specific to improvement in the clinical setting, an understanding of the types of measures that may be developed and evaluated will be defined. There are structure, process, outcomes, and balancing measures. Each measure may seem somewhat self-explanatory; however, the definitions may vary (Langley et al., 2009). Structural measures are related to components of the infrastructure of a unit or microsystem, such as a daily census or nursing staff mix. Process measures quantify processes, such as provider adherence to a protocol or time to discharge. Outcome measures may quantify the outcome of a process or a patient outcome, such as a fall rate or a pressure ulcer rate for a nursing unit. Balancing measures are factors that may be impacted by the improvement intervention, such as provider satisfaction with a new process (one thing may be negatively impacted when something else is improved).

In defining each of these types of measures, operational definitions are developed. An operational definition clearly defines all aspects of the measure, including the numerator and denominator in such specific terms that there is little question about what is included in the calculation of the measure or metric.

SPC knowledge is imperative for measuring improvements in processes. Tools called run and control charts that measure over time can be analyzed for process variation that is either a common cause (inherent in the process) or a special cause (something that is out of the ordinary in either a positive or negative fashion). SPC provides a perspective that is not evident in a traditional measure of statistical significance (Langley et al., 2009). For example, knowing that there is a statistically significant difference in the rates of infection at two points in time does not address the stability of the measure over time. Has the phenomenon been stable over time, or is there some special cause over time? In this case, SPC will show variation in the stability of the measure over the course of time.

Application to Practice: Measurement for Improvement

Using the CAUTI example in the MICU, an outcome measure may be the CAUTI rate per month. To operationally define this measure, a denominator must be developed. The nurse leader asked a number of questions and engaged the staff. What patients are included? What patients are excluded? Do we include all adult patients with a Foley catheter? Does the catheter need to be placed on the unit? Are patients excluded who transfer to the unit with an indwelling Foley catheter in place? For the numerator, the same type of questions should be asked. How is a CAUTI defined? Is there a particular laboratory confirmation that will be used? Will symptoms be used to diagnose?

In this example, one may also develop a process measure. The use of a protocol in treating CAUTI becomes a process that can be measured for variation. Do all providers adhere to the protocol? If not, what components of the protocol or process are lacking, and what is the rate of adherence based on all providers who use the protocol?

As you can see, a variety of metrics may be developed based on the type of improvement project that is developed. However, measuring for improvement requires an understanding of a variety of statistical methods.

COMPONENTS OF A QUALITY MANAGEMENT PROGRAM

A quality management program is composed of the following (Koch, 2013):

1. Clear and concise written statements of purpose, philosophy, values, and objectives
2. Standards or indicators for measuring the quality of care
3. Policies and procedures for using such standards for gathering data; these policies define the organizational structure for the program
4. Analysis and reporting of the gathered data, with isolation of problems and variances
5. Use of the results to prioritize, plan action, and correct problems and variances
6. Monitoring of clinical and managerial performance and ongoing feedback to ensure that problems stay solved
7. Evaluation of the quality management system

These components may be conceptualized in many different ways. One component builds on another. Batalden and Stoltz (1993) describe a framework for the continual improvement of health care that incorporates underlying knowledge, a policy for leadership, tools and methods, and daily work applications.

The mission, vision, guiding principles, and integration of values are critical to the policy for leadership. As quality and safety initiatives have taken off, it is not surprising to see a vast array of strategies, structures, and tools developed in the evolution of improvement work. Tools and methods can be grouped into four major categories: process and system, group process and collaborative work, statistical thinking, and planning and analysis. Daily work applications include developing models for testing change and making adjustments as well as reviewing improvements. Conceptualizing quality management principles provides nurses with tools to help the nursing department with the overall quality management process.

Standards for Measuring the Quality of Care

Standards define nursing care outcomes and nursing activities, as well as the necessary structural resources. They are used to plan and evaluate nursing care. Outcomes include positive and negative indexes. Standards are directed at structure, process, and outcome issues and guide the review of systems function, staff

---

BOX 13-1 Framework for the Continual Improvement of Health Care

Underlying Knowledge

Professional knowledge:
- subject
- discipline
- values

Improvement knowledge:
- system
- variation
- psychology
- theory of knowledge

Policy for Leadership

Mission, vision, and quality definition
Guiding principles
Integration with values

Tools and Methods

Process, system
Group process and collaborative work
Statistical thinking
Planning and analysis

Daily Work Applications

Models for testing change and making improvement
Review of improvement

Source: Batalden, P. B., & Stoltz, P. K. (1993, October). © Joint Commission Resources: The framework for continual improvement of health care. *Joint Commission Journal on Quality and Patient Safety.* Reprinted with permission.

---

performance, and client care. A number of healthcare organizations issue indexes. Annually, the Centers for Medicare and Medicaid Services discloses projected and actual hospital select indicator rates by diagnosis-related groups. A number of tools and methods are used to evaluate quality.

Root Cause

An analysis is conducted to understand how and why an adverse sentinel event occurred and to prevent its recurrence. A sentinel event is an unexpected, unwanted occurrence involving death or serious physical injury. It is called *sentinel* because it signifies immediate attention. A root-cause analysis includes assigning a team to assess the event as soon as possible (within 72 hours). The team should include staff members at all levels who are closest to the specific case, including those with decision-making authority. The process involves a review of events, process failure, action plans, implementation of plans, and follow-up review (Batalden & Davidoff, 2007).

The Joint Commission is not the only group that collects quality data for measurement. Other organizations include the American Hospital Association, Voluntary Hospitals of America, the National Committee for Quality Health Care, and the National Association of Health Data Organizations (Batalden & Davidoff, 2007). These organizations gather, analyze, and publish data on the quality of health care for consumers, employers, and the federal government. The standards include performance standards for providers. The objectives are to achieve improvement in the health status of clients, reduce unnecessary use of healthcare services, and meet specifications of clients and purchasers. These standards address the improvement of healthcare quality, functions, and processes that must be carried out effectively to achieve good patient care outcomes, governance, and management. Quality management theory has been applied in the form of identifying common causes and special causes of performance variation.

Policies and Procedures

The third element of a quality management program is the development of policies and procedures for using standards or indicators for gathering data to measure the quality of care. Batalden and Davidoff (2007) describe guiding principles that reflect an organization's assumptions about the responsibilities and desired actions of leaders who create positive work environments. Integrating leadership policy with the values common to healthcare professionals and underlying healthcare work is essential to contribute to shared ownership of the policy by everyone in an organization (Batalden & Davidoff, 2007). The policies and procedures define the organizational structure for the quality management program and prescribe the tools for gathering data.

DATA COLLECTION

Data collection tools may be in the form of questionnaires, rating scales, or interviews. Reliability and validity are important concepts in determining the worth of instruments used to measure variables in a study. Reliability is the extent to which an experiment, test, or measurement procedure yields the same results on repeated trials. Interrater reliability refers to the degree to which two raters, operating independently, assign the same ratings for an attribute. Validity is the degree to which an instrument measures what it is intended to measure. Content (face) validity is the degree to which an instrument adequately represents the universe of content (Langley et al., 2009).

QUALITY MANAGEMENT TOOLS

Statistical Techniques

Statistical techniques include measures of central tendency and variability, tests of significance, and correlation. Central tendency refers to the middle value and general trend of a set of numbers. The three most common measures of central tendency are the mean, the median, and the mode. Measures of variability look at the dispersion of the measures. Three common measures of variability are the range, the standard deviation, and interpercentile measures (Langley et al., 2009). Correlation refers to the extent to which two variables are related. The Pearson product-moment correlation coefficient of determination (r^2) is a method whereby cause and effect, or relationships, may be evaluated. This statistical analysis tool may be found in various computer software programs and is used with scatter diagrams. The coefficient of determination (r^2) is helpful in determining the percentage of variance on one variable that can be predicted by the variance on another variable (Spuck, 1999).

Data Analysis

Data analysis tools may be divided into three types: decision-making tools, data analysis charts, and relational charts. Brainstorming and multivoting are types of decision-making tools that involve groups or teams.

Brainstorming

Brainstorming is a free-flowing generation of ideas. This approach can generate excitement, equalize involvement, and result in original solutions to problems (Mukherjee, 2006). Ideas are not discussed as they are generated, but the team can build on the ideas of others. No judgments are made concerning an idea's worth or its feasibility. This discussion comes at a later point in the process. Brainstorming is useful when a list of possible ideas is needed. This technique works well to generate ideas for such tools as cause-and-effect diagrams.

Multivoting

Multivoting is a method to determine the most popular or important items from a list, without a lot of discussion or difficulty. This method uses a series of votes to cut the list in half each time, thus reducing the number of items to be considered (Mukherjee, 2006). This technique is used after a brainstorming session to identify the key items on which the group will focus.

Nominal Group Technique

This is a group decision-making process for generating a large number of ideas in which each member works alone. This technique is used when group members are new to one another or when they have different opinions and goals. This approach is more structured than brainstorming or multivoting (Mukherjee, 2006).

Delphi Method

The Delphi method is a combination of the brainstorming, multivoting, and nominal group techniques. It is used when the group is not in one location, and it is frequently carried out through mail or email (Mukherjee, 2006). After each step in the process, the data are sent to one person who compiles the data and sends the next step for the participants to complete.

Prioritization Matrix

A prioritization matrix organizes tasks, issues, or actions and prioritizes them by agreed-upon criteria. The tool combines a tree diagram and an L-shaped matrix diagram to display the best possible effect. A prioritization matrix is often used before more complex matrices are needed. The matrix applies options under discussion to priority considerations (Mukherjee, 2006). This is used when issues are identified and options must be narrowed down, options have strong relationships, or all options need to be done but prioritization or sequencing is needed.

Run Chart or Trend Chart

Run charts are graphic displays of data points over time (**Figure 13-3**). Run charts are control charts without the control limits. Their name comes from the fact that the user looks for trends in the data or a significant number of data points going in one direction or to one side of the average (Langley et al., 2009).

Trends generally indicate a statistically important event that needs further analysis. The tendency to see every variation in the data as significant should be resisted by waiting to interpret the results until at least 10 (preferably 20) data points have been plotted. These charts are used to display variation, detect the presence or absence of special causes, or observe the effects of a process improvement.

Control Chart

Control charts are run charts to which control limits have been added above and below the mean. Generally, upper and lower control limits are statistically determined by adding and subtracting three standard deviations from the mean. Assuming a normal distribution and no special-cause variation, a majority of the data points are expected to fall within the upper and lower control limits. Variance within the control limits results from aggregate common causes, and one should not tamper with a process that is performing as expected. As discussed earlier with regard to Deming's model, special-cause variance (data points outside the control limits) occurs in less than 10% of cases and requires evaluation. These charts are used to distinguish variations from common and special causes, assist with eliminating special-cause variations, and observe effects of a process improvement.

FIGURE 13-3   Example of a Run Chart

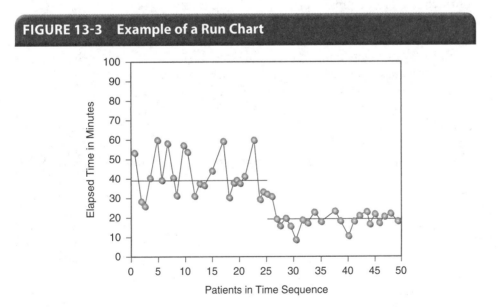

Source: Batalden, P. B., & Stoltz, P. K. (1993, October). © Joint Commission Resources: The framework for continual improvement of health care. *Joint Commission Journal on Quality and Patient Safety.* Reprinted with permission.

Process Flowchart

A process flowchart is a graphic display of a process as it is known to its authors or team. The flowchart outlines the sequence and relationship of the process components. Through management of data and information, the team comes to a common understanding and knowledge concerning the process. Information is discussed about the structure (who carries out the specific step in the identified process), what activity is occurring, and the outcome or the results (Langley et al., 2009).

Fish Bone Cause-and-Effect Diagram

A cause-and-effect diagram is used to analyze and display the potential causes of a problem or the sources of variation. There are generally at least four categories in the diagram. Some of the most common categories involve the Four Ms—manpower, methods, machines, and materials—or the Five Ps—patrons (users of the system), people (workers), provisions (supplies), places (work environment), and procedures (methods and rules). The diagram is used to identify and organize possible causes of the problem or identify factors that will lead to success (Langley et al., 2009).

Histogram or Bar Chart

Before a set of measured data is analyzed, the distribution of values is reviewed for each variable. The optimal tool for reviewing a distribution depends on how many data are available. A bar graph with a separate bar for each value may be used when data are sparse (fewer than 12 values), but as the data increase it becomes necessary to organize and summarize. A histogram, the most commonly used frequency distribution tool, does this by presenting the measurement scale of values along the x-axis (broken into equal intervals) and a frequency scale (as counts or percentages) along the y-axis. Plotting the frequency of each interval reveals the pattern of the data, showing its center and spread (including outliers) and whether there is symmetry or skew. This information is important because it may signal problems in the data and should influence the choice of measures of central tendency and spread. An important distinction must be made regarding bar charts and histograms. The x-axis consists of discrete categories, and each bar is a separate group. This chart is used to show the data distribution or spread, whether the data are symmetric or skewed, or whether there are extreme data values (**Figure 13-4**).

Pareto Chart

A Pareto chart displays a series of bars in which the priority can easily be seen by the varying height of the bars (**Figure 13-5**). The tallest bar is the most frequent. The bars are always arranged in descending height. A Pareto chart is related to the Pareto principle (named after the 19th-century economist Vilfredo Pareto), which states that 80% of the problems or effects come from 20% of the causes. This chart is used to identify the most frequent or the most important factors contributing to costs, problems, and so on (Langley et al., 2009).

FIGURE 13-4   A Histogram of Errors

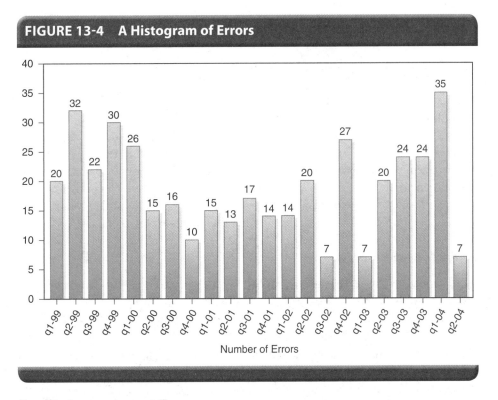

Number of Errors

Quality Improvement Teams

One method of implementing a quality management program is through a team or council. This team functions with a team leader, team members, and a facilitator.

FIGURE 13-5   Generalized Pareto Chart

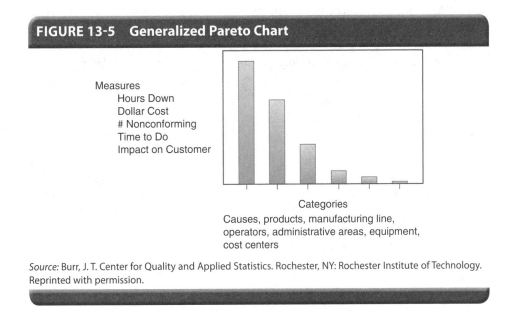

Measures
    Hours Down
    Dollar Cost
    # Nonconforming
    Time to Do
    Impact on Customer

Categories
Causes, products, manufacturing line,
operators, administrative areas, equipment,
cost centers

Source: Burr, J. T. Center for Quality and Applied Statistics. Rochester, NY: Rochester Institute of Technology. Reprinted with permission.

The team supports management in developing and implementing a quality management program and may follow group dynamics (Langley et al., 2009).

PROBLEM IDENTIFICATION

Analysis and reporting of data gathered from the evaluation process lead to problem identification and isolation. Evidence comes from primary sources, such as clients and nursing personnel, and from secondary sources, including clients' charts and families. Active client and family participation should be part of the process. Quality management addresses current problems. Nurses look for patterns or trends of deviation from normal. They also identify deficiencies that stem from other departments and affect nursing care. If one takes a systems approach, problem identification is a team approach, with clients and families as major team players.

Problem Resolution

After problems have been defined and isolated, plans are made to solve them on a priority basis. Critical problems are addressed first, and plans are immediately made and implemented to resolve them. Those involving the safety and welfare of clients take first priority. Other factors used in determining priority include severity, frequency, benefit, cost effectiveness, elimination, reduction, association with professional liability, and impact on accreditation. The first consideration is always based on the impact on client care. Solutions and corrective actions for problems are assigned to appropriate nursing departments, services, and units. The goal is to resolve problems, not just evaluate them.

MONITORING AND FEEDBACK

The quality management process is cyclic and requires monitoring of clinical and managerial performance and feedback to ensure that problems stay solved. Follow-up can be expensive and difficult. Problems of a multidisciplinary nature, such as those involving occupational therapy, physical therapy, speech pathology, and nursing, can be one consideration. The cyclic process will continue to set standards of care, take measurements according to those standards, evaluate care from multiple sources, recommend improvements, and, above all, ensure that improvements are carried out (Langley et al., 2009).

Involvement of Practicing Nurses

Practicing nurses can be motivated to embrace quality management by a direct behavioral experience. Nurse managers should find out why nurses view quality management unfavorably. Negative connotations may exist because of a lack of executive administrative support, views that the process is futile and changes in practice do not occur, and lack of physician involvement. Changing a negative viewpoint may be accomplished by using the following strategies:

- Ask clinical nurses to identify areas that need improvement.
- Provide release time for clinical nurses to participate in quality management activities, including attendance at committee meetings and time for quality management audits.

- Provide rewards, such as performance results achievement records, that can lead to pay raises, promotions, educational opportunities, or special assignments.
- Target quality management to patient care outcomes, the essence of nursing practice.
- Involve clinical nurses in management through such techniques as quality circles, employee involvement programs, participatory management, decentralization, adhocracy (a flexible, informal organization that can respond quickly to change), and quality of work life.
- Establish a peer review program involving nursing staff at all levels of patient care. Such a program can identify outcome criteria based on established standards for nursing practice. Peers determine whether outcomes have been met based on ongoing and retrospective audits. Corrective action is determined by peers based on the outcome being adequately met.

Efficiency

Efficiency is concerned with the cost-to-benefit ratio. Can the appropriate standard be met with a cost that is acceptable to both consumer and provider? The computer is an example of a labor-saving device for developing and conducting a quality management program. Nurse managers use it and teach other practicing nurses to use it. Standards will be kept up to date and accessible to all units in paper or electronic files. Standards should be cross-referenced.

Charts can be labeled for easy retrieval for nursing quality management evaluation. In addition, the Long-Term Care Minimum Data Set can be an efficient quality management tool for nursing homes. The Minimum Data Set is a collection of baseline data (physical, social, and psychological factors) that can be used to assess, analyze, and plan care for residents in nursing homes.

The following are some elements of efficiency and effectiveness:

- Identify the impact of nursing care on the health of the patient; that is, results or outcomes should be measured in terms of the patient's health status. Does nursing documentation meet such a standard?
- Implement a program that is practical enough to be used in all clinical nursing settings.
- Collect random, unannounced samples.
- Nursing personnel should serve on committees long enough to be proficient.
- Grading of standards should be done by each person who administers criteria.
- Higher patient acuity should be combined with shorter hospital stays.
- Conduct interdisciplinary programs so nurses will not do the work of other disciplines. Nursing is ethically and operationally interdependent with other groups and organizations.
- Plan for an uncertain future by blueprinting scenarios for managing the future, changing the culture of nursing organizations, developing interpersonal skills, and responding creatively to risk taking.
- Hold each nurse responsible for self-improvement and for delivering a high standard of patient care.

Customer Satisfaction

Customer satisfaction is an integral part of quality management. The satisfaction of not only external clients and their families but also internal customers (an organization's staff and departments) should be assessed. Patient rights and human resource standards specified by The Joint Commission and Centers for Medicare and Medicaid Services warrant measurement of these factors.

Consumer satisfaction as an outcome of quality management can be assessed through methods such as patient, family, and nurse interviews or surveys and observation checklists of nurse–patient interactions.

Quality in the healthcare marketplace is defined by employers, employee benefit consultants, physicians, and consumers—not by providers (even though physicians are providers, as are hospitals, nurses, and other caregivers). The reason physicians determine quality is that they have control over orders for diagnosis and treatment procedures. Only one-half of consumers, employers, and employee consultants differentiate between high- and low-quality hospitals.

Good employee relations and consumer relations programs are necessary for success in the healthcare marketplace, and their good quality must be communicated. Consumers want quality factors in the following order:

1. Warmth, caring, and concern
2. Expert medical staff that is concerned, thorough, and successful
3. Up-to-date technology and equipment
4. Specialization and scope of services available
5. Outcome

Training and Communication

Training and communication are important elements of a total quality program. Training includes interpersonal skills, stress management, and conflict management. Learning is a cyclic or continuous process. Nurse managers who play educator roles develop self-awareness by applying learning principles to their own behaviors. Patient education requires an interdisciplinary team approach.

Communication of quality management findings, including problems, resolution of problems, and results, must be clear. Both physicians and nursing employees need to be kept up to date. Quality must be provided and communicated to be successful. This means that providers as well as consumers will know the status of the quality of care being rendered.

RESEARCH AND QUALITY MANAGEMENT

Nursing quality management programs can be combined with research programs. Nursing research is being done in clinical settings to improve patient care outcomes. Research can provide prestige, advanced knowledge for nursing professionals, and a database for clinical nursing practice for nurse managers.

Nursing research can be used to evaluate management issues such as staffing, cost management, and staff retention. It produces new knowledge of the relationship between processes and outcomes. Combining quality management with research makes efficient use of personnel and other resources to link research with a mandatory process, to increase the probability that research will relate to patient care, and to increase sharing of successful quality management programs with others outside the institution.

Anticipating Risk as a Strategy to Mitigate Loss

As individuals and systems continue to master core competencies that are necessary to anticipate and manage risk and mitigate loss, opportunities are available to create value-added care models. As the care models are implemented, risk is commonplace. What follows are system leaders becoming accustomed to anticipating and managing risk. Quality, safety, value, sustainable patient outcomes, and tort reduction result in risk anticipation and management.

Various definitions of risk are presented in the literature (Chassin & Loeb, 2013; Corrigan & McNeill, 2009). A simple but comprehensive definition is as follows: Risk = Probability × Impact. Because health care has become increasingly complex, it is more difficult to anticipate, analyze, and interpret future trends that create risks and threaten opportunities. The concept of strategic foresight can be useful for reducing risk and mitigating loss as the healthcare arena becomes more regulated, unpredictable, and globalized (Habegger, 2009).

Remaining transparent and reporting incidents publicly will aid systems and leaders to become more risk intelligent. Risk-intelligent individuals and organizations are recognized as a value proposition in which vulnerability is identified and variability is reduced through data capture. Preventing and mitigating loss are realized as systems complete risk assessments, set priorities, and take corrective actions. Similarly, organizations that assess the relationship and synergistic effects of risk anticipation and management create solutions that produce organizational value.

SUMMARY

Quality management programs ensure that quality control standards are maintained and that care delivery continually improves. Quality management requires careful planning, development, data collection, resource allocation, and evaluation. Ideally, quality management programs should be founded on total quality management, a proven theory for broad application. Leadership is paramount for successful integration of total quality management into quality management programs; leadership will change the organizational culture and climate to give workers the training they need to affect planning and productivity. Through the effective use of quality management tools, the efficiency of nursing interventions or actions can be demonstrated. Quality management programs may lend efficacy of results to research in support of establishing best practices for nursing.

REFLECTIVE QUESTIONS

1. You are a new nurse manager on an acute medical nursing unit and note variation in the way patients are being discharged. Your noting this is due to trying to determine reasons why patients are being readmitted fewer than 30 days after discharge. What are your first steps in developing a plan to improve the quality of your discharge planning process?

2. As the director of the outpatient orthopedic services, you are asked to create a referral system for your clinic for women who are high risk for osteoporosis. How would you approach this project? How would you determine the effectiveness of your project?

CASE STUDY 13-1 Patient Safety

Sheree C. Carter

Southwest Kentucky Rheumatology Associates (SKRA) is a 10-year-old private practice consisting of four rheumatologists, one office manager, one nurse practitioner, two registered nurses, one laboratory technician, one radiology technician, and three medical assistants. In addition to seeing clients with various rheumatologic diseases, SKRA maintains an infusion suite in a corner of the office consisting of 10 infusion chairs, a small desk for mixing IVs, a small storage closet, and a refrigerator. The infusion suite averages 5,000 infusions of biologics and disease-modifying agents per year at the rate of approximately 20 to 25 infusions per working day. The physicians have been concerned about the number of medication errors, the lack of certifications and prior authorizations for administration of the various infusible medications, and the increase in the amount of medication waste or lack of available medication for clients who are receiving care.

The general responsibility and management of the infusion suite at SKRA have been assumed by one of the medical assistants who has been in practice with one of the rheumatologists for more than 20 years. This self-appointed chief medical assistant orders all supplies pertaining to the infusion suite and is responsible for preparing clients and cleaning the suite at the end of the day. The chief medical assistant works exclusively for her particular rheumatologist and does not conduct any work for the other three rheumatologists in the practice. The other two medical assistants rotate between the three remaining rheumatologists and the nurse practitioner in caring for patients within the infusion suite and in the general office practice. One of the registered nurses or, on rare occasions, the nurse practitioner is called into the infusion suite to start patients' IVs and initial infusions and then quickly returns to the office practice.

At the last practice management meeting, one of the rheumatologists loudly voiced concern about the infusion suite experiencing an increasing number of issues regarding medication shortages and errors, as well as negative client satisfaction reports. The rheumatologist demanded that the practice immediately hire a registered nurse to be solely devoted to managing the infusion suite. An ad was placed in the local newspaper for a registered nurse with the idea that the practice manager would interview and hire a nurse as soon as possible. Seven nurses were hired over the next 7 months. Three were fired because they did not have IV skills, and the other four left, citing various reasons, such as a hostile work environment, unreasonable work hours, unsafe practice management, unmanageable workload, lack of support, and resistance to change.

You are asked by one of the rheumatologists to drop by the office and offer advice to fix the problem.

Case Study Questions

1. What would your first steps in this process be?
2. What information will be most useful to you?
3. What is the evidence for the safe practice of an infusion suite?
4. Are there state or professional scope of practice issues at hand?
5. How would you handle personnel issues?
6. What would be your recommendations for this practice, and what do you base your recommendations on?
7. What management theory or theories apply before and after your recommendations?

CASE STUDY 13-2   Creating a Culture of Safety within a Microsystem

Joseph White

Patient safety is of paramount importance to the operations of any nursing unit. Nurses who work in direct patient care must be trained in patient safety techniques and need a curriculum to help guide their development and acquisition of these skills. An important component of the nurse leader's role is to positively influence the culture of safety within the nursing environment to promote optimal outcomes. Nurse leaders must help their nurses be empowered to recognize and report potential patient safety and quality issues.

The Heart and Lung Transplant unit identified opportunities in their annual employee survey that addressed issues surrounding the culture of patient safety. The unit experienced low scores in the following areas: "this organization is committed to patient safety," "this organization makes every effort to deliver safe, error-free care or service," "I feel empowered to report patient safety and quality issues," and "my unit works well as a team to promote patient safety." Further assessment of the unit allowed the nurse leaders to identify that many nurses who were employed in the unit were not trained in patient safety techniques and skills as part of their formal nursing education. This created an opportunity for nurse leaders to introduce new patient safety ideas and techniques into the nursing unit.

The Heart and Lung Transplant ICU is a complex environment where many different healthcare disciplines interact to provide care for vulnerable patients. One issue identified by leadership involved nurses who were not speaking up to voice a suggestion or observation when a key safety practice was not being observed by someone. For example, nurses felt that they could not speak up to other healthcare workers when they observed that someone did not wash his or her hands.

At the same time, patient safety goals identified by The Joint Commission were being implemented in the unit to improve how healthcare workers hand off patients to each other and use a time-out during high-risk procedures to safeguard patient care. The leadership identified that some nurses were frustrated by the lack of understanding and appreciation for how these practices could transform care when they are implemented as intended. Many nurses lacked the attitude and ongoing commitment needed to prevent adverse patient safety and quality events from happening.

To transform the culture of patient safety, the unit leadership identified a patient safety curriculum called Team Strategies and Tools to Enhance Performance and Patient Safety (TeamSTEPPS). This program was developed by the Agency for Healthcare Research and Quality and the U.S. Department of Defense. TeamSTEPPS is a comprehensive program that includes a set of modules and exercises designed to engage healthcare workers in understanding how they can assume their roles in a more collaborative teamwork approach that supports and promotes patient safety. The program teaches healthcare workers skills like situation monitoring and mutual support to promote a culture that embraces patient safety. In addition, important concepts, such as communication and conflict management negotiations, are taught to all disciplines to instill a common language surrounding patient safety.

A strategic plan was written to implement the TeamSTEPPS program. The plan was shared with key hospital and medical leadership, and support was given to develop a set of TeamSTEPPS master trainers. The strategic plan included a training budget and plan. The nursing unit leadership decided to implement the complete TeamSTEPPS modules in a 1-day training class.

As a result of implementing TeamSTEPPS, pre- and postsurvey assessment measurements included in the program indicated that the nurses' attitudes toward teamwork and perceptions of teamwork improved. The unit leadership observed that the nurses were able to use a common language surrounding patient safety to make a difference in patient care. For example, as a result of learning about and practicing huddles and debriefings in the TeamSTEPPS class, nurses were able to identify when these activities should be included to promote patient safety.

(continues)

CASE STUDY 13-2 Creating a Culture of Safety within a Microsystem (Continued)

Reflecting back, the unit leadership was proud of the adoption of TeamSTEPPS to improve teamwork and patient safety. The leadership recognized that the adoption of such a program requires ongoing attention to on-board new employees with the teamwork curriculum and to continue to develop the entire team's knowledge and attitudes of teamwork.

Case Study Questions

1. What obligations do nurse leaders have to develop their own understanding of patient safety within their areas of responsibility? How could nurse leaders position themselves to demonstrate ongoing support for teamwork and patient safety?
2. Research materials on programs such as TeamSTEPPS. How could a teamwork intervention program make a difference within your microsystem?
3. What evidence should nurse leaders look for that could indicate their teams and microsystems could benefit from improving their culture of patient safety?
4. Describe how a nurse manager could develop a plan to have his or her staff participate in a teamwork intervention program. What key elements would need to be included in the plan?

CASE STUDY 13-3 Healthy Work Environments

Kristen Noles and Terri Poe

Establishing a healthy work environment is important to optimize safe and quality care for patients and their families. According to the American Association of Critical-Care Nurses' (2005) standards for establishing and sustaining healthy work environments, six standards have been identified: skilled communication, true collaboration, effective decision making, appropriate staffing, meaningful recognition, and authentic leadership.

After assessment, reflection, and discussions with all members of the healthcare team, the new nurse leader on the Acute Trauma Care Unit (ATCU) established a healthy work environment as the top priority. The unit had a high turnover rate with a 40% vacancy rate. Employee engagement was down, and not one staff member was involved with hospital committees. After talking with the staff and patients and their families, and after reviewing quality metrics, it was evident that accountability for nursing practice was lacking.

As simple as it may sound, policies and procedures were enforced, and consistency was maintained. In the first month, additional vacancies occurred. Purposeful leadership rounding on staff, patients, and families occurred daily. Information obtained from the rounding process identified quick ways to improve both the work environment and the clinical care provided to patients. Needed supplies, resources, and education provided the nurse manager with a blueprint to make positive changes.

As new staff entered the environment, they brought newness, positivity, and a passion to make a difference. The staff created a purpose statement for the unit that is posted for patients, families, and staff members to see. A unit-based, employee-led team was created. It provides a forum for staff members to bring issues and concerns forward. The team discusses the staff's concerns and works with individuals on solutions. Currently, there are five initiatives being led by frontline staff members. Several of these teams are interprofessional. The nonlicensed staff created a process improvement team that focuses on their practice and their role in the team.

CASE STUDY 13-3   Health Work Environments (Continued)

With a current vacancy rate of 0%, the staffing is adequate. The unit has transformed into a healthy learning environment that promotes staff development, mentoring, and individualized coaching. The staff owns their quality patient outcomes and uses various tools to evaluate processes. One staff nurse completed a Failure Mode Effect Analysis (FMEA) about the current discharge process. Nurses complete an RCA for every never event on the unit, including central line–associated bloodstream infections (CLABSI), cathether-associated urinary tract infections (CAUTI), and pulmonary embolisms (PE). More than 75% of all staff members completed an additional certification course specific for trauma. Several staff members voluntarily completed a Collaborative Educational Program with the School of Nursing: Quality and Patient Safety: Developing Unit-Based Interprofessional Competencies for Improvement. Establishing a healthy work environment is crucial for creating a foundation to promote a safe culture to care for patients and their families.

Case Study Questions

1. If you were to describe your leadership style, what would it be? Do you feel that it promotes team building, or is it a barrier at times?
2. Each of us has been a part of a team. Reflect on the most positive team experience you have had. What qualities of the team made it so special?
3. Have you heard the saying, There is no I in *team*? As a leader, what key characteristics would you look for when building a team?

CASE STUDY 13-4   Developing a Successful Culture of Safety and Point of Care

Lisa Keegan

Consider a scenario in which there are sister units with 24 beds each. One cares for patients who have complex GI issues and patients who require colorectal, gynecological, and urological surgery. The other cares for patients who are listed for, or who have had, kidney, liver, or small bowel transplants and patients who have had bariatric or other complex surgical procedures. The units have the following staff mix: registered nurses (RNs), patient care assistants, health unit coordinators, environmental coordinator, care manager, RN educator, outcome manager (shared), and unit leadership.

The nursing leader is aware of the essential elements of a safety culture as defined by the IOM:

- Commitment of leadership to safety
- All employees empowered and engaged in ongoing vigilance
- Organizational learning from errors and near misses (precursor events)

The nurse leader must use the components of a healthy work environment as she works to determine how to offer support. In this case, the nurse leader chose to implement the following components:

- Commitment to high-reliability processes
- Organizational safety briefs
- Rounding to influence
- Unit huddles
- Charge nurse huddles (flow, staffing, safety issues)
- Senior leader walks rounds
- Medical response team
- Safety team

(continues)

CASE STUDY 13-4 Developing a Successful Culture of Safety and Point of Care (Continued)

- Interdisciplinary shared governance
- Clinical systems improvement (CSI)
- Improvement science training
- Rapid cycle improvement collaborative (RCIC)
- Crucial conversations training
- Safety coach training

The nurse leader considers methods and strategies that provide structure for a safe environment, and a safe passage for patients from admission to discharge. An example of a strategy would be shift huddles, which would be completed at specified times; for example, 0700 and 1900, and would last no longer than 5 minutes. Information covered in the shift huddle could include: review of safety data, current status of patients (census, watchers, staffing), forecasting (admits, discharges, potential problems, and regulatory visitors), retrospective review (concerns from the prior shift), and tracking of safety issues. Along with shift huddles, another strategy is reporting between outgoing and incoming shifts. Reporting could include in-room safety checks, particularly during walking shift reports, introduction of staff to patients and family, checking identification bracelets, monitoring fluids and medication, being assured that emergency equipment is accessible and up-to-date, and review of the patients' plan of care (PPOC).

Clinical rounds provide great opportunities for patient and staff engagement (**Figure 13-6**). Clinical rounds are generally nurse-led, family-centered, interdisciplinary, focused on patients' plan of care, including discharge goals, and medication reconciliation. Clinical rounding provides opportunity for mentoring and coaching staff, while engaging the patient in shared decision making about care delivery.

Managers review safety concerns daily and follow up as needed. Updates posted in a conference room may include referrals made to the unit's shared governance councils; ongoing communication among the unit's physical leaders, managers, and council members; and safety and family satisfaction data.

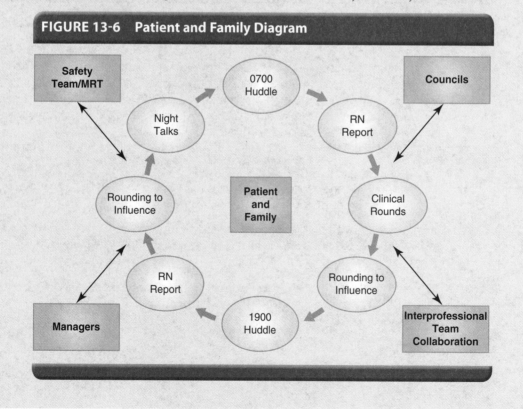

FIGURE 13-6 Patient and Family Diagram

CASE STUDY 13-4   Developing a Successful Culture of Safety and Point of Care (Continued)

The nurse leader used her knowledge of the healthcare environment and a culture of safety to determine metrics to demonstrate the following intended outcomes:

- Four months without a central line infection
- 1,764 days since the last medical response team (MRT) preventable code
- 1,602 days since the last Serious Safety Event (SSE) on nursing unit A4N

Case Study Questions

Based on this scenario and the knowledge gained to date, consider the following regarding your own practice setting:

1. Does our patient care delivery model ensure we are meeting our intended outcomes?
2. Do I understand the economics of the patient population for which I'm responsible?
3. Is my staff involved in effective decision making to the degree they are capable?
4. Are we using best evidence to inform our practice?
5. Have I internally and externally benchmarked my outcome measurements?
6. How am I using the principles of quality improvement to increase patient safety?
7. How is case management and care integration affecting readmission rates?
8. Do I know leadership's plan for stratifying risk and what their expectations of me are?

REFERENCES

American Association of Critical-Care Nurses (2005). *AACN Standards for establishing and sustaining healthy work environments, a journey to excellence.* Retrieved from http://www.aacn.org/wd/hwe/docs/hwestandards.pdf

Batalden, P. B. (2010). The leader's work in the improvement of healthcare. *BMJ Quality Safety Health Care, 19,* 367–368. doi:10.1136/qshc.2010.043745

Batalden, P. B., & Davidoff, F. (2007). What is "quality improvement" and how can it transform healthcare. *Quality and Safety in Health Care, 16*(1), 2–3.

Batalden, P. B., Nelson, E. C., Mohr, J. J., Godfrey, M. M., Huber, J. P., Kosnik, L., & Ashling, K. (2003). Microsystems in health care: Part 5. How leaders are leading. *The Joint Commission Journal on Quality and Safety, 29*(6), 297–308.

Birk, S. (2015). Accelerating the adoption of a safety culture. *Healthcare Executive.* Retrieved from http://www.jointcommission.org/assets/1/18/Healthcare_Executive_McKee_032015.pdf

Burr, J. T. Center for Quality and Applied Statistics. Rochester, NY: Rochester Institute of Technology.

Chassin, M. R., & Loeb, J. M. (2013). High reliability healthcare: Getting there from here. *The Milbank Quarterly, 91*(3), 459–490.

Corrigan, J., & McNeill, D. (2009). Building organization capacity: A cornerstone of health system reform. *Health Affairs, 28*(2), 205–215.

Davis, J., & Adams, J. (2011). The 'Releasing Time to Care—the Productive Ward' programme: Participants' perspectives. *Journal of Nursing Management, 20,* 354–336.

Dearmon, V., Roussel, L., Buckner, E. B., Mulekar, M., Pomrenke, B., Salas, S., … Brown, A. (2012). Transforming care at the bedside (TCAB): Enhancing direct care and value-added care. *Journal of Nursing Management.* Retrieved from http://www.ncbi.nlm.nih.gov/pubmed/23409738

Deming, W. E. (1993). *The new economics.* Cambridge, MA: MIT Press.

Donabedian, A. (2002). *An introduction to quality assurance in health care.* New York, NY: Oxford University Press.

Eggenberger, T. (2012). Exploring the charge nurse role: Holding the frontline. *Journal of Nursing Administration, 42,* 502–506.

Habegger, B. (2009). Strategic foresight: Anticipation and capacity to act. *CSS Analyses in Security Policy.* Retrieved from http://works.bepress.com /beathabegger/19

Institute of Medicine. (1999). *To err is human: Building a safer health system.* Retrieved from http://iom.edu/Reports/1999/To-Err-is-Human-Building-A -Safer-Health-System.aspx

Institute of Medicine. (2001a). *Crossing the quality chasm: A new health system for the 21st century.* Retrieved from https://www.iom.edu/~/media/Files /Report%20Files/2001/Crossing-the-Quality-Chasm/Quality%20Chasm%20 2001%20%20report%20brief.pdf

Institute of Medicine. (2001b). *Envisioning the national health care quality report.* Retrieved from http://www.iom.edu/reports/2001/envisioning-the-national -health-care-quality-report.aspx

Institute of Medicine. (2002). *Leadership by example: Coordinating government roles in improving health care quality.* Retrieved from http://www.iom.edu /reports/2002/leadership-by-example-coordinating-government-roles-in -improving-health-care-quality.aspx

Institute of Medicine. (2003). *Priority areas for national action: Transforming health care quality.* Retrieved from http://www.iom.edu/reports/2003/priority-areas -for-national-action-transforming-health-care-quality.aspx

Koch, M. L. (2013). Quality management: Key to patient safety. In *Management and leadership for nurse administrators* (6th ed., pp. 479–497). Burlington, MA: Jones & Bartlett Learning.

Langley, G. J., Moen, R. D., Nolan, K. M., Nolan, T. W., Norman, C. L., & Provost, L. P. (2009). *The improvement guide* (2nd ed.). San Francisco, CA: Jossey-Bass.

Lloyd, R. (2004). *Quality health care: A guide to developing and using indicators.* Sudbury, MA: Jones and Bartlett Publishers.

Marshall, D. A. (2013). Leadership rounding on the front lines. *Safer Healthcare.* Retrieved from http://myrounding.com/images/files/Best_Practice_-_Leadership _Rounding_-_2-19-2013.pdf

Melnyk, B. M., & Fineout-Overholt, E. (2015). *Evidence-based practice in nursing and healthcare: A guide to best practice* (3rd ed.). Philadelphia, PA: Lippincott Williams & Wilkins.

Microsystems Academy. (2015). *Transforming microsystems in healthcare.* Retrieved from https://clinicalmicrosystem.org/workbooks/

Moen, R., & Norman, C. (2010, November). Circling back: Clearing up myths about the Deming cycle and seeing how it keeps evolving. *Quality Progress,* 22–28.

Mukherjee, P. N. (2006). *Total quality management*. New Delhi, India: Prentice Hall.

National Center for Biotechnology Information. (n.d.). PubMed. Retrieved from http://www.ncbi.nlm.nih.gov/pubmed/

Nelson, E. C., Batalden, P. B., Homa, K, Godfrey, M.M, Campbell, C, Headrick, L.A, . . . Wasson, J. H. (2003). Microsystems in health care: Part 2. Creating a rich information environment. *The Joint Commission Journal on Quality and Safety, 29*(1), 5–15.

Porter-O'Grady, T. (2011). Leadership at all levels. *Nursing Management, 42*, 33–37.

Rutherford, P., Phillips, J., Coughlan, P., Lee, B., Moen, R., Peck, C., & Taylor, J. (2008). *Transforming care at the bedside how-to guide: Engaging front-line staff in innovation and quality improvement*. Cambridge, MA: Institute for Healthcare Improvement.

Siriwardena, A. N., Shaw, D., Essam, N., Togher, F. J., Davy, Z., Spaight, A., . . . Group, A. C. (2014). The effect of a national quality improvement collaborative on prehospital care for acute myocardial infarction and stroke in England. *Implementation Science, 9*, 17.

Spuck, J. (1999). Using the long-term care minimum data set as a tool for CQI in nursing homes. In J. Dieneman (Ed.), *Nursing administration: Managing patient care* (2nd ed., pp. 95–105). Stamford, CT: Appleton and Lange.

Thompson, P. A. (2009). Creating leaders for the future: TCAB is helping to redesign hospital care by developing new nursing leaders. *American Journal of Nursing, 109*, 50–52.

U.S. National Library of Medicine. (2013). Medical subject headings (MeSH). Retrieved from http://www.nlm.nih.gov/pubs/factsheets/mesh.html

U.S. National Library of Medicine. (2015). Medical subject headings. Retrieved from http://www.nlm.nih.gov/mesh/meshhome.html

Leaders Achieving Sustainable Outcomes

James L. Harris

LEARNING OBJECTIVES

1. Describe the importance and attributes of leaders who transform care environments.
2. Define values and attributes that support achievable and sustainable outcomes.
3. Discuss how meaningful outcomes are required to engage champions who lead others to ensure that outcomes are achieved and sustained.
4. Describe how staff engagement and satisfaction define models of sustainability and information infrastructure.

AONE KEY COMPETENCIES

I. Communication and relationship building
II. Knowledge of the healthcare environment
III. Leadership
IV. Professionalism
V. Business skills

AONE KEY COMPETENCIES DISCUSSED IN THIS CHAPTER

II. Knowledge of the healthcare environment
III. Leadership
IV. Professionalism

II. Knowledge of the healthcare environment
- Clinical practice knowledge
- Patient care delivery models and work design knowledge
- Healthcare economics knowledge
- Healthcare policy knowledge
- Understanding of governance
- Understanding of evidence-based practice
- Outcomes measurement

- Knowledge of, and dedication to, patient safety
- Understanding of utilization and case management
- Knowledge of quality improvement and metrics
- Knowledge of risk management

III. Leadership
- Foundational thinking skills
- Personal journey disciplines
- Ability to use systems thinking
- Succession planning
- Change management

IV. Professionalism
- Personal and professional accountability
- Career planning
- Ethics
- Evidence-based clinical and management practices
- Advocacy for the clinical enterprise and for nursing practice
- Active membership in professional organizations

FUTURE OF NURSING: FOUR KEY MESSAGES

1. Nurses should practice to the full extent of their education and training.
2. Nurses should achieve higher levels of education and training through an improved education system that promotes seamless academic progression.
3. Nurses should be full partners with physicians and other health professionals in redesigning health care in the United States.
4. Effective workforce planning and policy making require better data collection and information infrastructure.

Introduction

Mandates for quality, safety, and sustainable outcomes within a cost-contained structure remain hallmarks of healthcare success. Leaders who are transformative innovators are required if healthcare outcomes are to be meaningful, value based, and sustainable. Hard wiring environments that transform systems for sustainable quality and safe, economically based care outcomes can be a daunting task, but it is achievable.

Sustainable outcomes will be evident in direct and indirect savings and in a reduction of variability. Sustainability could provide Medicare a new lease on life, underwrite biomedical research, reduce debt, support education, and inform public and private purposes (Litvak & Fineberg, 2013).

This chapter will provide an overview of leadership qualities, sustainable outcomes, value and sustainability, approaches to managing variability, and tools that are available to healthcare leaders for sustaining data-driven outcomes. Clinical case examples are also included for reflection by students and administrators who are confronted with the myriad challenges of healthcare reform.

LEADERSHIP QUALITIES FOR ACHIEVING SUSTAINABLE OUTCOMES

The U.S. healthcare system requires leaders who are visionary, transformative, and accountable. As healthcare costs spiral upward and the population continues to require significant care to contain the magnitude of chronic illness, one may question what role leaders play in combating a growing epidemic. Although there is no easy answer, one solution is a leader who engages all stakeholders and remains mindful of the Institute for Healthcare Improvement (IHI, 2013) Triple Aim, which describes an approach that optimizes healthcare system performance. The IHI unwaveringly posits that new care designs must be developed in which systems simultaneously pursue the three dimensions of the Triple Aim:

1. Improving the patient experience of care (including quality and satisfaction)
2. Improving the health of populations
3. Reducing the per capita cost of health care (IHI, 2014b, p. 1)

Being mindful of the Triple Aim requires leaders to maintain a state of action and be attentive to the present, rather than revisiting the past or focusing on the future. When leaders are mindful, they are open to observing thoughts and feelings without judgment of right or wrong. Mindful leaders in health care help one to cope with stresses, connect with the patient experience, and improve the quality of life for others. Negative emotions and anxiety are reduced, and positive emotions and feelings of self-compassion increase (Kabat-Zinn, 2012).

Leaders can no longer rely on past practices and individual accomplishments; they must engage others in the creation of healthy communities, position patients and families to be at the center of care, expand the role of primary care by all providers, and ensure a seamless continuum of care. Such actions result in positive outcomes that remain sustainable and achievable by others. Contemporary leaders must be able to lead and engage others so new financial approaches create processes and structures that are replicable as evidence is spread and individual systems remain a sustainable and viable option for care.

A useful tool for leadership teams to use prior to implementing change is force field analysis. This tool compares driving and restraining forces in the context of resources, staff engagement, education, and more (Mitchell, 2013). For example, door-to-electrocardiogram is a moderate driving force that is necessary to perform quick patient registration and triage. The restraining force is resistance from the registration staff to completing only a partial intake on initial patient contact. Such an approach may be beneficial for teams considering bedside registration versus the traditional method in which an improved workflow is possible and patient needs are readily met. Driving and restraining forces are inherently important as leaders increase their awareness of work processes and anticipate issues that may be associated with change in the workplace.

What Makes a Leader?

Everyone knows an individual who is highly skilled and is promoted into an executive leadership position only to fail. Conversely, everyone knows someone who may have solid, but not extraordinary, intellectual and technical skills who is promoted into an executive leadership position and is highly successful.

Numerous anecdotes identify the qualities of leadership, but the question remains, is leadership an art or a science? Skills and individuals vary, as do leaders and followers. Healthcare mergers, acquisitions, and turnarounds may require a sensitive negotiator and forceful authority. This often depends on the situation. Leadership strength, emotional intelligence, team champions, and cultural sensitivity are essential for leadership success, quantifiable outcomes, and sustainability.

Gallup Inc. has worked with many leadership teams and identified four distinct domains of leadership strength: executing, influencing, relationship building, and strategic thinking (Rath & Conchie, 2008). **Table 14-1** provides a clinical example for each type of leader.

Executing focuses on making things occur. Leaders with executing skills implement solutions, and ideas become reality. Influencing leaders take charge and sell a team's idea to internal and external stakeholders. Individuals who lead through relationship building have a distinct ability to create and engage a group whose sum is greater than its parts. Strategic thinkers keep a group focused on the primary aim and stretch thinking toward future possibilities (Rath & Conchie, 2008).

Beyond the leadership domains, other quality attributes and actions reinforce sustainable outcomes. Emotional intelligence is the first attribute. According to Goleman (2004), emotional intelligence is a process of self-awareness, regulation, motivation, empathy, and social skills that are necessary for an effective, transformative leader who has multiple followers. Goleman has repeatedly discussed that the most effective leaders have one common denominator: they all have a high degree of emotional intelligence, the sine qua non of leadership. He further identified five components of how emotional intelligence operates at work. The components include self-awareness, self-regulation, motivation, empathy, and social skill. Each of the components has distinct but related parts that are twice as important as cognitive and technical skills and result in high-performing individuals within organizations.

The second action is engaging and coaching teams. Talent without teamwork can result in unsustainable outcomes. High-functioning teams in the workplace require employee engagement. Employees who are engaged are committed to

TABLE 14-1 Leader Strength Clinical Examples	
Leader strength	**Clinical example**
Executing	The executive leader simultaneously readies the healthcare system for a successful Magnet and Joint Commission survey.
Influencing	Upon the loss of revenue when skin assessments are not completed and documented on admission and patients develop hospital-acquired pressure ulcers, an influencing leader sells the idea of how to change practice and eliminate the loss of revenue while eliminating pressure ulcers.
Relationship building	Multiple staff vacancies remain consistent, in excess of 60%, on a medical unit. A relationship-building leader engages staff to build and maintain a harmonious work environment, thus reducing the sustained rate to less than 10% annually.
Strategic thinking	A strategic-thinking leader redesigns care delivery toward a patient-centered care environment in which interprofessional collaboration is fostered.

organizational goals and values, are motivated toward success, and are able to enhance their sense of well-being (Noreen & MacLeod, 2014). Leaders who are driven to succeed often engage championship team building using seven techniques: a common goal, commitment, complementary roles, clear communication, constructive conflict, cohesion, and credible coaching (Janssen, 1999). Although this is a complex process that requires consistent monitoring and improvement, the use of these techniques is evident as a motivated, committed, and cohesive team emerges that is dedicated to accomplishing goals and building coalitions.

Finally, being culturally sensitive as a leader is paramount because the world is increasingly more global and diverse, and healthcare leaders are becoming more cognizant of the deleterious effects of insensitivity (Johnson, 2011; Kokemuller, 2014). Cultural belief systems interact with all aspects of information processes (Seibert, Stridh-Igo, & Zimmerman, 2002). This notion is not surprising when one considers the importance of culture in designing care processes and related recovery periods after medical procedures. Culturally competent leaders and healthcare workers are exceedingly relevant because quality of care has become central to improvement initiatives and sustainable outcomes. The one-size-fits-all mantra is obsolete in healthcare delivery in an era of reform when patients are the center of care. Without understanding the cultural context in which individuals build their understanding of information, high-quality outcomes that are safe and sustainable are easily jeopardized (Kalnins, 1997; Seibert, Trejo, & Zimmermann, 1999).

Leaders must be positioned to manage complexities in health care and harness a range of determinants to be successful in today's environment. Leaders who embrace teamwork and diverse viewpoints, while remaining emotionally intelligent, have greater potentials for success and are able to implement activities that remain sustainable in the most turbulent of times. Culturally sensitive leaders become exemplars for others in the organization by setting examples and establishing norms of behavioral activity that engenders the importance of cultural awareness.

SUSTAINING OUTCOMES

Owing to its complexity, sustaining care outcomes can be a dynamic process with many related concepts and actions operating in tandem. Understanding the importance of sustainable care outcomes can be beneficial to any organization as quality, safe, and value-based initiatives are implemented and sustained. The broad array of challenges in any organization—including how to define and assess quality, evaluate services, and use technology effectively—can place considerable burden on managers and staff. One tool that has been used by leaders in meeting the challenge to sustain care outcomes is cognitive mapping. Cognitive maps are useful because they represent the concrete, operational, and theoretical notions that are already known (Lourdel, Gondran, Laforest, Debray, & Brodhag, 2007). The ultimate goal is realized as managers and staff members identify what is occurring (antecedents), the consequences, and the overall outcomes that are reflected in positive and sustainable care practices. For purpose of this discussion, **Table 14-2** is an example of a cognitive map related to sustainable quality care outcomes.

Sustainability in care delivery is widespread in health care and is a direct link between improved care and lower operating costs. Sustainability is no longer a fleeting trend, but rather a business approach being adopted to maintain

TABLE 14-2 Sustainable Quality Care Outcomes: A Cognitive Map

Antecedents	Consequences	Outcomes
■ Care practice changes	■ Care compromised by adverse event	■ Quality, safe, and value-driven care delivery initiated and sustained
■ Restrictive practice environment	■ Risk (potential and actual) increases	■ Practice change occurs
■ Social, cultural, ethical, technology, environmental, competency, and skill deterrents	■ Staff and patient dissatisfaction	■ Risk minimized or eliminated
■ Risk potential increased	■ Blaming and staff splitting	■ Practice governance and ownership
■ Adverse care event occurs	■ Disciplinary potential increases	■ Staff competency and skill enhancement
	■ Root-cause analysis initiated	■ Culture of quality, safety, and value
		■ Collaborative practice and engagement
		■ Satisfied staff and stakeholders

competitive operations. Integrating sustainability in clinic and hospital operations can be challenging as one links the mission of care to sustainable quality and safe, value-based initiatives (Boone, 2012). A cognitive map is one tool that can assist managers in sustaining positive outcomes.

VALUE AND SUSTAINABILITY

The healthcare industry has been hard at work since the late 1990s. Upon release of the Institute of Medicine's report *To Err Is Human: Building a Safer Health System* (1999), a series of changes in healthcare delivery, quality, and reimbursement followed. Specifically, the following transformative events and actions occurred:

- The Leapfrog Group began rating hospitals on technology and safety
- The Joint Commission introduced 10 starter set core measures
- The Malcolm Baldrige National Quality Award was presented for the first time
- Transforming Care at the Bedside was launched
- *The Future of Nursing: Leading Change, Advancing Health* report was released (Institute of Medicine, 2010)
- Healthcare reform passed

Change is inherent in any organization, and health care is not exempt. Value and sustainable outcomes have never been more important. As Porter-O'Grady and Malloch (2015) so pointedly stated, understanding the value of work has shifted. Previously, excellence in care focused on process. Process, however, is not consistently linked to outcome, value, or sustainability. A process can lose its value, and sustainable outcomes are diminished, which are the essence of the interrelationship. Process derives value from desired outcomes, and if outcomes do not inform and discipline the process, much is lost. Today's leaders must reformulate actions and engage in modern imperatives where health care is valued, measured, and reimbursed. It is the moral compass, however subtle, that must underpin leaders' actions (Holden, 2005). Leadership demands as much conviction as diplomacy in the transition to value-based, responsible care delivery (Sturmberg & Martin, 2012).

Improving performance and accountability depends on a shared goal that joins the actions and interests of all stakeholders. This is requisite for change in health care and for organizational solvency. In health care, stakeholders have conflicting goals due to the myriad issues related to access, profitability, satisfaction, cost containment, and safety. Unclear goals lead to divergent approaches in which systems are gamed and improvement processes are diminished (Porter, 2010).

Of the multiple transformations reshaping health care, none is more profound than the shift toward value. Achieving high value for patients is an overarching goal of healthcare delivery where value is defined as the health outcomes achieved per dollar spent (Porter & Teisberg, 2006). Value must define the framework for performance improvement in health care. However, measuring value in health care remains largely misunderstood. It is elusive for many reasons. First, there is no clear consensus definition of what constitutes quality among providers, let alone purchasers, due to variations in age, expectations, and general health. The Centers for Medicare and Medicaid Services has developed core measures that focus on processes that may be indicators of clinical treatment and are largely removed from actual outcomes. The outcome metrics emphasize either mortality or readmission rates within certain time periods after procedures or admissions. Adverse events inform outcome metrics versus positive outcomes that purchasers expect from care. Second, the full amount paid for health care is not transparent. Payments are fractionally distributed to several providers and multiple purchasers. Third, providers are not typically reimbursed for producing value, but for volume. This leads one to question if the value equation needs to be reconsidered for health care where value equals quality divided by payment. Quality is measured by a composite of patient outcomes, safety, and experiences, and payment is the cost to all purchasers of purchasing care.

How does a leader respond to the demand for value? The Healthcare Financial Management Association (2014) identified four capabilities that organizations should consider, based on extensive interviews with provider organizations in the United States:

- Instilling a culture of collaboration, creativity, and accountability of staff
- Collecting, analyzing, and connecting quality and financial data that supports decision making (business intelligence)
- Developing and managing data to reduce variability and improve performance
- Developing and managing care networks that are predictive and anticipate risk (contract and risk management)

The convergence of multiple factors will assist leaders to create sustainable value in turbulent and ever-changing environments. Creating a sense of responsibility among individuals in organizations that connect to strategic imperatives can balance the value equation that creates sustainable value (Porter-O'Grady & Malloch, 2015).

MANAGING VARIABILITY: AN IMPERATIVE FOR ACHIEVING AND MAINTAINING SUSTAINABLE OUTCOMES

Scientists view the universe as linear; causes affect applications. This view is predictable and can be controlled. As societal changes and dynamics unfolded, scientists from all disciplines shifted focus. Such has been the case, over time, in healthcare management and practice. How to control for variability while sustaining quality, safe, and value-based outcomes remains a significant challenge for managers today. Although many factors are attributed to variability in care, unmanaged variability in patient flow remains constant in all systems and challenges the best systems to develop equitable solutions (Litvak, Vaswani, Long, & Prenney, 2007).

During recent decades, complexity theory evolved as a new opportunity to view how relationships and systems adapt to change within various environments. Complexity theory is based on relationships, emergence, patterns, and iterations (Plesk & Greenhalgh, 2001). It holds that the universe is full of systems, regardless of type, and the systems are constantly adapting to their environments. Considering that many healthcare systems are unable to manage variables associated with patient flow, one may contemplate the importance of the theory to remedying care dilemmas and controlling for variability, actions to sustain profitable outcomes, and properties that are associated with complex adaptive systems.

Complex adaptive systems and associated properties have significant relevance to this discussion. Complex adaptive systems refer to agents in a system and all components of that system. Agents interact with one another and connect in unpredictable ways. From multiple and variable interactions, regularities emerge and a pattern evolves that provides feedback to the agents (Fryer, 2014). As patterns evolve and agents are informed, leaders have new choices and the freedom to engage in change processes.

The Institute for Healthcare Optimization introduced variability methodology as another approach to manage the variability associated with patient flow. The methodology is based on a three-phase approach (Institute for Healthcare Optimization, 2014):

Phase I: Separate groups (such as inpatient and outpatient) that are specific to procedures (for example, emergent and nonemergent).
Phase II: Reduce the nonemergent procedures and reschedule them, leaving options for add-ins.
Phase III: Estimate what resources are needed to ensure flow.

Regardless of the method used, leaders can manage variability in practice so sustainable outcomes can become commonplace. Sustainable savings are possible, waste is reduced, and both patient and staff satisfaction increases.

MANAGING SUSTAINABLE OUTCOMES

The need to improve work environments and the unprecedented national efforts to use any methods or tools to enable leaders to manage and achieve sustainable quality and safe and valuable outcomes remain constant. Managing outcomes is neither linear nor unilateral, but it is multifocal and interactive among various healthcare teams. Ellwood (1988) stated that managing sustainable outcomes includes a technology of patient experience designed to assist patients, payers, and providers to make rational decisions based on relevant and evidence-based information. A common health outcomes language, a national database that includes the relationship between interventions and outcomes, the relationship between outcomes and finances, and access to information are imperatives for quality care and sustainable outcomes. In the advent of technology and interconnectivity in health care, Ellwood's notion is attainable as access, improvement, and sustainment become the cornerstone for purposed action by healthcare leaders.

Although the healthcare industry is acutely aware of the reality that human error is part of daily practice, one must remain cognizant of the need to engender a culture of safety. This is amplified when one reviews landmark cases, such as the near-death of the twins of actor Dennis Quaid and his wife due to an overdose of heparin and the infant who succumbed to a tenfold overdose of arginine (Hernandez, 2008; Word, 2014). To counter such tragedies in the future, the healthcare industry has adopted an array of methods developed by industry to reduce the frequency of errors. Methods by Deming, Juran, and Ohne are proving effective. While such methods are effective, the challenge of escalating healthcare costs and mandates to manage outcomes that are sustainable have caused leaders to question how quality relates to performance.

Measurement is central to managing performance and outcomes that are sustained over time. Common process models and tools used in health care today that assist managers to analyze issues related to low performance and unstable outcomes are included in the following discussion. Applying these improvement tools can be challenging, but they are effective in reducing and preventing future errors and managing outcomes.

FADE Model

This model shares the common threads of analysis, implementation, and review with other quality improvement models. The four prongs of the FADE model include focus, analyze, develop, and execute. Each of these prongs involves two additional steps to develop a model for change. For example, focus refers to identifying the problem. Within the focus domain, the process of determining the focus includes creating a problem list, selecting one problem, verifying and defining the chosen problem, and producing a written statement describing the defined problem. Analyze refers to data collection and root-cause analysis and includes the following: deciding what information is needed, collecting baseline data, listing influential factors, further synthesizing useful baseline data, and prioritizing influential factors (Duke University Department of Community and Family Medicine, 2014). Develop refers to action plan and solution development. Within this domain, the process includes listing possible solutions, selecting a solution, and developing an implementation plan. Execute refers to the implementation and monitoring of action plans. Within this domain, the process includes gaining commitment, executing the plan, and monitoring the impact of the plan. As with any tool or process, evaluation is an additional step that continuously evaluates the change and impact.

Situation Background Assessment Recommendation (SBAR)

This tool is used in most organizations to promote optimal communication between nurses and physicians. The SBAR tool provides a useful outline for framing critical conversations that require a physician's immediate attention (Institute for Healthcare Improvement, 2014a). According to Labson (2013), the tool is used to explain a situation in a clinical area, such as obstetrics, so a nurse can provide relevant information to a physician to obtain a medication order. The tool, when used effectively, can alleviate potential clinical issues.

Flowcharts

Similar to blueprints, flowcharts guide continuous improvement. Readiness teams dissect a situation, related processes, and event sequences in great detail (Lighter, 2011). For example, flowcharts can be useful in understanding the factors contributing to bottlenecks, redundancies, and inefficiencies within an emergency department. This graphic representation illustrates the inputs and outputs and helps the team consider actions that can improve process measures, such as utilization, cost, and satisfaction. A flowchart is also useful as the genesis of a root-cause analysis and a preventive tool called failure mode effects analysis (FMEA).

Root-Cause Analysis

A root-cause analysis is a retrospective method of evaluating an event due to an error or incident. It assists in identifying what, how, and why an event occurred. Findings from a root-cause analysis are central to developing improvement recommendations (Rooney & Heuvel, 2004).

Although this tool is not limited to health care, it has much applicability due to the number of actual and potential medical mistakes that are documented daily. The basic tenets of a root-cause analysis are grounded in the belief that correcting and eliminating the root cause will correct the identified problem. Through a series of reviews, drilling down, and asking why, teams identify root causes that are related to an event and recommend improvement actions that are directed at the underlying causes. This is accomplished using a four-step process: data collection, causal factor clarity, root-cause identification, and recommendation development and implementation. As corrective actions are initiated, monitoring the impact over time may ensure the event does not reoccur. This is an important step that organizations may overlook; without such information, organizations may lose opportunities for efficiency, quality, and safe practices in the future. Common examples of root-cause analyses within healthcare agencies include defective or shortages of materials or equipment, hazardous environments, lack of communication and procedures, and lack of skill sets and competency validation.

FMEA

FMEA is used to ensure that potential problems have been considered and addressed during product and process development cycles. Specifically, FMEA assists in the following:

- Discovering potential failures, causes, and risks
- Developing actions that reduce risks and failures
- Evaluating the results of actions taken based on identified risk (Stalhandske, DeRosier, Wilson, & Murphy, 2009)

In 2002, The Joint Commission began requiring FMEA as an accreditation standard. Severity index scores, ranging from 1 (low) to 10 (catastrophic), are assigned to organizations based on the event (The Joint Commission, 2004).

Matrices

Matrices provide a systematic approach for identifying relationships and opportunities for improvement among groups of information (Lighter, 2011). The data offer valuable information in health care; namely, how a learner perceives information, competencies of individuals, team efforts, and information about how the organization functions. This provides support for mandatory measurement and reporting of results as the healthcare system is reformed and managers transform systems of care.

Decision Trees

A decision tree is an excellent tool to help managers choose from several actions based on a highly effective structure that allows them to identify and investigate all possible options. The tool helps managers form a balanced picture of the risks and rewards of each option. A common decision tree in health care is a sensitivity analysis of risk coefficients, where the organization may prefer the risks and payoffs of one product versus another. This is commonly measured in dollars.

As with any tool, there are advantages and disadvantages. The advantages of decision trees include the following:

- Simple to understand and interpret
- Have value with minimal data whereby insights are generated
- Possible scenarios can be added
- Expected valuation can be determined from possible scenarios
- Easily combined with other decision tools.

The disadvantages include the following:

- Bias possible when there are attributes with numerous options and levels
- Calculations may become complex due to multiple linked outcomes

Cause-and-Effect Analysis

Cause-and-effect analysis is a diagram-based technique combining brainstorming with mind mapping that forces the consideration of all possible causes of problems, instead of just the obvious ones. Cause-and-effect diagrams are also called fish bone, Ishikawa, herringbone, and fishikawa diagrams. The analysis allows individuals and teams to identify the root cause of a problem, uncover bottlenecks, and identify where and why a process is not working (Ishikawa, 1990).

BENCHMARKING

Multiple sources for benchmarking outcomes and performance have been developed by accrediting bodies, government entities, and private entities. The websites of various healthcare agencies provide charts, graphs, and tables that illustrate performance. Benchmarking is common in the quality literature, but one may question if the process is fully understood. Benchmarking should move beyond comparing one hospital with national averages; it is more informative to look at the best-in-class hospitals to see what may be learned (Sower, 2007).

One of the most popular benchmarking approaches is Six Sigma, which is a systematic method of using information and statistical analyses to measure an organization's performance, practices, and systems by identifying and preventing defects in production and service-related processes to improve effectiveness (George, 2002). Some sources for benchmarking data and operational definitions are provided in the following sections (Lighter, 2011).

National Quality Forum

The National Quality Forum is a voluntary standards-setting organization that recommends metrics and endorses standards, performance measures, quality indicators, preferred practices, and reporting guidelines used by healthcare industry stakeholders.

The Joint Commission

The Joint Commission's ORYX program requires quality improvement initiatives and developed sets of core measures that must be reported. Hospitals must report four sets of criteria to be accredited through a measurement system that is evaluated and approved by The Joint Commission. The measures include the following:

- Acute myocardial infarction
- Heart failure
- Children's asthma care
- Pneumonia
- Pregnancy and related conditions
- Surgical care improvement project
- Hospital-based inpatient psychiatric services
- Hospital outpatient measures

National Committee for Quality Assurance

The National Committee for Quality Assurance is an adopter of performance measures for healthcare payers through the Healthcare Effectiveness Data and Information Set (HEDIS). Examples of these measures include antibiotic utilization, outpatient drug utilization, and flu shots for older adults. They are applicable to commercial insurance, Medicare, and Medicaid.

Medicare Data Sources

Information that is relative to Medicare utilization and quality data includes Medicare Provider Analysis and Review (MEDPAR) data.

SUMMARY

The healthcare environment during this decade and beyond will continue to present opportunities for leaders to examine multiple options for achieving excellence. Outcomes must be sustainable and replicable. By evaluating evidence that guides change in practice environments, leaders must embrace opportunities to adopt new and novel ways of thinking and acting.

Environments must become hard wired to promote quality, safe, and value-based care. Cultural sensitivity has never been more relevant in care environments given the global nature of society. Various cultures live, act, and interact in tandem. Leaders and care providers must remain cognizant of cultural differences and remain sensitive to each of them.

Healthcare organizations must revisit their value proposition and its context within each environment. Answering what constitutes value in a responsible healthcare organization has never been more important for thought and reflection. Being aware of one's emotional intelligence will prove useful in answering the question, as will utilizing various techniques that are yet to be determined as changes evolve.

This chapter has provided a brief overview of leader attributes that are necessary to transform care environments, as well as tools for sustaining quality, safe, and value-driven outcomes in a rapidly changing healthcare landscape. As leaders drive change and respond to the array of mandates imposed by external stakeholders, they must remain cognizant of how one action will directly and indirectly affect the whole.

REFLECTIVE QUESTIONS

Sustainability within any healthcare environment today requires skillful leaders. Being a full partner in the identification, resolution, and sustainment of issues is required. As a current or future healthcare leader, consider the following questions and your impact on achieving sustainable outcomes.

1. What qualities must a contemporary leader possess to be a valued contributor and partner in achieving organizational effectiveness in rural and urban healthcare settings?
2. What impact does a transformational leader have on achieving excellence in an organization?
3. Consider the structures required for meeting the impending changes imposed by healthcare reform legislation.
4. A variety of tools and techniques are available for leaders to achieve goals. Which of these can be beneficial to you as a leader in a practice area?
5. Identify how the value equation drives quality, safe, and value-driven outcomes.

6. Identify techniques that are used by leaders to engage staff in improvement activities, and identify techniques that are suited for individual use.

7. What measurement tools provide consistent outcomes in your area of practice, and what techniques are used to communicate findings to other staff members?

CASE STUDY 14-1   Cultural Awareness and Sensitivity: Imperatives for Healthcare Providers

James L. Harris

Achieving cultural awareness and sensitivity is one of the many arts that healthcare providers must master. Quality care and patient satisfaction will follow. Being culturally aware and sensitive to patients and their families has become increasingly constant in daily practice, given the global nature of communities. Consider the following clinical case and reflect on the issues and cultural dynamics as they relate to your current practice setting and the need to be aware and sensitive to the needs of others from different cultures.

Jose, a 16-year-old Hispanic male, traveled by bus from rural Mexico to southern Alabama to work on a farm during the spring and summer harvest seasons. Jose speaks limited English and has a rural Spanish dialect. Upon arrival to Alabama, Jose and his traveling companion, who speaks some English and Portuguese, were met by the farm owner at the local bus station. The two would be part of a group of 50 workers during spring and summer. The group members speak a variety of languages and are from different cultures.

Work began immediately upon their arrival. Their work days were Monday through Saturday from 5 a.m. to 7 p.m. After the third week of work, Jose fell from a moving tractor and struck his head on a concrete slab. He was unconscious and was taken to the local trauma center by air flight, where he was diagnosed with a traumatic brain injury (TBI). No family was available, and the farm owner knew nothing about Jose's medical history or how to contact his family members.

In the following weeks, Jose's condition continued to deteriorate, and little to no verbal communication was possible even though several Spanish-speaking staff members were consulted. Jose's traveling companion visited him weekly on Sundays. The attending physician, nurse, and social worker spoke with the traveling companion using an interpreter and questioned if he knew of any family member or anything that may aid in Jose's recovery. The traveling companion recalled that during their trip to the farm, Jose spoke of the importance of family during healing, and he recalled that Jose mentioned that a brother lived somewhere in northern California. After several days of research by a social worker, the brother was located and was able to visit Jose.

The brother stayed with Jose for 3 weeks and communicated to the treatment team the importance in their culture of having family at their side when someone is ill. When his brother arrived, Jose started to respond to therapy. After several months of rehabilitation, he was able to leave the facility and relocate to California with his brother, where he started a vocational training program that he successfully completed. Jose had few residual effects from the TBI, and a California-based company employed Jose.

Case Study Questions

1. How would an interdisciplinary team work with Jose and his family to best transition his care from the hospital to home?

2. In considering outcomes, how would the team set priorities? What priorities would you establish with the family if you were the team leader working with Jose?

CASE STUDY 14-2   Universal Protocol and Time-Out: What Is Being Measured?

Shea Polancich

In 2009, the National Patient Safety Goals for universal protocol and time-out (UP/TO) expanded the coverage of these procedures to areas outside the perioperative arena. During this time period and thereafter, it became imperative to have a robust measurement for assessing adherence to this important process. However, what exactly does adherence to the UP/TO process mean? UP/TO is a comprehensive process for ensuring that all safeguards prior to the performance of a procedure are examined prior to initiation of a procedure. The final time-out is initiated prior to entry into a site and concludes with the final safety net of ensuring the correct patient, procedure, site, and side by the entire procedural team. Since the inception of UP/TO, the goal has always been to safeguard patients against procedural harm. However, the traditional use of the procedural checklist may or may not be producing the desired outcome.

In 2009, many medical centers developed procedural checklists to integrate all aspects of UP/TO. In one academic medical center, the process was developed into an electronic smart form with hard stops. The form was used in the operating room and in other procedural areas, including procedures performed on an inpatient unit. The electronic process was implemented with resource allocation for technology support and provider education. At the end of the implementation, the outcomes were analyzed, and the results showed 100% compliance with UP/TO. But was that really the case? What exactly did 100% adherence to UP/TO mean?

After the results of the UP/TO electronic process were reported, the results were questioned from the perspective of behavior modification. Did the process result in behavioral adherence to the process, or did the outcomes represent 100% documentation of a checklist? To answer this question, observers were deployed into procedural areas. These trained observers were like secret shoppers whose identities were not compromised because they were not considered outsiders. The observers were competent to observe and perform the observations, and they were trained in a standard fashion for the observations. Armed with pocket observation forms, the observers were able to navigate the procedural areas and observe the UP/TO process.

The results of the observational assessment were analyzed, and a roughly 15% difference was noted in random observations from the electronic checklist process. Upon review, the first assessment ensured that there was no danger to the patient. Deficiencies were noted primarily in the use of identifiers for patient identification (variations in what identifiers were used) and the participation of all team members in the process. After the nonadherent elements were reviewed, the leadership had to reevaluate the use of the checklist and exactly what was being measured. It was determined that the electronic checklist provided a method of assessing documentation of the process. However, observational assessment was considered necessary to confirm behavioral modification of the UP/TO process.

In developing measures of adherence to behavioral changes, a checklist approach may not adequately address behavior modification. A checklist may address documentation, but it will be necessary to compare both quantitative and qualitative approaches to confirm the desired change.

Case Study Questions

1. What is the leader's strength in managing outcomes of the National Patient Safety Goals for UP/TO in this organization?
2. Describe the antecedents, consequences, outcomes, and leader's responsibility to the team.
3. This case study suggests ways to manage variability in evidence-based protocols. Identify other ways to manage variability and anticipated outcomes.

REFERENCES

Boone, T. (2012). Creating a culture of sustainability. Centre of Health Care Management, University of British Columbia. Retrieved from http://read.chcm.ubc.ca/2012/04/16/creating-a-culture-of-sustainability/

Duke University Department of Community and Family Medicine. (2014). FADE—what is quality improvement. Retrieved from patientsafetyed.duhs.duke.edu/module_a/methods/fade.html

Ellwood, P. (1988). Shattuck lecture—outcomes management: A technology of patient experience. *New England Journal of Medicine, 318*, 1549–1556.

Fryer, P. (2014). What are complex adaptive systems? Retrieved from http://www.trojanmice.com/articles/complexadaptivesystems.htm

George, M. L. (2002). *Lean six sigma: Combining six sigma quality with lean speed.* New York, NY: McGraw-Hill.

Goleman, D. (2004). What makes a leader? Retrieved from http://hbr.org/2004/01/what-makes-a-leader/ar/1

Healthcare Financial Management Association. (2014). Learn, analyze, apply. The healthcare management association can change the world of healthcare finance. Retrieved from https://www.hfma.org

Hernandez, G. (2008). Quaid fights common medical errors. *Los Angeles Daily News.* Retrieved from http://www.dailynews.com/20080315/quaid-fights-common-medical-errors

Holden, L. M. (2005). Complex adaptive systems: Concept analysis. *Journal of Advanced Nursing, 52*(6), 651–657.

Institute for Healthcare Improvement. (2013). IHI Triple Aim Institute. Retrieved from http://www.ihi.org/Engage/Initiatives/TripleAim/pages/default.aspx

Institute for Healthcare Improvement. (2014a). SBAR technique for communication: A situational briefing model. Retrieved from http://www.ihi.org/resources/Pages/Tools/SBARTechniqueforCommunicationASituationalBriefingModel.aspx

Institute for Healthcare Improvement. (2014b). The IHI Triple Aim. Retrieved from http://www.ihi.org/Engage/Initiatives/TripleAim/pages/default.aspx

Institute for Healthcare Optimization. (2014). IHO variability methodology services. Retrieved from http://www.ihoptimize.org/

Institute of Medicine. (1999). *To err is human: Building a safer health system.* Retrieved from https://www.iom.edu/~/media/Files/Report%20Files/1999/To-Err-is-Human/To%20Err%20is%20Human%201999%20%20report%20brief.pdf

Institute of Medicine. (2010). *The future of nursing: Leading change, advancing health.* Retrieved from https://www.iom.edu/~/media/Files/Report%20Files/2010/The-Future-of-Nursing/Future%20of%20Nursing%202010%20Recommendations.pdf

Ishikawa, K. (1990). *Introduction to quality control.* New York, NY: Productivity Press.

Janssen, J. (1999). *Championship team building.* Tucson, AZ: Winning the Mental Game.

Johnson, S. (2011). What globalization means for diversity and inclusion efforts. *Profiles in Diversity Journal, 1.* Retrieved from http://www.diversityjournal .com/4919-what-globalization-means-for-diversity-and-inclusion-efforts/

Kabat-Zinn, J. (2012). *Mindfulness for beginners.* Boulder, CO: Sounds True.

Kalnins, Z. P. (1997). Cultural diversity and today's managed health care. *Journal of Cultural Diversity, 4,* 43.

Kokemuller, N. (2014). Negative effects of diversity in the workplace. Retrieved from http://smallbusiness.chron.com/negative-effects-diversity-workplace-18443 .html

Labson, M. (2013). SBAR—a powerful tool to help improve communication! Retrieved from http://www.jointcommission.org/At_home_with_the_joint _commission/sbar_-_a_powerful_tool_to_help_improve_communication /default.aspx

Lighter, D. E. (2011). *Advanced performance improvement in health care.* Sudbury, MA: Jones & Bartlett Learning.

Litvak, E., & Fineberg, H. V. (2013). Smoothing the way to high quality, safety, and economy. *New England Journal of Medicine, 369,* 1581–1583.

Litvak, E., Vaswani, S. G., Long, M. C., & Prenney, B. (2007). Managing variability in healthcare delivery. Retrieved from http://www.ihoptimize.org/knowledge -center-publications.htm

Lourdel, N., Gondran, N., Laforest, V., Debray, B., & Brodhag, C. (2007). Sustainable development cognitive map: A new method of evaluating student understanding. *International Journal of Sustainability in Higher Education, 8*(2), 170–182.

Mitchell, G. (2013). Selecting the best theory to implement planned change. *Nursing Management—UK, 201*(1), 32–37.

Noreen, S., & MacLeod, M. D. (2014). To think or not to think, that is the question: Individual differences in suppression and rebound effects in autobiographical memory. *Acta Psychologica, 145,* 84–97.

Plesk, P. E., & Greenhalgh, T. (2001). The challenge of complexity in healthcare. *British Medical Journal, 323,* 625–628.

Porter, M. E. (2010). What is value in health care? *New England Journal of Medicine, 363,* 2477–2481.

Porter, M. E., & Teisberg, E. O. (2006). *Redesigning health care: Creating value-based competition on results.* Boston, MA: Harvard Business School Press.

Porter-O'Grady, T., & Malloch, K. (2015). *Quantum leadership: Building better partnerships for sustainable health.* Burlington, MA: Jones & Bartlett Learning.

Rath, T., & Conchie, B. B. (2008). *Strengths based leadership: Great leaders, teams, and why people follow.* New York, NY: Gallup Press.

Rooney, J. J., & Vanden Heuvel, L. N. (2004). Root cause analysis for beginners. *Quality Progress, 37*(7), 45–53.

Seibert, P. S., Stridh-Igo, P., & Zimmerman, C. G. (2002). A checklist to facilitate cultural awareness and sensitivity. *Journal of Medical Ethics, 28,* 143–146.

Seibert, P. S., Trejo, L. S., & Zimmerman, C. G. (1999). *The importance of communication and cultural awareness when treating TBI patients: Cultural sensitivity checklist.* Poster presented at Third World Congress of Brain Injury, Quebec, Canada.

Sower, V. E. (2007). Benchmarking in hospitals: More than a scorecard. *Quality Progress, 40*(8), 58–60.

Stalhandske, E., DeRosier, J., Wilson, R., & Murphy, J. (2009). Healthcare FMEA in the Veterans Health Administration. *Patient Safety and Quality Healthcare, 6*(5), 30–33.

Sturmberg, J. P., & Martin, C. M. (2012). Leadership and transitions: Maintaining the science in complexity and complex systems. *Journal of Evaluation in Clinical Practice, 18,* 186–189.

The Joint Commission. (2004). The Joint Commission press kit. Retrieved from http://www.jointcommission.org/accreditation/accreditation_publicity_kit.aspx

Word, R. (2014). Parents of Florida boy killed by hospital error hope to prevent similar accidents. *Associated Press.* Retrieved from http://www.nctimes.com/articles/2008/03/16/health/9_56_273_15_08

CHAPTER 15

Messaging and Disseminating Excellence in Leadership and Ethical Implications

Linda Roussel, Patricia L. Thomas, and Cynthia King

LEARNING OBJECTIVES

1. Outline strategies that enhance thinking and learning and invite disruptive innovation, strategic messaging, and facilitate stakeholders' abandoning outdated approaches to leading.
2. Describe the mechanisms for achieving organizational outcomes that are replicable and applicable to advancing nursing knowledge, practice, and policy development through messaging.
3. Identify ethical leadership and principles for guiding ethical behavior.
4. Outline the components of an executive summary.

AONE KEY COMPETENCIES

I. Communication and relationship building
II. Knowledge of the healthcare environment
III. Leadership
IV. Professionalism
V. Business skills

AONE KEY COMPETENCIES DISCUSSED IN THIS CHAPTER

I. Communication and relationship building
II. Knowledge of the healthcare environment
III. Leadership
IV. Professionalism

I. **Communication and relationship building**
   - Effective communication
   - Relationship management
   - Influence of behaviors
   - Ability to work with diversity
   - Shared decision making
   - Community involvement

- Medical staff relationships
- Academic relationships

II. Knowledge of the healthcare environment
- Clinical practice knowledge
- Patient care delivery models and work design knowledge
- Healthcare economics knowledge
- Healthcare policy knowledge
- Understanding of governance
- Understanding of evidence-based practice
- Outcomes measurement
- Knowledge of, and dedication to, patient safety
- Understanding of utilization and case management
- Knowledge of quality improvement and metrics
- Knowledge of risk management

III. Leadership
- Foundational thinking skills
- Personal journey disciplines
- Ability to use systems thinking
- Succession planning
- Change management

IV. Professionalism
- Personal and professional accountability
- Career planning
- Ethics
- Evidence-based clinical and management practices
- Advocacy for the clinical enterprise and for nursing practice
- Active membership in professional organizations

FUTURE OF NURSING: FOUR KEY MESSAGES

1. Nurses should practice to the full extent of their education and training.
2. Nurses should achieve higher levels of education and training through an improved education system that promotes seamless academic progression.
3. Nurses should be full partners with physicians and other health professionals in redesigning health care in the United States.
4. Effective workforce planning and policy making require better data collection and information infrastructure.

Introduction

As leaders have progressed during their careers, there are memorable moments that guide actions. Memorable moments provide great fodder for stories, and great messages. We all have a story to tell. Great leaders understand the power, influence, and leverage created by great messaging. They are able to constantly reinvent themselves and rediscover their creative genius. We are no longer able to use our current way of thinking and doing to resolve issues, let alone come up with better, more efficient ways to work. Daniel Pink, journalist and futurist, states, "The future belongs to a very different kind of person with a very different kind of mind. . . . The era of left-brain dominance, and the information age that it engendered, is giving way to a new world in which creative and holistic right-brain abilities mark the fault line between who gets ahead and who falls behind" (Pink, 2005, pp. 5–6).

Have you ever been starstruck by leaders who always seem to have the right words to say? Compare this with the feelings you have when you hear an inane sound bite that makes a leader look uninformed, unintelligent, or irrelevant. The difference is that great leaders excel at the art of finding the right message regardless of the medium, market, or constituency being addressed. Great leaders are able to communicate in ways that pack a punch.

Behavioral scientists Martin, Goldstein, and Cialdini, in *The Small Big: Small Changes That Spark Big Influence* (2014), note that successful influence is governed more by context than cognition and by the psychological environment in which information is presented. They state, "Anyone can significantly increase their ability to influence and persuade others by not only attempting to inform or educate people into change, but also by simply making small shifts in their approach to link their message to deeply felt human motivations" (p. xviii). In their work on influence and persuasion, the authors report that a small change in the timing, setting, or context of how information is communicated or conveyed can dramatically alter how it is actually taken in and acted upon.

Without action for sustainable outcomes, it does not matter what messaging strategy is used. Martin and colleagues (2014) provide a number of small changes that can be impactful. These changes include commitment and consistency, which translates into active involvement to an action or goal and requires real-time participation and effort on our part (versus passively receiving information) and making it public. The authors give an example of patients committed to a plan of action when they are engaged, including writing down specific time frames, and measurement. Over a 4-month period, when patients were asked to write down the time and date of their next appointment (versus the receptionist writing it down), there was an 18% reduction in no-shows in a medical group. This resulted in a savings of $180 million, with zero cost to the medical group (Martin et al., 2014).

The authors say that commitment and consistency are followed by owning the decision and subsequent action. "In fact, there are two other aspects that are also crucial ingredients to the likelihood of a commitment made being fulfilled: how action-oriented that commitment is and how publicly it is made by the person or group committing to it" (Martin et al., 2014, p. 43).

The authors cited challenge and attainability as other small changes. These two factors are important influences on individuals pursuing goals. Reconnecting to goals that have realistic possibilities enhances the probability of greater impact. An example is when the World Health Organization adopted a 5 A Day program encouraging citizens to consume five portions of fruits and vegetables every day. The results revealed mixed success. Making a small change to four or five portions per day increased the success of meeting the goal (Martin et al., 2014, p. 75).

Why is strategic messaging so critical? In the business world, for a chief executive officer or entrepreneur, organizational messaging is the key to both a personal and professional positioning strategy. A leader's message has a direct impact on personal and corporate brand equity, how a crisis is managed, marketing initiatives, stakeholder relations, press and public relations, team building, and staff engagement. Communicating the mission and strategic aims of the organization is a critical responsibility of the chief executive.

Keeping messages succinct also has merit. Speaking in the present and speaking authentically are acts of courage. Goss, in *What Is Your One Sentence?* (2012), describes three steps to develop a memorable message. Step 1 involves the content of the message by identifying the people, action, and drama that is to be communicated. Consider the people involved in the issue, your audience, and how you, the leader, will be portrayed. What actions are important to the goals, and what dramatic elements need to be included in the messaging? Step 2 involves the process of messaging, including the clarity of goals, the focus, and the value added to the communication. What do you want to achieve, and what special value is distinctive and inspiring in what is to be conveyed? Step 3 is about the leader's style and the importance of "saying it with flair" (p. 44). If the message is to be memorable, it should be authentic, concrete and visual, easy to understand, and memorable. Goss notes it is essential to use concrete and visual examples or the message will be abstract and "poetic and soaring" (p. 45).

The logic of the leader's message rests on the main sentence and contains three elements: simplicity (easy to grasp, hopeful, passionate); relevance (popular appeal, differs from competitors' messages); and repetition (repeated messages allow the audience to remember) (Goss, 2012).

The reality is that your messaging will often have a greater impact on your career than your performance. Many have witnessed leaders with average, or even subpar, performance histories who have enjoyed success because they practiced exceptional messaging skills. Message execution skills do not take the place of form over substance. Great communicators understand how to message their shortcomings and flaws to critical spheres of influence while gaining confidence in planning for corrective measures (Goss, 2012; Keller & Papasan, 2012; Wiseman, 2010).

Nurse executives who are seen as great leaders are prepared, articulate, consistent, and succinct in their messaging. Their messages convey authority, clarity, and certitude. A great leader's message never conflicts with his or her values. Executive leaders will not compromise their core values and beliefs to manipulate the outcome of a specific situation. Great leaders are confident that they are doing and saying the right things that will ultimately put them in a favorable position. Likewise, if the consequences are negative, they are comforted in knowing their messages come as a result of right thinking and decision making.

MANAGING MESSAGES

Hamm (2006) describes five messages leaders must manage: organizational structure and hierarchy, financial results, the leader's sense of his or her job, time management, and corporate culture. Messages about these subjects could produce extraordinary influence within the organizational system. It is unwise for managers and leaders to assume that stakeholders within the system know and share their mental models regarding the structure, hierarchy, finances, time management, and culture. If an executive team makes these assumptions, they may lose their perspective and become insulated. Paying attention to details in the messaging, disseminating and controlling communication, and the five areas of focus provide executive leadership with an opportunity for organizational alignment, increased accountability, and substantially better performance. According to Hamm (2006), the five topics provide an excellent place to start and are highly representative of the kinds of difficulties that exist for leaders as they speak to their teams every day. The topics provide keen examples of the perils of imprecise communication. Likewise, when messages are competently executed, they produce the greatest leadership leverage.

Constructive Messaging

When it comes to the construction of messaging, noted researchers tend to fall into the following groups (Goss, 2012; Hamm, 2006; Neffinger & Kohut, 2013; Wiseman, 2010):

- The medium is the message: Communicators who believe the medium is the message hold that the reach and power of the medium can overcome any flaws in the message. That is, if you reach enough people, using a numbers-based approach in the business logic, an acceptable percentage of the people who are reached will embrace the message.
- The market is the message: This messaging approach views the target market and audience as front and center and focuses on specific content. With this level of specificity, those inside the target population would likely be misunderstood by those on the outside, as communication may be guarded, and limited to only those internal to the system.
- The message is the message: The content is central to this type of messaging. The belief is that if the message is inspiring enough, or if it provides value, nothing else matters. This concept of messaging is about the calls to action, the design, the concept, and the information to be communicated.
- The messenger is the message: This messaging approach values the person delivering the information; it is a branded approach to messaging. It relies on the credibility and influence of the messenger. This is an egocentric approach to messaging that places a high premium on the spokesperson. Examples of this type of messaging are famous and infamous persons selling a product, even though the person may have no connection to the product. The wow factor influences the sale.

When considering these four messaging methods, the total value is greater than the stand-alone value. There are any number of genres of marketing, branding, positioning, and messaging; a collaborative and cross-disciplined approach provides a holistic impact. The messaging content can create credibility, and credibility can advance the perception of the content. Blending approaches to craft the right message does not happen independently of the other approaches. Even with superior content, a credible messenger communicating to the wrong audience with the wrong message or through the wrong medium will not add value or have the intended impact. Approaches must be balanced to craft the right message. Consider the following when crafting your message and approach:

- Always be truthful: If your message is not authentic and does not pass public scrutiny over time, you have the wrong message.
- A multiple-medium approach can have the greatest impact: Multiple approaches that consider various points in time with different audiences create multiple connections with various constituencies and demographics.
- Know and prepare your talking points: Craft a succinct message and do not get lost in the medium. Strive for clarity and precision, making sure the main points are consistently communicated. This will facilitate conviction in your messaging and your positions. Be clear, concise, and confident on key points.
- Know your audience: Tailor messages to the audience and do not compromise your stance. Keep your message relevant, timely, and significant. Your messaging points need to remain the same and also address the concerns and areas of interest of those in the audience.
- There will be critics in the audience: Know all aspects of your message because critics will likely test your theories and positions. Be prepared to consider all sides of the issue and provide logical, reasoned responses. Be matter-of-fact in your approach to responding.

Messaging and the Creative Process

Messaging requires a thorough thinking process and a delivery that will inspire and ignite the workforce. Futurists encourage us to unthink, think like a freak, and show our work (Kleon, 2014; Levitt & Dubner, 2014; Wahl, 2013). In a 2010 IBM survey, chief executives were asked to name the most crucial factor for success. Interviews with more than 1,500 executives from 60 countries and 33 industries worldwide noted that—more than rigor, management discipline, integrity, or even vision—successfully navigating an increasingly complex world requires creativity (IBM, 2010). The executives did not believe their organizations were adequately prepared to take on new endeavors. When the executives were asked to identify activities that define successful creative leaders for the future, they observed that inviting disruptive innovation and encouraging others to abandon outmoded approaches and taking balanced risks were front and center. Drastic changes that are not mainstream were encouraged, and being comfortably uncomfortable with ambiguity and experimentation in creating new business models was also identified. Changing mental models and inventing new business models that are based on different assumptions, along with being courageous enough to make decisions that alter the status quo, were also identified.

Wahl (2013) suggests ways to unthink and emphasizes that being provocative, intuitive, committed, accelerated, spontaneous, surrendered, and original are key skills to learn along the way. Wahl considers improvisation to be a competency that opens white space for creative thinking (Brafman & Pollack, 2013; Brockman, 2013). Wahl states, "Fill your mind with information, but move forward with an objective mind-set that allows you to trust what the facts say *and* what your senses are telling you. Creative genius lies in the ability to juggle both facts and feelings until the right path is found" (Wahl, 2013, p. 109).

For each of the suggested ways to unthink, Wahl provides a number of strategies. On being intuitive, Wahl describes knowing what is under the surface, loosening your processes, and making discoveries. For example, three simple ways to keep discovering is remaining self-critical, submitting to regular outside critique, and listening while you work (Wahl, 2013). On having conviction, Wahl suggests doing the next thing in your heart and being a catalyst. Spontaneity means acting through fear and leaving room for interruption. On surrendering, Wahl suggests that recognition be surrendered, along with labels, the moment, and outcomes. "Enjoy your daily journey at work—enlist the unexpected humor, adventure, and beauty of your interactions and regular duties—and the monthly outcomes will often take care of themselves" (p. 182).

Kleon, in *Show Your Work* (2014), suggests a number of new ways to operate, include thinking processes (not products), sharing something small every day, opening up your cabinet of curiosities, telling good stories, teaching what you know, learning to take a punch, selling out, and sticking around. For example, in telling good stories, Kleon says, "Your work doesn't exist in a vacuum. Whether you realize it or not, you're already telling stories about your work. Every email you send, every text, every communication, every blog comment, every tweet, every photo, every video—they're all bits and pieces of a multimedia narrative you're constantly constructing. If you want to be more effective when sharing yourself and your work, you need to become a better storyteller. You need to know what a good story is and how to tell one" (p. 95).

Strategic Planning and Messaging

Drucker describes strategic planning as making decisions in a consistent, systematic way by taking risks and taking into consideration the impact the decisions will have on the future, then determining the results by measuring outcomes and feedback (Drucker, 1999).

Nursing administrators can increase effectiveness through strategic planning, which can promote professional nursing practice and the long-term goals of the organization and the nursing division. Clear, complete plans are developed in seven areas of key results, which are designed to include standards of performance that challenge and inspire (Sherman, 1982):

- Client satisfaction
- Productivity
- Innovation
- Staff development
- Budget goals
- Quality
- Organizational climate

Strategic planning in nursing is concerned with what nursing should be doing. Its purpose is to improve the allocation of scarce resources, including time and money, and to manage the agency for performance. Strategic planning includes forecasting from 1 to more than 20 years; organizations that change rapidly may need to strategically plan more often. This activity should involve top nurse managers and representatives from all levels of the nursing hierarchy, including clinical nursing personnel, to promote professional satisfaction throughout the nursing department and increase the likelihood of successful implementation. The process includes analyses of factors such as expected technological advances, internal and external environments, the nursing and healthcare market and industry, the economics of nursing and health care, the availability of human and material resources, and the judgments of top management.

Marketing and Messaging

Marketing identifies and meets both human and social needs. It provides a means for an organization to assess the needs of healthcare consumers. A needs assessment helps develop and deliver services to meet the needs of a specialty market.

There are several benefits of marketing, including increased customer satisfaction, improved resource attraction, improved operational efficiency, and becoming the hospital of choice. Ten steps to strategic market planning are outlined in **Box 15-1**. Nurses and nurse leaders should be involved in developing the strategic marketing plan because they have direct involvement with patient services (Scott, 2010).

COMMUNICATION AND RELATIONSHIP-BUILDING COMPETENCIES

Competencies related to communication and relationship building are important for nurse leaders. There are several competencies that nurse leaders need to develop, including effective communication, relationship management, the ability to influence behaviors, the ability to work with diversity, shared decision making, community involvement, and creating staff and academic relationships (Bianco, Dudkiewicz, & Linette, 2014).

BOX 15-1 Steps to Strategic Marketing Plans

- Analyze the organization mission, objectives, goals, and culture.
- Assess the organization strengths, weaknesses, opportunities, and threats by completing a SWOT analysis.
- Analyze the future environment in regard to the public served; competition; and the social-cultural, political, technologic, and economic environment.
- Determine the marketing mission and objectives. Also, determine specific goals for the planning period.
- Develop the marketing strategy that will allow achievement of the goals.
- Implement the necessary structure in the organization to ensure follow-through.
- Establish detailed programs to carry out the strategies; create a timeline of activities and responsibilities.
- Execute the planned programs.
- Monitor and evaluate performance; make adjustments as needed.

Source: Scott, 2010

Effective Communication

Effective communication is essential for nurse leaders and is the heart of business in healthcare systems. With a variety of individuals to communicate with daily, nurse leaders need to have basic communication skills that drive collaboration and teamwork toward the goals of the strategic plan and the overall organization. These basic skills include the ability to communicate via technologies such as email, instant messaging, text messaging, and communication software within the organization. In addition, leaders must know how to articulate ideas and understand the audience (Bianco et al., 2014).

Communication may occur through verbal interaction or through technology. Communication with technology is highly effective, and many organizations have internal communication technologies. Examples include email, social media, video conferencing, and other technologies that enable fact-to-face communication via the Internet.

Caring for patients requires many individuals who need to share information to discuss care management. As a result, there is an increasing interest in, and use of, information and communication technologies to support healthcare services. Simple communication technologies, such as voice mail and email, are commonplace. Email is used internally both for communicating announcements and information that needs to be pushed out from various business departments in healthcare settings, such as the human resources department or training department, and for communicating patients' care needs.

Nurse leaders are positioned to point out issues, ask for changes, seek improved performance, and other tasks that involve approaching staff and other administrative personnel. In doing so, nurse leaders should consider the following factors when communicating with others both verbally and via technology:

- Monitor your defenses
- Understand your audience
- Consider using metaphors and stories to help with understanding
- Lighten up the message
- Listen to yourself (Bianco et al., 2014)

Monitoring Defenses

Whether you are communicating verbally or via technology, care should be taken to monitor your defenses. This is crucial because when a person becomes defensive, they not listening; they are focused on defending their position. Communication does not work when the listener is defensive. Avoiding defensive situations in both verbal and technical communication is important. Ask neutral questions—such as, Does this make sense?—throughout the conversation to help alleviate defensiveness.

Understand Your Audience

It is important to understand your audience. Communicating with staff nurses on the unit about performance and patient care will be different from communicating with the information services department about implementing a new system.

Many times, realizing who you are talking to makes a difference in how effectively you understand the need. For example, nurses understand the importance of documenting at the point of care. Application developers may not understand the necessity; they just need to know that nurses must be able to document at the time an intervention occurs. The same applies if a system is being designed. Application developers do not necessarily need to understand a process; they just need to know what the process is so they can develop it electronically.

Using Metaphors and Stories to Help with Understanding

Nurse leaders need to develop communication skills that allow them to be effective with any audience they may encounter on a daily basis. In some situations it may be necessary to use metaphors and stories to help individuals understand what is being presented to them. For example, it may not be enough to say that something will not work. You may need to explain that it is like putting a square in a circle. Such a statement communicates the concept more effectively. Using a metaphor makes the information more memorable and less personal. Using stories is another effective way to convey information you want others to understand. The stories do not have to be real, but they should get to the point and portray what needs to be done.

Lighten Up the Message

Often we take ourselves and our jobs too seriously. The stress of daily work tends to weigh people down, and everyone likes a stress reliever. Lightening up before a conversation and making others laugh may improve communication. Using humor to relieve stress demonstrates comfort with yourself and conveys humility. Often humor removes the intimidation that individuals feel when they deal with managers.

Listen to Yourself

Individuals want to be heard. People often feel that they cannot communicate if they are not respected. Listening to your tone of voice is very important; it is crucial when communicating respect. If your tone of voice is accusatory, demanding, or overbearing, the person you are talking to is likely to respond with hostility or defensiveness. This can happen even if the words themselves are not hostile. The first step is to listen to yourself and pay attention to how others perceive you (Bianco et al., 2014).

Imaging, Messaging, and Dissemination

Wocial, Sego, Rager, Laubersheimer, and Everett, in a qualitative study (2014), explored the meaning of the phrase "image of the nurse" in the context of the desired brand experience of patients' perceptions that they will be well taken care of by the nurse. A focus group strategy provided insights into the perception of nursing in various facilities within the organization. Some coding schemes became apparent when participants discussed examples of how not to convey assurance of care. Sharing negative examples reinforced the opportunity to redefine the brand of nurses and set expectations for appearance and conduct. The methods used to collect data for this study were instrumental in engaging direct care nurses in thoughtful reflection about their impact on patients' experiences. A number of themes were revealed: appearance, behavior, character, accountability, application, and dissemination.

Appearance

When respondents were asked about how nurses should look, the number one response was that nurses should be clean, well groomed, and wear understated makeup, jewelry, and perfume. Participants also identified the importance of being able to easily identify a nurse. Participants had significant difficulty identifying tangible things that represented the nurse. The nurse's name tag—complete with the company logo and "RN" in large red letters—and the uniform were the only tangible items that were consistently identified.

Behavior

The most significant factors related to behavior were being genuine (approachable) and being an advocate (professional). Being respectful, attentive, and caring were also identified as genuine behaviors. Being an advocate included being informative and reliable and collaborating with other members of the healthcare team.

Character

Character traits that were identified as ideal included being compassionate, approachable, attentive, and caring. The major indicators of character were being genuine and service oriented. Having good manners and being gracious were other ways participants described nurses who assured patients they were cared for.

Accountability

An unexpected finding from the focus group participants revealed that nurses expect to be treated by their peers and leadership the same way they are expected to treat patients and families. The themes also described leaders who demonstrate respect, compassion, and integrity toward frontline nurses in their ability to communicate safe, quality care to patients. The expectation from participants is that leaders should hold everyone accountable to uniform codes of conduct. Mutual support, respect, and accountability work in tandem to convey assurance. Participants also identified a need to hold one another accountable.

As the abstraction process of the study continued, assurance was identified as the unifying theme of the data. For example, the unexpected and prominent message of nurse accountability had a significant influence on the task force recommendations. Members of the task force interpreted accountability as representative of nurses' desire to reconnect with what it means to be a nurse in the best sense of the profession and to be part of an organization that is focused on comforting patients during their care.

The most significant and consistent meaning found in the data was that, rather than a specific color, it is a nurses' overall appearance—being clean, well groomed, and wearing a modest, well-fitting uniform—that establishes tangible elements of assurance. The intangible elements of assurance cannot be defined by any one trait or behavior. Comments from participants suggested that character and behavior traits are mediated by interpersonal skills, confirming what has been reported in the literature. Interpersonal skills can reinforce the skills and behaviors of nurses and communicate assurance.

Application and Dissemination

The study provided data that supported the importance of paying attention to the details of how the image of nursing is communicated and messaged. Establishing a clear policy outlining the specifics of a uniform, including consequences for failing to uphold the standard, supported strategies for accountability. Some recommendations were to have one standard uniform style, not just a single color scheme, and bold, easily identifiable uniforms with specific colors that are branded with the system's logo. This meant new uniforms for all 9,000 nurses in the system.

Conclusion of the Study

The research revealed that it is not just the color of the nursing uniform that influences the image of nurses. The color and style of uniform were identified; however, a uniform must clearly communicate to patients and families that the wearer is a nurse. No matter the uniform color, the nurse must be clean and well groomed. Every aspect of the nurse, uniform, behavior, attitude, and overall appearance reflects on the nurse and promotes the brand promise of an organization. Health systems should communicate the promise of assurance, which is accomplished through actions and is influenced by the nurses' presentation and overall appearance. More than uniforms, nurses' behaviors (what they do, how they act, and the care they provide) influence the patient experience.

The evidence gathered in this work also served as a foundation for the implementation of an initiative to improve the professional image of nurses in the authors' organization (Wocial et al., 2014). The nurses' ethical behavior has a significant impact on influence and messaging.

Ethical nursing leadership promotes behaviors that guide professional practice and influence patient outcomes for safe, quality care. True professional status implies a code of ethics, which has always been significant in professional nursing practice. This commitment has been further intensified with the establishment, in 1990, of the Center for Ethics and Human Rights under the umbrella of the American Nurses Association (ANA). The center's guiding mission is to address the complex ethical and human rights issues confronting nurses and to designate activities and programs that serve to increase ethical competence and the human rights sensitivity of nurses (Baker, Salas, King, Battles, & Barach, 2005). Professional integrity reinforces the Code of Ethics for Nurses with Interpretive Statements and can be defined as strict adherence to a code of conduct.

Standard 12 in the ANA Scope and Standards of Practice for nurse administrators describes the decisions and actions made by nurse administrators that are based on ethical principles. Measurement criteria are identified as follows:

1. Incorporates Code of Ethics for Nurses with Interpretive Statements (ANA, 2001) to guide practice.
2. Ensures the preservation and protection of the autonomy, dignity, and rights of individuals.

3. Maintains confidentiality within legal and regulatory parameters.
4. Ensures a process to identify and address ethical issues within nursing and the organization.
5. Participates on multidisciplinary and interdisciplinary teams that address ethical risks, benefits, and outcomes.
6. Informs administrators or others of the risks, benefits, and outcomes of programs and decisions that affect healthcare delivery.
7. Demonstrates a commitment to practicing self-care, managing stress, and connecting with self and others. (American Nurses Association [ANA], 2009)

This standard and the code of ethics provide a framework for decision making and managing healthcare systems.

DEVELOPING A HEALTHCARE ETHICS PROGRAM

A healthcare ethics program can be instrumental in developing ethical competence and creating a climate that is conducive to ethical practice. Clinical practice, research, and administration can reinforce ethical competence. Competence in ethics requires moral sensibility, moral responsiveness, moral reasoning, and moral leadership (Bandman & Bandman, 2002). A sound healthcare ethics program should support the mission, philosophy, strategic plans, and policies related to human resource management and patient care. The Joint Commission standards address ethical issues, specifically focusing on respect for patients, responding to patient values and preferences, and patient responsibilities (Turner, 2003).

Elements of an ethics program include education, consultation, and policy development and review (Turner, 2003):

- Education includes classes and information on topics such as natural law, deontology, utilitarianism, emotionalism, feminist ethics, and others. Developing a glossary of terms that is useful for understanding the vocabulary of an ethics committee is also important and may include principles such as autonomy, justice, beneficence, no maleficence, veracity, and confidentiality. Discussing clinical topics related to services offered in the facility helps make the disseminated information applicable to the management of ethical dilemmas within the organization.
- Consultation on ethics requires individuals skilled in assessment, process, and interpersonal competencies when dealing with ethical dilemmas. The American Society for Bioethics and Humanities provides core competencies for successful ethics consultation.
- Policy development provides guidance to organizations in addressing ethical dilemmas. Developing policy entails a deep understanding and ability to write clear guidelines and protocols on possible areas of ethical dilemmas such as withholding/withdrawing treatment, surrogacy, organ transplant, futility, and conflict of interest (Turner, 2003).

Ethical Implications for Managing a Clinical Practice Discipline

Many ethical issues are directly related to the provision of patient care services. These issues have become more important since the 1990s because of several factors: the increased sophistication of medical science and technology;

interprofessional relationships; organ donations and transplants; special concerns relating to patients with AIDS, uninsured persons, aged persons, and high-risk neonates; concern about practical limits on financial resources for health care; changes in society; and a growing emphasis on the autonomy of individuals (Jones & Fowler-Dixon, 2004).

Professional nurses implement the employer's policy concerning the moral responsibility of health care. Nurses have responsibility for supervising and reviewing patient care, meeting quality standards, making certain that decisions about patients are based on sound ethical principles, developing policies and mechanisms that address questions of human values, and responding to social problems and dilemmas that affect the need for healthcare services.

To fulfill this responsibility, professional nurses support other nurses who are confronted with ethical dilemmas and help them think through situations in an open dialogue. Nurse managers establish the climate for this discussion. Ethics rounds as a means of discussing ethical dilemmas is recommended as way to incorporate critical thinking and a moral environment. Such discussions can stem from hypothetical cases, case histories, or a case based on a current patient. Ethical reasoning requires participation by a knowledgeable person. Ongoing awareness and reinforcement of ethical principles and reasoning increase the organization's awareness of the nature of professional practice.

Nurse managers need to know the legal framework for their actions. They should help clinical nurses balance teaching, research, clinical investigation, and patient care. Practicing from an evidence-based framework provides a strong foundation for ethical work. All nurses should work for social justice to ensure a desirable quality of life and healthcare services. Nurses may promote compassion and sensitivity through protest of public policies that reduce the quality of or access to health care for the poor. Nurses should pursue human values, wholeness, and health values. This does not mean that nurses must subsidize health care by working for lower salaries; rather, they should work to have the cost shared by all of society.

Among the ethical dilemmas seldom addressed by nurse managers are ethical boundaries, particularly those involving sex. Nurse managers and administrators should provide continuing education to increase nurses' awareness of improper nurse–patient relationships, including accepting gifts and favors, doing business with patients and their families, being coerced or manipulated by patients, visiting patients at home while off duty, and making nontherapeutic disclosures. Risk environments include inpatient psychiatric services and chemical dependency treatment programs.

Ethics committees should be established to prevent burnout. Their goals should include being a forum for expressing concerns, promoting awareness and education, participating in clinical decision making and policy and procedure development, developing professional identity, and communicating with other committees. Communicating ethical decisions to executive committees and community partners requires skillful articulation in oral communication and writing. Writing an executive summary, a formal report, can provide an efficient and effective way to share salient points, for follow-up, and next steps in the ethical decision-making process.

WRITING AN EXECUTIVE SUMMARY

One of the most difficult skills for leaders and administrators to learn is communicating successfully in formal reports. Most individuals need to learn the proper style, tone, organization, flow, and mechanics for many different types of formal documents. For nurses, this can be a challenge after learning to communicate in written care plans, patient case studies, and other clinical papers. Writing business reports can certainly be taught, but it is neglected in the nursing curriculum. The most difficult portion of learning to write any formal business report is developing the skills to write an executive summary to accompany the business report. This section outlines key aspects for nursing leaders and administrators to consider when writing effective executive summaries, and it provides examples to help leaders succeed in this area.

What Is the Purpose of an Executive Summary?

The purpose of an executive summary is to provide a concise overview or preview to an audience who may or may not have time to read the whole report carefully. This group could account for 90% of the people who will receive a copy of the report. In many ways, an executive summary highlights a report much like an abstract summarizes a manuscript (Guffey, 2003). Therefore, it is critical that an executive summary accomplish three things:

1. Explain why you wrote the document.
2. Emphasize your conclusions or recommendations and any financial considerations.
3. Include only the essential or most significant information to support those conclusions.

Who Is the Audience for an Executive Summary?

It is important to know who you are writing the executive summary for. Different audiences and plans require different summaries, but they all have one thing in common: the readers are busy individuals and are usually most interested in the bottom line (Guffey, 2003; Thompson & Way, 2000). For example, the executive summary of an internal plan, such as an operations plan, annual plan, or strategic plan, does not have to be as formal. Make sure the highlights are covered, but it is not necessary to repeat the location, product or service description, or other details. After reading the executive summary, your audience should understand the main points and the evidence for those points without having to read every part of the report. Never waste words in an executive summary.

If you are looking for investments, resources, or decisions, state your request explicitly and specify the amount needed or decisions that are required. Also add some highlights about the management team, your competitive edge, and how your skills are unique. If you are looking for a loan, ask for it directly and specify the required amount, but loan details do not need to be stated in the executive summary.

Advantages of Writing an Executive Summary

It is essential for leaders, managers, and administrators to include an executive summary when submitting a report to high-level executives. A concise, informative executive summary allows readers to identify the important aspects of the report without reading all the details. The executive summary also helps readers identify whether to examine the details of the entire report or to delegate that task to another individual (Guffey, 2003; Roach, Tracy, & Durden, 2007).

What Should an Effective Executive Summary Include?

All executive summaries should be brief; the best length is one or two pages. Emphasize the main points of the problem, issue, or plan, and keep it brief. The goal is to entice the audience to read more of the plan, not explain every detail. Highlight the contents of the full report. You may start by stating the issue or problem and then summarizing how it will be addressed (Thompson & Way, 2000).

For a standard executive summary, the following should generally be included:

- An introduction with the unit, department, or organization name and location
- The grab (briefly, the opportunity or recommendations you are presenting)
- Purpose of the executive summary
- The problem, issue, or question that prompted the research and summary
- The competition (if any)
- Solutions or recommendations (address the need or opportunity) and highest priorities
- The individual or team that will do the work
- Return on investment and financial considerations (what it will cost and what the outcomes will be)
- Brief conclusion

Include the most important points you do not want the audience to miss. Summarize the key points of the report, including the purpose (Guffey, 2003). This is a good place to put a small chart or table. Also cite and explain the numbers in the text.

Provide a summary that may be a bulleted list instead of a narrative. The full report will provide supporting details, so do not waste the readers' time if they cannot commit to reading the full report or do not need to.

It may be helpful to use headings in the executive summary. Follow the order of the report so readers are not confused if they decide to read the entire report. Be sure to use consistent terms that all audience members will understand. Use strategic words or sentences from the report. You may use tables, graphs, or bullet points as long as the executive summary remains brief (Guffey, 2003; Hynes, 2008; Thompson & Way, 2000).

Proofread and polish the executive summary several times. Read it aloud or have colleagues read it. Does it flow, or does it sound choppy? When you are happy with it, ask someone who knows nothing about your business to read it and make suggestions. Most importantly, remember that an executive summary should communicate independently of the report. Be sure it is concise compared to the report.

In general, one to two pages are enough; however, if the report is 100 pages the executive summary may need to be 8 to 10 pages. Gauge the length according to the length of the report (Guffey, 2003).

Writing Tips and When to Include an Executive Summary

Nurses often have little experience writing formal business reports. This skill needs to be taught to all nursing leaders and administrators. Formal business reports and executive summaries take considerable effort and should not be undertaken lightly. Before writing the report and executive summary, the author should spend time analyzing the problem (e.g., root-cause analysis or Plan-Do-Study-Act), anticipating the audience, writing a draft, revising, proofreading, and evaluating the final product. The following tips may help nurse authors during this process:

1. Allow enough time to be successful. Develop a time line and adjust it as needed.
2. Do not start writing until you have completed the research and data collection concerning the problem or issue.
3. Start with a good outline and revise it as needed. You may want to use bullets to insert key points that you do not want to forget.
4. Plan quiet, uninterrupted time and a dedicated space to write.
5. You may want to write in sections so you can save difficult material until after you have developed confidence by working on easier sections.
6. Use a consistent verb tense.
7. In formal reports, avoid using "I" and "we."
8. Revise the report for coherence and conciseness. Read it out loud. Does it make sense and flow?
9. Proofread the report several times or have someone help you proofread it.

In addition to knowing how to write an executive summary, nurses need to know when to include an executive summary with a report. An executive summary and table of contents can be included with any lengthy report that will be submitted to administrators and executives. Examples of such reports include strategic plans, annual budgets, annual reports, and reports that focus on root-cause analyses or failure mode analyses.

Examples of Executive Summaries

It is vital for future nursing leaders and administrators to be trained on how to write a successful executive summary. In addition to didactic content and specific tips, it is important for nurses to practice these skills through assignments. **Box 15-2** is an example of an assignment for clinical nurse leader (CNL) students related to quality improvement initiatives. An example of an effective introduction to an executive summary was written by Leah R. C. Ledford (**Box 15-3**). An executive summary written by Kyla Slagter focuses on the lack of documentation for evening snacks for diabetic patients. To explore the issue and write the executive summary, Slagter initiated a Plan-Do-Study-Act (PDSA) to identify the problems, plan the interventions, and study the results. It is included in the executive summary (**Figure 15-1**).

BOX 15-2   An Assignment for Writing an Executive Summary Related to a Quality Improvement Initiative

Directions: This project will be written as an Executive Summary format. You will be given information on how to write an executive summary. As clinical leaders, learning how to write an executive summary for administrators and executives is as important as completing the quality improvement project. For executive summaries it is best to use headings, a mixture of narrative, and either bullet points and/or tables.

  I. Title Page (5 pt)
 II. Introduction (very brief) (5 pt)
III. Identify the Clinical Quality Issue (very brief—including how you discovered the issue, e.g., from staff, nurse manager, your daily or weekly logs, etc.) (15 pt)
IV. Describe the Root Cause(s) (briefly and how you found the root cause) (15 pt)
 V. Summary of aggregate data you looked at in evaluating this issue (15 pt) (brief and how you got data—like from risk management, finance, NDNQI, etc.)
VI. List of several barriers and facilitators within unit/organization (15 pt)
VII. Recommendations (brief list or description of potential actions to resolve) (15 pt)
VIII. Conclusion (very brief) (5 pt)
IX. References (at least 3) (10 pt)

Kasia Kudla chose to assess the increased use of restraints as a quality and safety issue. Kudla completed her assignment with an executive summary template using roman numerals to highlight and summarize key aspects of the issue (**Box 15-4**).

Marie D. Litzelman discovered that there was a low compliance rate with the venous thromboembolism (VTE) protocol. In her executive summary, Litzelman used bullets to effectively summarize barriers and facilitators (**Box 15-5**).

BOX 15-3   Introduction to Docosahexaenoic Acid (DHA) Recommendations in Pregnancy by Leah R. C. Ledford, MSN, RN, CNL

Introduction

Docosahexaenoic acid (DHA) is a part of the omega-3 fatty acid family. Most obstetric providers are recommending to their pregnant patients to take a daily supplement of DHA to ensure adequate ingestion. This is because most Western pregnant women do not get sufficient amounts from their diet. Lack of enough DHA in pregnancy has been linked with several adverse maternal and neonatal outcomes, including pre-eclampsia, preterm labor and delivery, and developmental delays in the fetus, especially related to brain and vision maturity.

FIGURE 15-1   PDSA for documentation of evening snack for diabetic patients

Documentation of Evening Snack for Diabetic Patients

PLAN a change or improvement

The Problem

Evening snacks for diabetic patients are not being documented consistently. If snacks are not documented it is assumed they are not being given.

Aim/Goal

1. Determine documentation of evening snacks for diabetic patients.
2. Staff on 3T will understand what to provide as an appropriate snack for a diabetic patient.
3. Staff on 3T will understand the importance and rationale of documenting evening snacks for diabetic patients.
4. Improve the documentation of evening snacks for diabetic patients.

Team

John Schooley, RN, AVP
Kyla Slagter, RN, PCL

DO the improvement, make the change

The Interventions

- Audit 20 charts from 3T to determine the documentation of evening snacks for diabetic patients. Charts audited must be from patients with a history of diabetes and a current order for a consistent carbohydrate diet.
- Educate staff on appropriate evening snack options for the diabetic patient.
- If evening snacks are not being documented consistently, educate staff on the importance and rationale for documenting evening snacks on diabetic patients.
- Create a process map specific to the documentation of evening snacks for diabetic patients.
- Audit 20 charts during and post education period.

STUDY the results and examine data

Graphs/Data

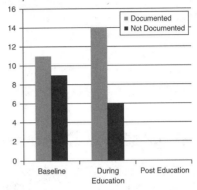

Lessons Learned

- Evening snacks are calculated into the patient's daily caloric intake. If snacks are not documented and assumed not given, the prescribed caloric intake is not being provided for the diabetic patient.
- Appropriate evening snack for a diabetic patient is ½ turkey sandwich on whole wheat bread with 240 ml skim milk.
- Baseline data determined evening snacks were **documented** on 55% of patients and **not documented** on 45% of patients audited. During education evening snacks were **documented** on 70% of patients and **not documented** on 30% of patients.

ACT to sustain performance and spread change

Next Steps

- Monthly chart audits × 3 months to evaluate documentation of evening snacks.
- If an improvement is not noted, determine the next step of action.

Executive summaries generally conclude with recommendations. Sara Pratt assessed the quality and safety issue of large amounts of maternal caffeine consumption and the negative effects on the fetus and neonate. In her executive summary, Pratt provides brief recommendations for nurses and other healthcare professionals (**Box 15-6**).

An executive summary is a vital part of a formal report or proposal because most of the audience will read it, and some may read only this section. Busy executives and members of advisory boards have decision-making authority in the organization, but they rarely have time to read anything other than the executive summary. Because the executive summary is such a crucial part of the report, it is essential for nurses who will be leaders and administrators to learn to write effective executive summaries.

BOX 15-4 Example of Executive Summary Template Used by Kasia Kudla, MSN, RN, CNL

I. Reducing restraint prevalence on 4C, a progressive cardiology unit.

II. Restraint usage can be a major barrier to improving the safety of patients at Presbyterian Hospital. Increased restraint prevalence is of major concern on 4C. Methods of patient restraint include physical/chemical restraints, and seclusion. The most common methods of patient restraint on 4C include physical and chemical restraints. The purpose of this report is to decrease restraint prevalence on 4C.

III. The nursing staff and the management team on 4C have identified that restraint prevalence is a major clinical quality issue. Daily restraint logs not only identify the number of restraint occurrences but also confirm that among the patients who are restrained, there is frequently an increased length of stay.

BOX 15-5 Example of Executive Summary Using Bullets by Marie D. Litzelman, MSN, RN, CMSRN, CNL

Barriers/Facilitators

Barriers for this quality issue on the unit include:
- No one group or person taking responsibility for outcome (pointing fingers at others)
- Nurses feeling overworked as it is, not wanting to take on further task of making sure VTE protocol is on the chart
- No printed out protocols on unit
- Physicians not signing protocols placed on chart by nurses

Facilitators for this quality issue on the unit include:
- Patient Care Leader/Clinical Nurse Leader Role
- Quality Council initiatives

Interdisciplinary team meetings to discuss how to achieve better outcomes

BOX 15-6 Caffeine Recommendations in Pregnancy by Sara Pratt, MSN, RN, CNL

It is important to provide recommendations to high-risk obstetric patients to prevent negative outcomes to a fetus or neonate as a result of excessive intake of caffeine. Two recommendations could include:

1. Provide proper education to all nursing staff, dietary staff, and all patients admitted to the Obstetrical High Risk Unit at Carolinas Medical Center—including a reference sheet that displays the quantity of caffeine that is in different dietary and herbal products.
2. At the Carolinas Medical Center's Obstetrical High Risk Unit, place all patients on a dietary restriction of less than 200 milligrams of caffeine a day as suggested by the March of Dimes in 2008. Patients should then be held accountable for their own consumption of caffeine after receiving the proper education.

SUMMARY

Nurse leaders who are recognized as great leaders are prepared, articulate, consistent, and succinct in their messaging. These messages communicate authority, clarity, and certitude. Conflicting messages that confuse the leader's core values and mission can weaken the leader's influence. Executive leaders will not compromise their core values and beliefs to manipulate the outcome of a specific situation. Great leaders are confident that they are doing and saying the right things to ultimately put them in a favorable position. Working from an ethical lens is important to authentic messaging. Likewise, if the consequences are negative, they are comforted knowing their messages are a result of right thinking and decision making. Executive summaries are another means of messaging and communicating influence. Ethical leadership guides the development of an environment that supports moral decision making.

REFLECTIVE QUESTIONS

1. A nurse leader must present to the staff a major change needed to align resources with current patient care needs. This will involve rethinking the current patient care delivery model. Using content from constructive messaging and strategic management, what are the first steps and the next steps the nurse manager can take in conveying critical messages?
2. How might the nurse leader use the qualitative study to address image issues in the nursing department? Using messaging strategies and creative thinking, how might the nurse leader work closely with the nursing staff to find the most creative and efficient solutions?

CASE STUDY 15-1   How Will They Know?

Kathleen E. Ebert

At the completion of a research project, K. E. was trying to determine how to disseminate the findings to the hospital and all the staff. Historically, research that had been done across the system was well known on the unit or service line that was involved with the study; however, other units and sites had little to no knowledge of the research findings. The system had an evidence-based practice and research council and system meetings, but neither were well attended. The colleagues who attended these meetings were typically involved in the research and already had knowledge of the studies that were occurring across the system.

The system was made up of three full-service regional medical centers, an orthopedic surgical hospital, and a freestanding emergency room. The health system was also affiliated with a college of nursing that was located on the campus of the main medical center. The college of nursing has a large robust library that serves the college and the health system, so resources for research are readily available within the system.

Communicating findings and current projects has always been difficult for the system. Councils have had campaigns to raise awareness, sent emails and newsletters, held seminars, and attempted other ways to disseminate the findings, but the majority of colleagues are not aware of projects within the system.

(continues)

CASE STUDY 15-1   How Will They Know? (Continued)

Within the same city, there is a large university-based medical center that is renowned for the research that is done there and how it is disseminated into practice. The university medical center hosted a research symposium that highlighted work done within their system and other systems, including K. E.'s health system, and they presented their current research. The idea then came to a professor at the college to host a similar event. A team consisting of members from both the college and the health system came together to plan a research symposium for their own system. The idea was to help disseminate and highlight all the projects that had been done. The team planned to find projects that had been translated into practice within the system. The college liaison for research was aware of many of the projects, so the team created a list and started with those projects. They then determined the resources staff would need to participate in research. The chief nursing officers were approached to support the financial aspects of the project, along with members of the alumni association and contacts from local professional nursing organizations.

After the budget was defined and the staffs' needs were assessed, the committee began to plan the agenda for the day. Presenters were selected and invited to participate in the event. The agenda included a national expert on translating research into practice, ethical considerations for research, and an editor from the state who was a faculty member at another college and whose expertise was journal publishing. The emphasis for the day was staff members who were active in the research that was done on their units. Many of the presenters had attended the college of nursing and had completed these projects as part of their graduate work.

The day was targeted primarily at direct care providers, and secondarily at management. The attendance was about half direct care providers and half management staff. The staff was very engaged and felt a new energy to participate in research and evidence-based practice projects. Many of the managers were already familiar with the work that had been done. The chief nursing officers recognized the importance of the work being presented and offered comments during introductions of the presenters about the impact of the work on the health system and the discipline. The attendees left with a knowledge of the current work, the tools needed to be successful, and resources available to support research and evidence-based projects.

Case Study Questions

1. How can you ensure that more direct care providers than managers attend research conferences?
2. Would a formal needs assessment survey provide more clarity to define the agenda?
3. How can you engage staff in process improvement if the managers and leaders are not engaged?
4. What is the best form of communication for direct care providers?
5. Does staff know where to find resources to support process improvement projects?

CASE STUDY 15-2   Where Do I Get Started?

Kathleen E. Ebert

K. S. is the professional practice coordinator at a 60-bed orthopedic surgical hospital. In an attempt to increase the interest and participation in evidence-based practice and research projects, K. S. set out to identify an area of potential improvement. K. S. surveyed many of the nurses and physicians looking for potential ideas.

CASE STUDY 15-2   Where Do I Get Started? (Continued)

One identified area was the noncompliance of lumbar fusion postoperative patients using ice therapy for pain relief. K. S. joined one of the orthopedic neurosurgeons as a coinvestigator to identify a way to increase compliance. The facility had been trialing a product from a commercial manufacturer that provided cold therapy in a flat pad. The feedback from the patients was that they loved the product, and it appeared to help reduce their pain. It was hypothesized that by reducing pain, the amount of narcotics could be reduced.

The first step was to conduct a thorough literature review to determine if there is a current body of knowledge. A small team was created, and they discussed who was going to lead the research and what the goals would be. The study was to be a random controlled trial (RCT). The interdisciplinary team included representatives from respiratory therapy, physical therapy, nursing, and case management. All members of the team completed ethics training to qualify for institutional review board (IRB) approval. The team met several times before the IRB application was submitted. During the team meetings the question needed to be defined, but before that could happen, the objectives of the study needed to be clear. What did the team want to prove? The variables that were to be measured needed to define the question. The challenge with defining a question was making sure that the issues the team wanted to prove were clear, concise, and measureable. When they were measureable, clearly defined variables were determined, then the group could start their work.

The team defined the roles and expectations of each team member and their respective departments. The team was very active in planning, executing, and monitoring the progress of the study. Maintaining patient confidentiality and assuring complete randomization were challenges for the group. Many different approaches were considered (home phone numbers, medical record numbers, patient ID numbers, etc.), but a decision was ultimately made to use a randomly generated number and have staff select a sealed envelope containing a number.

The population of the study then needed to be defined. The inclusion and exclusion criteria were based on historical findings of the patient populations. The inclusion and exclusion criteria were broad to try to reduce any potential bias in the study.

The consent process then needed to be defined and communicated to the staff and physician offices. The design of the study was completed with a plan to run the study for one calendar year and to have 500 participants. The protocols were defined, and the research plan was completed. The study was submitted to the IRB for expedited consideration, and it was approved because there was minimal potential risk to the patients.

The final stage in the planning process was to educate the staff about the study. The staff would collect the data, so it was vital that they understood the process for the study. The study was presented at a staff meeting, and protocol sheets were distributed and posted on the unit. The research team made rounds on the unit to educate the staff, and the coinvestigator was available for any questions.

Data were collected and statistically analyzed to determine whether the intervention had affected the patient outcomes. The team then came together to determine the next steps to disseminate the findings. The findings were presented at a site-based education session and in print literature to the physicians and their assistants.

Case Study Questions

1. What could have been done during the planning phase to better prepare the team and staff for the study?
2. Many staff members did not understand the difference between trialing a product and conducting research. Could this affect the outcomes?
3. In a review of the process, it was determined that the planning phase needed to be more comprehensive. How could the coinvestigators have planned the format of the study to be more precise?

CASE STUDY 15-3   New Director Challenges

Jennifer L. Embree

Mary Carroll, MSN, RN, is new to the organization. She self-identified as a servant leader and was a little anxious about her new role as the director of the critical care unit of the hospital. Two years after she earned her master's degree in health system nursing leadership, she was determined that she was up to the challenge and would be successful, but she was experiencing some trepidation. When Mary Carroll interviewed with the new chief nursing officer (CNO), who already envisioned the organization to be on the Magnet journey, she recognized that the CNO was relationship centered and was also a transformational leader.

When she reviewed the monthly budget and nurse-sensitive indicators, Mary Carroll noted the high turnover and vacancy rates (20% and 30%, respectively) on her unit, the high number of falls and hospital-acquired pressure ulcers, the high cost of overtime, and the use of traveling nurses. The mean age of the few seasoned nurses was in the upper 60s. The high number of nurses with less than 2 years of bedside experience alarmed Mary Carroll. Recognizing that the literature supports improved outcomes among nurses with higher education, Mary Carroll reviewed the number of diploma-, associate-, and baccalaureate-prepared nurses on the unit. She found that 30% of the nurses were diploma prepared, 45% were associate's degree prepared, and 25% were baccalaureate degree prepared. Mary Carroll recognized that, without some major changes, bringing additional new associate's degree nurses from the local community colleges into an environment with the current percentage of such nurses, a high turnover and vacancy rate, and poor nurse-sensitive indicators was not conducive to enhancing the strength of the nursing workforce. Patient complaints were frequent, and physician dissatisfaction was high. The quality and risk managers were demanding to meet with Mary Carroll regarding quality issues, patient complaints, and current litigation.

Prior to the first staff meeting, Mary Carroll spent time learning about the unit, dealing with daily operational issues, and formulating a plan to involve staff in enhancing care on the unit while decreasing turnover and vacancy and improving patient experiences. As she observed the staff on the unit, she noted that some were cool and noncommunicative, others were frantic and claimed they were too busy to talk, and others ducked into rooms to avoid having a conversation with their new director.

The first unit meeting was sparsely attended by a few seasoned nurses and several newer nurses. When she asked the attendees why they thought the meeting was poorly attended, they said that administration keeps cutting resources and everyone is exhausted and out looking for positions at other hospitals. As Mary Carroll continued to ask the staff to identify issues and discuss solutions to improve the critical care unit, many barriers to patient care were identified and potential solutions were listed. As she focused on positive topics after identifying issues and seeking solutions, nurses began telling their stories of why they had chosen a nursing career and how important and impactful they felt they could be to improve patient outcomes. Some of the seasoned nurses rolled their eyes during the storytelling, and others made negative facial expressions. Mary Carroll applauded the nurses who spoke up about the possibilities for nursing and the services they could improve on their unit. Mary Carroll asked for volunteers to begin working on improving a variety of aspects on the unit and asked the staff what kinds of teams they thought might be helpful in dealing with the current issues they had listed and how those teams could facilitate some of the solutions that were suggested. As the meeting adjourned, the staff expressed excitement about potential improvements and the unit issues that could be improved under the direction of their new leader.

As Mary Carroll left the meeting, she maintained hope that she could empower the staff to own their unit and improve the work environment, nurse satisfaction, the patient experience, and nurse-sensitive outcomes. She began to think about what resources she would need to further engage the staff in owning and improving their unit.

CASE STUDY 15-3   New Director Challenges (Continued)

Case Study Questions

1. Identify stakeholders who should be included in performing a needs assessment to help further identify core issues on the unit that must be addressed prior to being able to transform the unit culture.
2. Identify why each stakeholder should be included in the improvement process.
3. Discuss methods for identifying which stakeholders to engage, inform, and influence.
4. What are the issues in the case study?
5. What literature and theories can support resolution of the issues in the critical care unit?
6. What resources might Mary Carroll call upon to assist her in resolving the issues in the critical care unit.
7. What leadership and change theories might be helpful to Mary Carroll as she thinks about ways to successfully improve the nursing work environment and the nurse-sensitive indicators?

CASE STUDY 15-4   Effective Communication and Daily Briefings

Darla Banks

Texas Health Resources implemented daily care briefings in all inpatient nursing units on the medical–surgical, telemetry, progressive care, and intensive care units. The goal of these briefings is to increase communication between the disciplines to impact the patients' length of stay and readmission rates.

The focus of the briefings is to prepare for the transition of patients. The daily care briefings are led by a clinical nurse leader (CNL). The CNL is a new nursing role (the first new role in more than 40 years) and is being assigned in all units of the 14 wholly owned hospitals. The CNLs are responsible for the patients' care coordination as well as mentoring and implementing process improvement strategies.

All disciplines are welcome to attend the daily briefing. Personnel who are required to attend include the CNL, the case manager or social worker, the direct-care nurse, and the charge nurse.

The CNL implements the daily care briefing and is responsible for its quality. The CNL collaborates with the social worker or case management team, the unit's nursing leadership, and the unit-based council to determine a time and place for the briefings. The briefings take place before 11:00, and the discussion is limited to 1 minute per patient. When details for the briefing are established, the direct-care nurses are informed of the time and location.

Each nurse is assigned an online learning module to prepare for the briefing. Emails, flyers, and face-to-face conversations prepare the nursing staff. The direct-care nurses are given a report form to utilize during the briefing. The report form helps them give a focused report. The night shift assists the day nurses in filling out the report form. This allows the direct-care nurses to be prepared with information that focuses on the transition of the patients.

When the unit decisions are made and the time for the briefing is established, there are a few vital components needed to make the briefing successful:

1. The unit managers must communicate their support of the briefings. The managers' support empowers the nurses and encourages regular attendance.
2. The daily care nurses are required to rotate into the briefing and report on their patient, which takes 5–6 minutes. Every morning they sign up for a 5-minute time slot so there are no delays.
3. An announcement is made 10 minutes prior to the briefing. The briefing starts on time and with the required members present.

(continues)

CASE STUDY 15-4 Effective Communication and Daily Briefings (Continued)

4. Action items are assigned to individuals during the briefing to distribute the workload. In the afternoon, the CNL verifies that the action items have been completed.
5. A rating sheet is filled out for every briefing during the first 2 weeks of the go-live period. After the go-live period, the rating sheets are done monthly. The rating sheets are used to sustain the quality of the briefings and to ensure communication occurs in a timely manner.

Even though the process is new, daily care briefings result in a number of positive outcomes. The nurses appreciate having the information they are given in the briefings. It enables direct-care nurses to plan for their day and answer questions posed by families and physicians. In some briefings, physicians are present and orders can be given for patients without delays or multiple phone calls.

The results are positive. The readmission rates have decreased by 5% in the renal unit, and the length of stay has decreased on the medical–surgical units. For example, a patient was scheduled to have surgery in 3 days due to the need to hold aspirin therapy. The pharmacist attended the briefing and knew to draw blood to see if the patient could have surgery sooner. The lab work was ordered, and the patient went to surgery 3 days sooner than planned, which resulted in a 3-day shorter length of stay.

Case managers and social workers say their workload has decreased due to the information exchange. The daily care briefings have greatly enhanced communication among all health care disciplines at Texas Health Resources. This new process is promising great results.

Case Study Questions

1. Considering concepts from complex adaptive systems, how does the CNL integrate an understanding of complexity in the briefings?
2. How does the CNL promote healthy work environments, using briefings as a strategy to improve patient care continuity and staff satisfaction?
3. How does the CNL integrate informatics and technology into the daily patient briefings? How does this facilitate sustainability of this frontline strategy?

REFERENCES

American Nurses Association. (2001). *Code of ethics for nurses with interpretative statements*. Silver Springs, MD: American Nurses Association.

American Nurses Association. (2009). *Nursing administration: Scope and standards of practice*. Silver Spring, MD: Author.

Baker, D. P., Salas, H., King, H., Battles, J., & Barach, P. (2005). The role of teamwork in the professional education of physicians: Current status and assessment recommendations. *Joint Commission Journal on Quality Improvement and Patient Safety, 31*(4), 185–202.

Bandman, E., & Bandman, B. (2002). *Nursing ethics through the life span* (4th ed.). Upper Saddle River, NJ: Prentice Hall.

Bianco, C., Dudkiewicz, P. B., & Linette, D. (2014). Building nurse leader relationships. *Journal of Nursing Management, 45*(5), 42–48. doi:10.1097/01. NUMA.0000442635.84291.30

Brafman, O., & Pollack, J. (2013). *The chaos imperative: How chance and disruption increase innovation-effectiveness and success*. New York, NY: Random House.

Brockman, J. (2013). *Thinking: The new science of decision-making, problem-solving, and prediction.* New York, NY: HarperCollins.

Drucker, P. F. (1999). *Management challenges for the 21st century.* New York, NY: HarperCollins.

Goss, M. (2012). *What is your one sentence?* New York, NY: Prentice Hall.

Guffey, M. E. (2003). *Business communication: Process and product* (5th ed.). Mason, OH: Thompson Learning.

Hamm, J. (2006). The five messages leaders must manage. Retrieved from http://hbr.org/2006/05/the-five-messages-leaders-must-manage/ar/1

Hynes, G. E. (2008). *Managerial communication: Strategies and applications* (4th ed.). Boston, MA: McGraw-Hill Irwin.

IBM (2010). Capitalizing on complexity: Insights from the global chief executive officer study. Retrieved from http://www-304.ibm.com/easyaccess/fileserve?contentid=231014

Jones, M., & Fowler-Dixon, S. (2004). Ethical issues in human subjects research. *Human Research Protection Program (HRPP) Education.* Paper 6. Retrieved from http://digitalcommons.wustl.edu/hrpoed/6

Keller, G., & Papasan, J. (2012). *The one thing: The surprisingly simple truth behind extraordinary results.* Austin, TX: Relleck.

Kleon, A. (2014). *Show your work: 10 ways to share your creativity and get discovered.* New York, NY: Workman.

Levitt, S. D., & Dubner, S. J. (2014). *Think like a freak.* New York, NY: HarperCollins.

Martin, S. J., Goldstein, N. J., & Cialdini, R. B. (2014). *The small big: Small changes that spark big influence.* New York, NY: Grand Central.

Neffinger, J., & Kohut, M. (2013). *Compelling people: The hidden qualities that make us influential.* New York, NY: Penguin.

Pink, D. (2005). *A whole new mind: Why right brainers will rule the future.* New York, NY: Riverhead.

Roach, J., Tracy, D., & Durden, K. (2007). Innovating core knowledge through upper division report composition. *Business Communication Quarterly, 70*(4), 431–449.

Scott, D. M. (2010). *The new rule of marketing and PR* (4th ed.). Hoboken, NJ: John Wiley and Sons.

Sherman, V. C. (1982). Taking over: Notes to the new executive. *Journal of Nursing Administration, 12*(2), 21–23.

Thompson, R. W., & Way, M. L. (2000). How to prepare and present effective outcome reports for external payers and regulators. *Education and Treatment of Children, 23*(1), 60–74.

Turner, M. (2003). A toolbox for healthcare ethics program development. *Journal for Nurses in Staff Development, 19*, 9–15.

Wahl, E. (2013). *Unthink: Rediscover your creative genius.* New York, NY: Random House.

Wiseman, L. (2010). *Multipliers: How the best leaders make everyone smarter.* New York, NY: HarperCollins.

Wocial, L. D., Sego, K., Rager, C., Laubersheimer, S., & Everett, L. Q. (2014). Image is more than a uniform: The promise of assurance. *Journal of Nursing Administration, 44*(5), 298–302. doi:10.1097/NNA.0000000000000070

Leadership Matters

Linda Roussel and Patricia L. Thomas

LEARNING OBJECTIVES

1. Describe major themes identified by leaders in the field related to core competencies and qualities for future leaders.
2. Identify academic–clinical partnerships in preparing future leaders.

AONE KEY COMPETENCIES

I. Communication and relationship building
II. Knowledge of the healthcare environment
III. Leadership
IV. Professionalism
V. Business skills

AONE KEY COMPETENCIES DISCUSSED IN THIS APPENDIX

I. Communication and relationship building
II. Knowledge of the healthcare environment
III. Leadership
IV. Professionalism

I. Communication and relationship building
- Effective communication
- Relationship management
- Influence of behaviors
- Ability to work with diversity
- Shared decision making
- Community involvement
- Medical staff relationships
- Academic relationships

II. Knowledge of the healthcare environment
- Clinical practice knowledge
- Patient care delivery models and work design knowledge
- Healthcare economics knowledge

- Healthcare policy knowledge
- Understanding of governance
- Understanding of evidence-based practice
- Outcomes measurement
- Knowledge of, and dedication to, patient safety
- Understanding of utilization and case management
- Knowledge of quality improvement and metrics
- Knowledge of risk management

III. Leadership
- Foundational thinking skills
- Personal journey disciplines
- Ability to use systems thinking
- Succession planning
- Change management

FUTURE OF NURSING: FOUR KEY MESSAGES

1. Nurses should practice to the full extent of their education and training.
2. Nurses should achieve higher levels of education and training through an improved education system that promotes seamless academic progression.
3. Nurses should be full partners with physicians and other health professionals in redesigning health care in the United States.
4. Effective workforce planning and policy making require better data collection and information infrastructure.

Introduction

The impact and influence of nurse leaders have been major threads throughout this new edition of *Management and Leadership for Nurse Administrators*. Visionary leaders in a variety of healthcare settings informed and reinforced essential content in this text. We wanted to hear messages from those in the field who would guide future leaders and explore how the academic partners could best collaborate and integrate real-world experiences. We were privileged to have the opportunity to interview leaders and synthesize their messages into major themes. The purpose of this appendix is to share the results with readers and to connect the lived experiences from nurse leaders to themes and theory described in this text. The linkages between what we learn in the academic setting and the learned experiences of exceptional nursing leaders affirms the relevance and application of the content found in this text.

There are many documents to inform nurse executives in establishing a framework to guide and evaluate their practice as leaders. The Institute of Medicine's Future of Nursing report (2010), the American Organization of Nurse Executives' *Nurse Executive Competencies* (2005), the American Nurses Association's *Scope and Standards for Nurse Administrators* (2009), and the Advisory Board Company's nurse executive research roundtable reports (2015) are only a few.

Extending beyond the nurses' resources, the Advanced Leadership Initiative at Harvard University, a new third stage in higher education designed to prepare experienced leaders to take on new challenges in the social sector, is a think tank focused on ways to inspire leaders to make an even greater social impact. The members of the Advanced Leadership Initiative studied the decision-making process among business and personal leaders. The panel found that great leaders make choices within the framework of some common core strengths:

- Leaders are passionate. Passion is the engine that drives sustainability, even when it becomes difficult to remain enthusiastic to remain constant with challenging projects.
- Leaders know themselves. Being aware of your talents, skills, and strengths is essential to effective leadership. Leaders are reflective and are able to ask for help when needed, and they assert themselves when appropriate in the context of their work.
- Leaders have learned that context matters. They know that the why (as well as the what) matters to inclusive, holistic, and synergistic decision-making processes. Leaders are cognizant of the impact of various circumstances on their vision and strategic planning. Leaders are aware and are emotionally intelligent. They reflect on events and people that may trigger strong reactions within them and cause them to make reactive choices, rather than within the framework of a solid, flexible plan (The President and Fellows of Harvard College, 2015).

Covey (2013) provides a guiding framework for developing highly effective management skills. His seminal work, *The Seven Habits of Highly Effective People*, discussed the concept of paradigm shift, which described how different perspectives can exist; that is, two people can see the same picture and hear the same story, and yet their perspectives may differ. In reading through our notes and reflecting on the wisdom of our leaders, we found the seven habits to be a natural framework for discussing the themes.

Covey's first three habits focus on moving from dependence to independence (self-mastery). The habit of being proactive describes the various roles and relationships in a person's life. Beginning with the end in mind (habit 2) requires an envisioning of what you want in the future to begin proactive planning to make it a reality. Habit three, putting first things first, underscores the importance of self-management and self-discipline and implementing activities that aim to reach habit 2. Covey notes that habit 2 is the mental work, and habit 3 is the action orientation to carry out the mission.

Habits 4, 5, and 6 are about interdependence and working with others. Habit 4, think win–win, emphasizes the importance of developing mutually beneficial solutions or agreements in relationships. This habit speaks to the value and respect we show to others by understanding that a win for all is a better long-term resolution than if only one person, or a small group, ends up with the prize. Seek first to understand, then to be understood (habit 5) involves empathic listening to authentically and genuinely hear what is being said. It also means allowing yourself to be influenced. Empathic listening creates an environment of true caring and positive problem solving. Habit 6, synergize, combines the strengths of people through positive feedback. It is a holistic approach and is more than the sum of parts or different perspectives. Synergy means being able to achieve goals that no one person could have accomplished alone.

Habit 7, sharpen the saw, is about continuous improvement and has both personal and interpersonal spheres of influence. Covey notes that when people sharpen the saw, they balance and renew their resources, energy, and health to create a sustainable, long-term, effective lifestyle. For example, this habit focuses on physical renewal through exercise, prayer, yoga, good readings, and meditation as sources for spiritual renewal. Using the seven habits to examine what makes managers effective provided an overarching framework for understanding the context of nursing leaders' work.

INTERVIEWS

We conducted interviews with nurse managers, executive nurses, and directors of clinical services and service lines. The purpose of this qualitative work was to validate the revisions made in this text. Nurse leaders hailed from a number of clinical settings, including tertiary systems-level leadership, departments, acute nursing units, a public health setting, and home care services. Additionally, the leaders represent nonprofit, community, and academic institutions. The nurse leaders were located within the United States and in other countries. Three questions guided the interviews:

1. What messages would you give to aspiring nurse leaders and nurse managers as they decide on a career in management or leadership?
2. What experiences are important to being socialized into a nursing leadership or management role? How would the clinical partner set up these experiences? With a precepted type of experience, what should be included?
3. How should the academic partner prepare or position the student to maximize the clinical or field experiences?

THEMES

We reviewed our notes and transcripts of thoughtful messages from nurse leaders and identified the following themes. Chapter references were also identified because they reinforce the essential content that nurse leaders described in their daily work.

1. Lifelong learning; role modeling (Chapters 3, 4, 6, 9)
2. Self-reflection; appreciate inquiry; learning from self (Chapters 3, 4, 7)
3. Coaching and mentoring (seeking experiences outside of comfort zone) (Chapters 3, 4)
4. Cross-pollination; going outside the box (Chapters 5, 10, 11, 12)
5. Value-added metrics; how to add value (value proposition) (Chapters 5, 6, 8, 15)
6. Practice of leadership; executive guide (Chapters 2, 4, 5, 7, 8, 9)
7. Stretching out of your comfort zone (Chapters 1, 3, 4, 5, 8, 9)
8. Care across the continuum; no longer about care of patient; development of associates (Chapters 2, 3, 9, 11)

9. Larger worldview; conceptualization of leadership practice (Chapters 4, 5, 7, 11, 13)
10. Clinical–academic partnership vital to enhancing students' experience; partnering on projects (Chapters 1, 3, 4, 9)
11. Value-added relevant projects during an immersion experience (Chapters 1, 5, 13, 14)

Theme 1: Lifelong Learning; Role Modeling

Theme 1 (sharpening the saw) means having a balanced program for self-renewal in four areas of life: physical, social and emotional, mental, and spiritual. Examples include nutrition, exercise, and sleep and rest (physical); meaningful relationships and connections (social and emotional); learning, reading, writing, and coaching (mental); and self-reflection through meditation, music, prayer, art, and service (spiritual). Lifelong learning is key to ongoing self-development. Being responsible for developing your skills and talents provides the opportunity to best serve as a coach and mentor frontline staff. Theme 1 is best exemplified by the following quotes by nurse managers and nurse executives:

"Remain open to constant learning; if you are not already one, become a 'lifelong learner.' Welcome change—learn to work with change to benefit your client/patients. Remember the principles of leadership, there are several, but one of particular importance to me is that leaders take action—learn to 'walk the talk' as you rally the team."

—Executive director, state health system

"In my case . . . today's healthcare system is located in Saudi Arabia . . . a country that has historically experienced a severe shortage of qualified Saudi nurses resulting in immense dependency on internationally-recruited nurses. The literature attests that this low number of qualified Saudi nurses is attributed to traditional, legislative, and occupational restraints of the country that often impede women from fully participating in the Saudi healthcare workforce. It is these factors that influence the prevailing negative images and perceived low status of nursing, resulting in nurses not always receiving the same level of professional respect that is attributed to other healthcare professions."

—Director of nursing, acute care setting

"CNE/CNO leadership today and in the future is largely about facilitating transformational change. All of the points above are very important—plus bringing the workforce along. Building or enhancing a culture of high reliability (to the Triple Aim) is vitally important as our industry/profession moves forward into the future."

—Vice president/Chief nursing officer, acute care hospital

"Take advantage of all leadership activities and opportunities. Volunteer to participate and demonstrate an eagerness to get involved in the community."

—Systems chief nursing officer

Theme 2: Self-Reflection; Appreciate Inquiry; Learning from Self

Theme 2 can best be illustrated by habit 5 (seek first to understand, then be understood) and habit 7 (sharpen the saw). The importance of communication is underscored in habit 5, primarily with empathic listening as a key to understanding and being understood. Nurse leaders described the importance of learning from the self and using appreciative inquiry as the best means of communicating for meaning. Sharpening the saw keeps managers renewed so they can practice the other six habits. Balancing all areas (physical, social, mental, and spiritual) will increase the capacity to produce and handle the challenges that leaders may face. Without renewal through self-reflection and appreciative inquiry, leaders can become stagnant and unable to be innovative and entrepreneurial. Theme 2 is illustrated through the voices of the following nurse leaders:

"My best advice for aspiring nurse leaders and especially nurse[s] working at the bedside is to look at their leadership role as a journey in which they will continue [to] learn on daily basis from their success and mistakes."

—Nurse manager, acute care setting

"Another concern for the future of nursing is health communication and collaboration. Nurses and healthcare providers do not work in isolation. Communication and true collaboration takes time, patience, self-awareness, and knowledge. Therefore, leadership must value knowing self, being honest, maintain a positive attitude, have a sense of humor, use open and respectful communication, and listen to others while listening to your 'gut feelings.' The balancing act is a challenge and requires thoughtful self-reflection. I do not believe these skills are never perfected; however, I keep working on improving and apologize when I make mistakes."

—Clinic manager, student-run clinic

"Be open to change and expect turbulence. That said keep your eye (vision) on where/what you desire—and keep going. Share your vision (over and over again) and rally/inspire your team. You are only as good as those around you."

— Vice president/Chief nursing officer, acute care hospital

"Don't be distracted; identify mentors from different backgrounds, in different roles throughout your career. You should vary your mentors throughout your career as you develop as an executive leader."

—System chief nursing officer

"It is important to engage in self-reflection and caring for yourself. You are 'always on stage,' and you must never miss opportunities to lead. For the example, at the end of every day plan 15 minutes (I do this on the drive home) without distractions (phone, radio), and reflect [on] your day . . . what you did, what you said, missed opportunities. It is important to learn from yourself."

—Chief nursing officer, acute care

"It's important to know what brings you joy? What brings you passion? What drags you down? Knowing yourself is critical to improving yourself, and being a good role model. You must be able to engage in polarity thinking. You're always making hard decision, and need integrity to carry out what is right for the system. Knowing yourself is the first step."

—Chief nursing officer, acute care

Theme 3: Coaching and Mentoring (Seeking Out Experience Outside of Comfort Zone)

Theme 3 can be described by habit 6 (synergize) and habit 3 (putting first things first). Habit 6 can be described as creative cooperation. Synergy involves teamwork, open-mindedness, and the capacity to find new alternatives to old problems. This does not happen on its own; it is a process through which individuals bring their personal experience and expertise. Coming together as a team can produce superior results that individuals may not create alone. The whole is greater than the sum of the parts. According to Covey, 1 plus 1 equals 3, or 6, or 60, or any number of opportunities. Nurse leaders share their perceptions of theme 3 in the following quotes:

"Finally, they need to know that all of this change will have an impact on you and how you feel as a leader. It is important to be able to be innovative with how you manage your career and maintain your mind-set for dealing with all of these complexities. Look for a health system who has demonstrated strong leaders to align with."

—Nurse manager, acute care unit

"I had the opportunity to participate in executive coaching, and learned much about myself, and the importance of using appreciative inquiry (AI) in my work . . . to be able to ask question[s], that guide decision making, to practice key communication skills. This coaching experience reinforced my ability to better coach and mentor those I guide, and lead."

—Chief nursing officer, acute care

"As a nurse manager, I have had the great fortune of being mentored and coached by great leaders, who have helped to develop me. It is my turn to coach and mentor, and I do as part of my responsibilities as a nurse leader. It is a privilege to be a servant leader; I take this responsibility very seriously, and see this as a primary role in leading to improve patient care. It is all that matters!"

— Director, clinical services, home care

Theme 4: Cross-Pollination; Going Outside the Box

Theme 4 can best be described by habit 6 (synergize) and habit 4 (think win–win). Synergizing and pursuing cooperative ends exemplifies theme 4. Pursuing a win–win means having a frame of mind and heart that continuously seeks mutual benefit in all human interactions. Agreements and finding solutions that are mutually beneficial and satisfying best illustrates a win–win. Vital character traits when approaching conflicts with a win–win mind-set are integrity, maturity, and abundance. Nurse leaders described the importance of expanding their horizons and integrating expertise across the continuum. The voices of nurse leaders are revealed through the following quotes:

"Nurse Executives need intelligent and dedicated team members who are willing to share ideas or brainstorm solutions to complex healthcare issues. High performing teams are empowered by their nurse executive to value relationships and explore the diversity of thinking, feeling, and behaving. Accepting diversity will keep team members talking and attempting to make improvements in the organization. Everyone wants respect, dignity, and [to be] honored for his or her participation. Appreciated teams will use their knowledge and expertise to go the extra mile for the cause."

—Clinic manager, student-run clinic

"Aspiring leaders need to have exposure and experience at all levels. For example, it has been my experience that many new nursing leaders have never been exposed to the board room. Nurse leaders also need to better understand the political environment around how policies are made. For example, where did the oversight for hospital readmissions come from and how did those decisions and regulations get implemented? Also, what policy changes are coming next? How do nursing leaders keep up with future policy changes that are being discussed so that they can be better prepared to deal with them?"

—Nurse manager, acute care unit

"Look for creative and entrepreneurial opportunities . . . this will help you make better decisions if you look outside of the healthcare industry. Look at aviation, manufacturing, and engineering to get ideas about performance improvement . . . systems thinking."

—Senior associate dean, clinical and community partnership

Theme 5: Value-Added Metrics; How to Add Value (Value Proposition)

Theme 5 exemplifies habit 1 (being proactive), habit 2 (begin with the end in mind), and habit 3 (putting first things first). Being proactive involves focusing efforts on the leader's circle of influence. Proactive managers put first things first and begin with the end in mind. They work on matters they can do something about—health, children, and problems at work. Proactive leaders focus their concentration on the work at hand. Beginning with the end in mind and putting first things first means to start each day, activity, and project with a clear vision of desired direction and destination. Leaders continue by proactively flexing their muscles to make things happen (Covey, 2013). Developing a personal mission statement is important to this end, as is focusing on what you want to be and do, and planning for success. Proactive leaders add value by affirming who they are, setting goals, and moving forward with a plan. Nurse managers and executives reflected theme 5 in the following statements:

"Become knowledgeable of our reforming healthcare industry. Pay particular attention to the massive shift in reimbursement methodology—from volume to value; and population health management. You must have core competence in nonclinical areas, i.e., finance, operations, HR, legal, public policy. Don't need to be the 'expert'—but does need a core level of competence. Include these sorts of learnings early on in your educational development."

— Vice president/Chief nursing officer, acute care hospital

"Aspiring leaders need to be able to critically examine each environment of healthcare and do an analysis of what is working correctly and what is not working correctly from a leadership standpoint and then be able to employ effective strategies."

—Nurse manager, acute care unit

"What adds value is working in interprofessional teams at the unit and larger level. Healthcare quality and safety are at the helm. At the center of all of our work is the patient. If we cannot communicate the why, we should not be doing it!"

—Nurse manager, acute care unit

"The executive leader brings the clinical focus as he or she understands the whole system, and stays connected with frontline, and wants to be the person that everyone turns to understand the clinical enterprise and the continuum of care."

—System vice president, integrated health system

"You add value by acknowledging the frontline and nurse managers. You do this by being a good role model. It is important to build credibility. It's important to actively engage in the continuum of care, working with multidisciplinary teams and learning through partnerships, and the academic agent."

—Vice president patient care services, chief nursing officer, acute care

Theme 6: Practice of Leadership; Executive Guide

Theme 6 (sharpening the saw) provides the balance that nurse leaders continually seek as they practice their craft. Serving as executive guides, nurse leaders take responsibility for their own development and seek coaching and mentoring opportunities. Nurse leaders expressed their perception of their leadership responsibilities and the importance of modeling these behaviors. Nurse leaders expressed the following, which best describe theme 6:

"Nurse administrative students need to have an experience as bedside nurses for a few years before joining the nurse administrative program. During their bedside experience the nurses will have a knowledge about the care delivery system, health care law and policy, how to work in teams/collaborating, and mentoring. Also nurses need to have knowledge about communication, conflict resolution and negotiating skills necessary to succeed in leadership and partnership roles."

—Nurse manager, acute care setting

"The emotionally intelligent nurse executive is in the best position to keep the high performing teams on track with the organization's strategic plan. Therefore, it is important to recognize conflict before it becomes a problem. When attempting to resolve conflict, I go back to my philosophies of life and nursing to guide my approach. As a phenomenologist, I attempt to gain insight into others' perspective. I may seek input from trusted peers that I know will tell me the truth even when my thinking is flawed. I use open and honest communication that may be considered a crucial conversation, which directly addresses the issue or concern. I do not address all issues or concerns because timing is critical after determining others' perceptions or agendas. Again, if I need to apologize I do so without hesitation; however, if I have the wrong person on my team then I make a replacement."

—Clinic manager, student-run clinic

"Financial acumen and a working knowledge of nursing informatics are also very important for the Nurse Leader to demonstrate. This experience may best be obtained by spending time with the personnel manager, financial director and nurse informatics."

—Director of nursing, acute care hospital

"It's important to have an executive guide, inside and outside of nursing as the nurse executive has the responsibility for many (or most) clinical services. It's important to strengthen professional nursing while promoting nursing as a good partner. The nurse executive needs to see the bigger picture, and has a unique opportunity to get to higher levels. Some chief nursing officers fail because they are not prepared for politics. You have to have a taste for politics."

—Systems vice president, integrated health system

Theme 7: Stretching Out of Your Comfort Zone

Theme 7 can be illustrated by habit 5 (seek win–win) and habit 7 (sharpening the saw). Nurse leaders described the essential responsibility of stretching themselves and finding opportunities to grow and develop. Coming out of their comfort zone required disciplined thought and action. Nurse managers and nurse executives described the following to illustrate theme 7:

"With massive change come tremendous opportunities. To 'take advantage' of this you must get active in public policy and advocacy. As noted above, understand HC reform . . . Read the IOM Future of Nursing . . . Know what is brewing in legislation . . . Meet your congress men and women . . . Engage with your professional organizations . . . Get involved! We can either be at the table—or on the menu."

— Vice president/Chief nursing officer, acute care hospital

"I would tell these aspiring leaders to absolutely be prepared to lead and live through change regardless. Healthcare inherently must change because the system is broken. These leaders need to be able to create synergy and motivation around change. However, most importantly they need to be able to genuinely and legitimately employ strategies that will help with the adoption of new ideas and processes."

—Nurse manager, acute care unit

"Challenging ourselves . . . learning outside the organization, having 'field trips' in acute and outpatient care broadens not only your horizons but your world view."

—Systems vice president, integrated health system

Theme 8: Care across the Continuum; No Longer about Care of Patient; Development of Associates

Theme 8 is illustrated by habit 6 (synergize) and habit 4 (think win–win). Nurse leaders shared that care across the continuum, and knowing the outpatient and the acute care side of the continuum, is critical to leading a healthcare system. Balance and collaboration support a healthy work environment and authentic leadership. Dealing with conflict can best be achieved by thinking win–win. Nurse leaders voiced their perspective in the following quotes:

"The key messages I would like to give to aspiring clinical or executive leaders in this country is to always promote the integral role that nurses play in the healthcare system. Acquiring knowledge of professional roles of other health care contributors is of importance. Nurse Leaders must promote the enhancement of the nurse practice environment and the nursing image through empowering a transformational leadership culture, promoting interdisciplinary partnerships, supporting professional development and ensuring that evidence based practice is a reality."

—Director of nursing, acute care setting

"It is critical to provide care across the continuum, and agree to partner with unconventional partners, such as accounting, attorneys, engineers and architects . . . all can offer perspectives that are important to patient care."

—Chief nursing officer, acute care setting

Theme 9: Larger Worldview; Conceptualization of Leadership Practice

Theme 9 is best illustrated by habit 6 (synergize) and habit 4 (think win–win). With a win–win perspective, team collaboration and cooperation are expectations and challenged when solo performance is manifested. The voices of nurse leaders are expressed in the following quotes:

"I would emphasize that because of their broad perspective on healthcare issues, nurse leaders must play a critical role in strategic decision-making at the highest level and in healthcare policy creation. They should see themselves as essential partners in the redesign of health care systems throughout the Kingdom and thus need to champion that their presence is visible."

—Director of nursing, acute care setting

"The learning experience for students is richer due to the cultural diversity between the students and patient. Students gain an understanding of life from the patients' perspective that results in empathy and compassion that is demonstrated in their interaction with the patient. For example, the medical and nursing students are now referring patients to the social work student or the social worker is referring back to the occupational therapy or community agencies. Furthermore, patients are coming back routinely to the health promotion clinic for information or just to talk with the students. The value of these relationships is helping the homeless person to start thinking about improving their health and life-style. As well as the students are learning to communicate respectfully with the patients. This is true patient-centered care that needs to be demonstrated by all healthcare professionals."

—Clinic manager, student-run clinic

Theme 10: Clinical–Academic Partnership Vital to Enhancing Students' Experience; Partnering on Projects

Theme 10 can best be described by habit 2 (begin with the end in mind). The ability to imagine is best illustrated by habit 2, which is the capacity to envision in the mind's eye and translate that vision to those being inspired to act. Clinical–academic partnership involves imagining a culture and environment (mental creation) and following up with the physical creation of the partnership. This mental picture empowers other people and circumstances to shape the vision. It is the connecting of the mental and physical that defines the personal, moral, and ethical guideline that makes this real for those in the system. Nurse managers and executives reflected theme 10 in the following statements:

"Of significant benefit for nurse administrative students/aspiring nurse managers in Saudi Arabia to have during their academy preparation strong clinical practicum experience. Creating new and innovative models for clinical learning that connects advanced nursing education with clinical practice is, I believe, an essential component for success. In Saudi Arabia, this involves forming academic/clinical partnerships in ways that differ significantly from the past. The University (bachelorette degree is the present entry level for nurses) and the health care agencies (which in the case of Saudi Arabia are predominately hospitals) must have thoroughly discussed and therefore must be cognizant of the mutual benefits and added value in forming these partnerships. To achieve success in this endeavor, which can be extremely time consuming and often difficult, there must be a shared vision, mutual trust, established goals and commitment."

—Director of nursing, acute care setting

"Nursing colleges should partner with health care organizations to develop competencies that can be added regularly to the academic curricula to ensure that nursing graduates from leadership programs are prepared to meet the current and future health needs. Nursing colleges should partner with health care organizations to foster a culture of lifelong learning."

—Nurse manager, acute care setting

Theme 11: Value-Added Relevant Projects during an Immersion Experience

Theme 11 describes the importance of taking on value-added projects, particularly though immersion experiences. Habit 1 (proactive) and habit 4 (think win–win) typifies theme 11, and nurse executives provided their perceptions:

"Experience working on a quality improvement project using proven methodologies such as Lean, PDCA etc. and in Risk management (i.e. adverse occurrence follow ups, how to investigate patient complaints, critical situation analysis) and in accreditation standards would be important. I suggest that the 'student' be given the opportunity to work alongside the Nurse Quality Team and/or Hospital Quality Team for exposure to this knowledge/skills. Other valuable experiences would be for the student to be included in team building, conflict resolution and employee management activities. As our organization is taking the Magnet journey . . . meeting with the Magnet Manager and participating in meetings/activities centering on enriching the practice environment to achieve better patient outcomes and more satisfied RNs would be of great value."

—Director of nursing, acute care hospital

"Collaboration and consensus building are key for project success—learn these skills well."

—Executive director, state health system

"Grad level internships are great . . . particularly when the academic institution allows collaborative experiential design. Traditionally, most hospital 'fellows' (paid fellowships) have been nonclinical grad students (MBAs, MHAs, etc.). I think we need to push for MSN hospital fellows."

— Vice president/Chief nursing officer, acute care hospital

"Schools of Nursing need to find ways to submerge aspiring nurse leaders to demonstrate outstanding leadership so that they can see how issues were effectively dealt with."

—Nurse manager, acute care unit

"It is important to expose students to content about the changing healthcare environment and financing care. Students need to understand that healthcare is moving to population health and the broader healthcare system. This is one aspect of a value creation equation."

—Senior associate dean, community and clinical partnerships

SUMMARY

Interviews with nurse executives and nurse managers served to validate the refinement of leadership and administrative content in this seventh edition. It was clear that nurse leaders believe in the importance of lifelong learning, self-reflection, and seeking diverse experiences outside of health care. The larger worldview, stretching beyond their comfort zone, and involvement in value-added projects were also reinforced through coaching and mentoring experiences. These experiences were important to self-development and for developing future nurse leaders as innovators and entrepreneurs.

Canton, in *Future Smart: Managing the Game-Changing Trends That Will Transform Your World* (2015), described top game-changers that are shaping future business (including health care). Innovation is the chief competitive advantage that needs to be embraced, or leaders and organizations will perish. Canton also notes the importance of disrupting and reinventing the business model, products, work processes, talent, strategy, and values. Lessons for building future smart organizations include being curious; paying attention; failing fast and frequently; getting the correct talent for the job; dealing with diverse cultural teams; managing complex information, knowledge, and data; among others. Game-changers of the future will serve in roles like "Coach of Creativity, Global Change Catalyst, Collaborator of Learning, Enabler of Bold Ideas, Facilitator of Discovery, and Whole-Systems Thinker" (Canton, 2015, p. 257).

The speed and complexity with which health care is delivered will not slow down, despite new technologies that enhance connectivity and create value that can be measured to demonstrate improved outcomes. Nurse leaders embrace their work and believe in the importance of sharing wisdom for successful transformational change.

REFERENCES

Advisory Board Company. (2015). Nursing executive center. Retrieved from http://www.advisory.com/Research/Nursing-Executive-Center

American Nurses Association. (2009). *Scope and standards for nurse administrators* (3rd ed.). Silver Springs, MD: Author.

American Organization of Nurse Executives. (2005). Nurse executive competencies. Retrieved from http://www.aone.org/resources/leadership%20tools/nursecomp.shtml

Canton, J. (2015). *Future smart: Managing the game-changing trends that will transform your world*. Boston, MA: Da Capo.

Covey, S. (2013). *The seven habits of highly effective people: Powerful lessons in personal change*. New York, NY: Simon and Schuster.

Institute of Medicine. (2010). *The future of nursing: Leading change, advancing health*. Washington, DC: National Academies Press.

The President and Fellows of Harvard College. (2015). Advanced Leadership Initiative. Retrieved from http://advancedleadership.harvard.edu/

Index

Note: Page numbers followed by *b*, *f*, and *t* indicate material in boxes, figures and tables respectively.